# Praise for *Tantra Yoga Sec*

MW00389816

"One of the beauties of Tantra is that, ......... ...........iduual is in charge of setting a goal, achieving it, and evaluating that achievement. Tantra is an experimental discipline, and those who follow the path of Tantra must carefully integrate each experience until experiencing itself is perfected, by uniting the experiencer with the Self. The lessons in *Tantra Yoga Secrets* provide a system of practices that can, when employed with determination, concentration, and discernment, open doors into rewarding perceptions of reality."

—**Robert Svoboda**, BAMS, Ayurvedic physician and author of *Ayurveda: Life, Health, and Longevity*; *Prakriti: Your Ayurvedic Constitution*; and *Ayurveda for Women*

"Preserving a deep spiritual lineage as well as appreciating the natural world, Mukunda Stiles offers a practical guide with useful tools to assist the spiritual seeker in achieving a profound transformation rather than superficial change. Anyone seeking self-awareness will benefit by following the step-by-step asana and meditation practices from this ancient path. I feel honored to have Mukunda in my life as he teaches on this Earth."

—**Ma Jaya Sati Bhagavati**, Kashi Ashram, founder of Kali Natha Yoga

"With this latest book, Mukunda Stiles has moved into the role of a spiritual yoga teacher. It is an excellent, lucid, skillful explanation that takes one beyond the illusionary misunderstanding that tantric practice/sadhana is about sexuality and raises it to its full value as a powerful way to wake up to the Self of all. Mukunda, as a wise and experienced yogi, reveals one of the deepest secrets of all yoga sadhana from Yoga Sutra I, 12. 'Persistent and earnest effort over a long period of time and dispassion from the results of practice gives success in yoga.'"

—**Gabriel Cousens**, MD, DD, diplomat of Ayurveda and acknowledged Kundalini and Shaktipat master; author of *Conscious Eating* and *Rainbow Green Live-Food Cuisine*

"It is refreshing to find a book on Tantra with genuine depth! *Tantra Yoga Secrets* is an invaluable manual for students ready to progress beyond yoga postures to expanded states of awareness. Tantra Yoga spiritualizes every aspect of life; *Tantra Yoga Secrets* shows you how."

—**Linda Johnsen**, author of *Daughters of the Goddess: The Women Saints of India*

"Mukunda has added to his deep study of yoga and ayurveda an innovative examination of Tantra. *Tantra Yoga Secrets* provides an insightful view of this fascinating yet misunderstood topic of how to balance the male and female energies of Shiva and Shakti within us to achieve *swastha* (the harmony of health with the inner Self)."

—**Dr. David Frawley** (Pandit Vamadeva Shastri), author of *Inner Tantric Yoga* and *Mantra Yoga and Primal Sound*

# TANTRA YOGA SECRETS

## Eighteen Transformational Lessons to Serenity, Radiance, and Bliss

MUKUNDA STILES

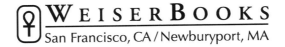
WEISER BOOKS
San Francisco, CA / Newburyport, MA

First published in 2011 by
Red Wheel/Weiser, LLC
665 Third Street, Suite 400
San Francisco, CA 94107
*www.redwheelweiser.com*

Library of Congress Cataloging-in-Publication Data
Stiles, Mukunda.
  Tantra yoga secrets : 18 transformational lessons to serenity, radiance,
and bliss / by Mukunda Stiles.
     p.   cm.
  Includes bibliographical references.
  ISBN 978-1-57863-503-0 (alk. paper)
  1. Yoga. 2. Tantrism. I. Title.
  B132.Y6S728 2011
  294.5'436—dc23

                                                        2011017730

Cover design by Jim Warner
Cover photograph and author photo by Chinnamasta Stiles
Interior photos by Sraddha Van Dyke; © SAYVA
Typeset in Garamond

Printed in Canada
TCP
10 9 8 7 6 5 4 3 2 1
The paper used in this publication meets the minimum requirements of the Ameri-
can National Standard for Information Sciences—Permanence of Paper for Printed
Library Materials Z39.48-1992 (R1997).

# Contents

# Devi Puja

Tara Mata ki Jay
Sarasvati Mata ki Jay
Lakshmi Mata ki Jay
Kali Mata ki Jay

The puja (ritual of submission) to the Devis has taken me to intimacy with the Goddess in the form of Tara as the sky, Saraswati as the dance of life, Lakshmi as the bounty and abundance of Mother's milk, and Kali as the remover of all that is no longer beneficial. From these subtle forms, grosser forms have been born, most especially Suptashring Devi—an expression of the Mother as the entire Earth—whom I was led to by my beloved tantric role model, Swami Prakashananda. These Devis in turn have transformed themselves into my blessed wife, consort, healer, and companion, Chinnamasta Devi, who has taken me to places others could not. She has only one mission—to dance the tandava, the eternal communion of Shiva and Shakti, merging and separating for the delight of being One and the enjoyment of being the worldly couple.

## Honoring Chinnamasta Devi

When I resist my Devi, life is difficult and dry; when I surrender to her, life flows. Devi naturally longs to live a life full of integrity. When the stress of life is accumulated through a lack of seeing what is truthful and honorable, Deva often has to swallow the bitter pill of seeing the truth about his foolishness and arrogance. Devi won't withhold in offering Deva darshan in order to help him return to the heart. It is my personal experience that the truth lies in the wisdom teachings given by my Devi. She only reveals them to me when I finally am ready to humbly submit and accept them. This often results in putting my head in her lap. Her thoughts are Divine Mother's flow running through her—there is no difference. She personifies the hidden meanings of the teachings that come naturally and intuitively to her. The serenity prayer and all other forms of prayer become juicy, and my confidence in infinite goodness and love are restored. The deepest acts of surrender are to believe and truly trust her way. For this is how the Divine Mother is naturally revealing and expressing herself as my Devi.

Teaching side by side with my Devi has enlivened our insights and has revealed more of the shakti hidden within the teachings. From the moment we met, there was an instant recognition. We were led to sit next to each other, and the teachings would flow naturally from Devi into Deva and vice versa without pause. Often, Chinnamasta Devi would reflect upon the words expressed by Deva. At the exact moment I would feel the stillness of the breath happening, Chinnamasta would say or do what was needed.

The ease of our interactions has naturally grown to become the living force supporting the integrity of the shakti which is manifested as the secrets of Tantra in this book. Our life together has greatly enhanced the final edits of this book.

While some students are more attracted to one of us, mature students feel an equal attraction and no separation.

Sharing and being with Chinnamasta is to me the living experience of the mysterious delight of Tantra, that is continuously arising and expanding as the sacred tremor of the tantric spanda.

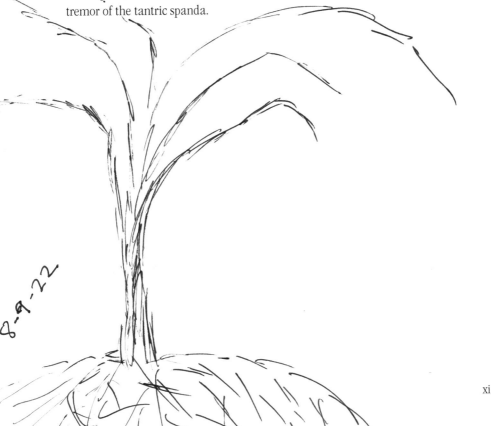

8-9-22

# Acknowledgments

I wish to give my gratefulness and gratitude to the forms of the formless: Deva has become Devi, the commonplace has become the unexpected, teachings have become my teachers.

First and foremost is to acknowledge Devi's path. My great respect and love go to my guru and teachers, the known, the unknown, and *the unknowable*.

Most profound gratitude to my guru Swami Muktananda Paramahansa and his guru Bhagavan Nityananda of Ganeshpuri, India and to my spiritual teacher Swami Prakashananda of Suptashring.

The known teachers include Paul Copeland, MD, Psychiatry; Rama Jyothi Vernon, BKS Iyengar; Mata Amrit Anandamayi Ma "Ammachi"; Professor Krishnamacharya, Indra Devi, Yogi Hall of the Redwoods; and Ma Jaya Sati Bhagavati, Bhadra Kali of Ganeshpuri. The many teachers and students with whom we shared both deep and superficial reflections of the nature of yoga. The texts that have inspired me—*Yoga Sutras, Guru Gita, Shiva Sutras, Vijnana Bhairava Tantra,* and, most especially, the *Yoga Vasistha*. My teachers and these texts have transformed the way I perceive the world and myself. All of these influences have totally captivated my life into one of seeking the mystery of form changing into formlessness. The known becomes unknown, the unknown becomes the unknowable.

The secret teachings have come to me since a vivid summer experience in 1979. Having been drafted into the army, I was on a bus headed from one section of Fort Ord to another. The Monterey Jazz Festival was happening nearby. While sitting on the bus, I began to notice that everything was breathing. Throughout the half hour bus ride, a formless undulating tide captivated my attention.

Many years later I would reflect back on this experience in light of tantric texts such as the *Tripura Rahasya* (the mystery of the trinity) and others that helped me understand the significance of the spontaneous arising of the Devi's triple forms coming in and out of the Oneness. We are all given experiences of the primal Mother, but without a text and a living teacher such a mystery goes unnoticed. The *Yoga Sutras of Patanjali* (II–1) reveals the secret that teachings can be given in such a way as to embody the Shakti as Devi. The first step is Sadhana Pada—the path of practice. The second step is Swadhyaya Pada—the path of understanding and inquiry. The third step, Isvara Pranidhana, is to seek a teacher who can elaborate and clarify the first two steps. In this way, such experiences turn into realizations.

Sitting on the bus, with everything undulating—this body space, the space surrounding the body, the space of the bus, the cornfield, the sky field—and yet, there is no difference. The experience of not seeing a difference is the culmination of practice and the study of the texts.

Chronologically speaking, the undulating bus experience took place years before texts were shown explaining the serenity, radiance, and bliss. At first, these three states of consciousness seemed to arise separately. After forty years of Tantrik Yoga, the three forms of the Devi undulate in and out of form and formlessness.

For all of the mistakes, for all the influences left without acknowledgment, I ask you forgiveness. May I realize as you do the significance of this great mystery called Life.

Sadgurunath Maharaj ki Jay. – Blessings to the true inner teacher, the Self.

Jagadambe Mata ki Jay. – Blessings to the Mother of the world.

# Introduction

These Tantrik teachings rest on a cornerstone of experiential knowledge gained over the ages by the men and women of this lineage. That knowledge can only be summarized and pointed to in book form. It is acquired through steady practice guided by a mentor, spiritual transmission from a teacher connected to a lineage, and reflections on a timeless text that will transform the mind. The mind needs to be transformed by each of these three factors. You cannot understand this writing unless your mind becomes free of thoughts, which happens when a guru's grace becomes God's grace. This is a crucial element; if you read this like any other inspirational book without that transmission, you will not get the full benefit and your awakening will remain incomplete.

When pranic, emotional, or mental energy is allowed its full and natural expression, it becomes neutral or *sattvic*. In this neutral state, all events of life are experienced as arising from a spiritual source. This fundamental shift—from an idea about omnipresence to an actual embodied awareness of the omnipresent nature of the Divine—brings you home to your Self.

I encourage you to commit yourself to completing the entire eighteen-lesson course. Without persistence, the transformations achieved in the early lessons will not produce long-lasting, sustainable results. If you wish more detailed information, see the recommended reading list on my website—*www.yogatherapycenter.org*. The best general book for those from a Hatha background is *Tantra: Cult of the Feminine* by André van Lysebeth (Weiser Books, 1995).

I wrote these lessons over a period of several years in response to questions from my students. These seekers have, in essence, been the source of this book. By reading and reflecting on this text, your inspirational mind will arise and resolve self-limiting thoughts, emotions, and energetic patterns that bind you. These eighteen lessons are specifically designed to *reveal your limitations* so that you can remove them by increasing the quality and quantity of your purifying pranic energy. When you get to a lesson that reveals your self-imposed limitations and lack of prana, *you will tend to stop.* That will be the crucial time to continue your practice and move through the lessons without concern for mastery. This will strengthen your detachment and discernment muscles and, in time, lead to true wisdom and spontaneously arising realizations.

Lesson 3 is the most powerful in allowing insights to arise so that illumination will naturally occur as a result of your reflections and practice. Use it repeatedly to encourage and build your prana. When suppressed emotional energy is allowed to build in this way, it transmutes, becoming neutral energy. If you persist, it will harmonize and be experienced as spiritual energy. Know that these lessons are for the singular purpose of moving to a higher consciousness.

The course consists of six parts:

> Part I: Lessons 1–4 cover how to engage your pranic energy and use it to transform energy blocks.
>
> Part II: Lesson 5–7 cover tools for Tantra in a yogic context, deepening experiences to a subtler dimension.
>
> Part III: Lessons 8–10 cover healing sexual wounds by opening to a devotional relationship with prana as the Divine Source.
>
> Part IV: Lessons 11–12 give my perspective on spiritual awakening.
>
> Part V: Lessons 13–15 show how to deepen your personal Tantrik practice through the Divine Presence or with another Tantrik practitioner.
>
> Part VI: Lessons 16–18 cover the awakening of devotional energies of God/dess that can move toward unity and spiritual illumination.

When you start each lesson, mark a date on your calendar that is two weeks out. Begin the next lesson no later than this date. Regardless of what you experience in your Tantrik practice, *it is enough just to read and reflect upon the lessons to complete the course.* It is common for students to experience blocks from doing the lessons. You may not experience freedom from your blocks merely from the first few lessons. By moving on, you will make significant progress in your spiritual *sadhana.* Complete this course in as few as eighteen weeks, but not longer than nine months. It is also important to note that it is not uncommon for Shakti to give lessons out of my sequence. Sometimes we get the harder lessons earlier and sometimes what seems a simple lesson doesn't reveal itself fully until later on.

Those who have had personal instruction from me, or who have an active Tantrik practice, will likely move through these lessons more quickly than others. Remember that spiritual awakening proceeds in its own manner, free of the sequences that are formed by the mind. You can more quickly review those lessons that you have received personally from me. If the name of a practice is familiar, but you did not learn it from me, be sure to read and follow the instructions carefully, as subtle-body anatomy distinctions do vary from one school of thought to another. I strongly encourage you to do the practices precisely as given here, as this will maximize your progress.

Tantrik Yoga, like all yoga paths, is an effective means of living a more fulfilling spiritual lifestyle. You cannot realize its full benefits, however, unless you receive a personal practice (sadhana) from a teacher who has been trained and authorized by their own teacher to uphold the blessings of the lineage. Both Classical and Tantrik Yoga are given from a lineage, not by teachers in isolation. These lessons and the author's spiritual mentoring consultations are available to you as my spiritual teachers have given them to me and directed me to share them with all who are motivated. If you would like me to serve you, you are welcome to schedule sessions via phone, Skype, email, in person, or by contacting me at *www.yogatherapycenter.org*.

If you find that some of the Sanskrit terminology used in these lessons is unfamiliar, consult the Glossary at the end of this book.


## Attainment as Realization

This book was written in a manner that seeks to pause the thought process and find the source of thought. With this in mind, it is important that you just read the text and let it work upon your mind. Don't concern yourself with repetition; any teaching worth giving is worth reflecting on again and again. The essence of tantric teachings can be given by the story of the crow and the coconut.

A crow in flight softly lands on a coconut at the very moment the coconut becomes ripe and falls. The mistake is that the crow made the coconut fall. The truth is nothing happened.

You will find a list of the Attainments for each lesson in the Appendix at the back of the book.

Finally, it is essential to begin and end each practice session with intentional focus using this prayer:

> ## With Great Respect and Love, I Honor
> ## My Heart, My Inner Teacher.

This entry and exit to sanctify your practice is of utmost importance; therefore, I have included the prayer at the beginning and end of each of the eighteen lessons.

## May God/dess bless and sustain your practice.

PART 1

12-27-16  —

# Engaging Your
# Pranic Energy

# The Energy Body and Tantrik Practice

With Great Respect and Love, I Honor
My Heart, My Inner Teacher.

The secret of success in yoga is given in the *Yoga Sutras* I, 12: *persistent and earnest effort over a long period of time and dispassion from the results of that practice.* Know that these lessons are for the purpose of moving through what the practices bring up, and persistently coming home—to your own True Self. If you persist in this spiritual tradition, all forms of your energy will be experienced as spiritual energy.

## The Tantrik Yoga Tradition

Let us consider the relationship of Classical Yoga and Tantra. Written around the time of Christ, Patanjali's *Yoga Sutras* offer this simple definition of Classical Yoga: "Yoga is experienced in that mind which has ceased to identify with its vacillating waves of perception." These waves are, in essence, prana. Tantrik Yoga seeks to attain communion by resolution of the states of mind into a singular form of prana. Yoginis find and eventually live in this stress-free state. Yoga seeks this state of equanimity and peace through mastery of the myriad forms of distraction that veil the pre-existing True Self.

Whereas Hatha Yoga attains this through stillness of breath as prana and Mantra Yoga through mastery of the mind as pranic sound vibrations, in Tantrik Yoga it is the polarities of Shiva/Shakti that are resolved into Communion.

Tantra has been greatly misunderstood, particularly in the West, where it is perceived primarily as sacred sexuality. This view is what I seek to transform with this book, so that the reader will not only understand but experience the wholeness of this path to communion. While Tantra does work with pranic energy, this energy is not merely sexual; it is the underlying energy of all forms of life. The key is to resolve all differences into the experience of spiritual reality. From this experience of unity arises a plethora of names and forms of sadhana that are the methodologies of communion. It is the communion that is important, not the discernment of their differences. Ultimately all spiritual practices reveal spirit as the fundamental ground of being and consciousness as the essence of the mind.

In the Vedic tradition, there are four arenas of life that must all be fulfilled in order to experience a meaningful life. The four areas are:

- Pursuing righteous duties (dharma)
- Abundance and wealth (artha)
- Sensual and sexual pleasure (kama)
- Spiritual liberation (moksha)

A balanced life depends on this foundation and leads to a peaceful existence, ultimately allowing one to meet death with contentment. Tantra as a yoga path can provide the means for fulfilling your destiny. The yoga texts point out that help is needed in three forms: reading and reflecting on a spiritual text, clarification of the mysteries revealed from that text by a spiritual teacher, and enhanced devotion to your chosen deity.

According to the first text on Classical Yoga, Patanjali's *Yoga Sutras*, the purpose of life is the dual experience of enjoyment of worldliness and spiritual liberation.[1] This arcane spiritual classic is poignant to the level of being terse in its 196 aphorisms. The same message is delivered in three sutras; no other topic is addressed with such deliberation.

> The seen world has the qualities of luminosity, activity, and stability.
> It is embodied through the elements and the sense organs.

---

1. See also *Guru Gita* introductory mantra, (SYDA Foundation: S. Fallsburg, NY, 1987), 7.

It exists for the dual purpose of sensory enjoyment and liberation of
the Self. (II, 18)

For the sake of the Self alone

does the seen world exist. (II, 21)

The mind accumulates countless desires,

although it exists solely for the sake of being close

to the True Self. (IV, 24)[2]

Self-realization is accompanied by one of two lifestyles: the renunciate path and the householder's path. The one renounces worldly activities and is celibate, while the other engages in fulfillment of worldly desires. Regardless of the path chosen, the *sattvic* (harmonious) way of being is predominant. The quest for sattvic balance needs to be foremost in our minds.

Sattva is the balanced state of mind, body, and prana that we wish to promote in all our yogic practices. Within this context, *tamasic* (lethargic) energies need to be stimulated or expressed to become sattvic. *Rajasic* (overactive) energies need to be somewhat sedated or neutralized to become balanced. In the highest expression of sattva, your energies will be elevated to a higher-dimension (*kosha*) expression. This will lead to finding Spirit in all your activities as the Tantrik process evolves all dimensions of pranic energies; over time, they will permeate all the dimensions. More on this in lesson 3, where I explain the Tantrik view of subtle anatomy.

The details of the Tantras are given in Shiva, Shakti, and Buddhist texts dating from the 9th century. Among them are:

- The Kularnava Tantra, which deals with concentration on the chakras and the supernatural powers (siddhis) that result
- Satchakra Nirupana, by Arthur Avalon (published under the title *The Serpent Power*), a text of Laya Yoga and Kundalini Shakti that explains the chakras
- Mahanirvana Tantra, which covers both socially acceptable (White Tantra) worship of your chosen deity and unorthodox or (Red) Tantrik practices
- Vijnana Bhairava Tantra, a text of non-dual Kashmir Shaivism, as taught by my own spiritual teacher.

---

2. Mukunda Stiles, *Yoga Sutras of Patanjali*, (San Francisco, CA: Weiser Books, 2001), 21, 53.

Hatha Yoga becomes more tantric by its mastery as the physical disciplines are trans-formed into energetic disciplines; this is expounded in texts like the *Hatha Yoga Pra-dipika, Gheranda Samhita,* and the *Shiva Samhita,* which date from the 14th to the 18th centuries. These texts are very Tantrik in nature, citing the ways in which the physical and subtle bodies may be transformed to create an experience of your Self as being made of an energetic blissful body, flowing with *amrita,* or nectar.

Tantra is complementary to Ayurveda and Classical Yoga practice. While Ayurveda is mainly a science of health, and Classical Yoga is a spiritual science, Tantra is a bridge between the two. The word Tantra comes from the word's root *tan,* meaning "energy," and *tra,* which means "to transform." The foundation practices of Tantrik Yoga heighten awareness of your energy body, elevating your prana to spiritual con-sciousness. Tantra's teachings focus on the energy body (emotions and mind), which is composed of the *chakras.* Distinct from neurological plexuses like the solar plexus, the chakras are the energy centers of desire.

Yogic anatomy depicts five dimensions. Most contemporary yoga practices only incorporate *asana,* which is one limb of the comprehensive eight-limb system. These practices serve wonderfully to transform the physical dimension, the first kosha. Tantrik Yoga is a spiritual practice for the transformation of each of your koshas, or multi-dimensions (see Stiles, *Structural Yoga Therapy,* pp. 43–46), through yogic energy practices. In contrast, Classical Ashtanga Yoga's teachings described in *Yoga Sutras* II, 28–55 focus on transforming the two most subtle of these dimensions (the wisdom and bliss body). Tantrik Yoga focuses on the next two dimensions (mind and pranic body). Ayurveda, the traditional medical system in India, emphasizes opti-mal health and longevity through lifestyle. An integration of these three systems, as described in my book *Ayurvedic Yoga Therapy,* can create optimal well-being and a spiritually empowered Presence.

Ayurveda describes a biological energy system composed of three *doshas* or pri-mal elements that are fundamentally unstable. They are *vata* (a combination of the elements of air and ether), *pitta* (water and fire), and *kapha* (water and earth). While Ayurveda seeks to harmonize these doshas, our efforts are unlikely to produce long-lasting benefits due to the fact that the doshas—by their very nature—do not retain stability. Therefore, our efforts need to be daily and seasonal, adapted to the individ-ual's constitutional makeup, so that the efforts made produce an underlying stability over time. Then, instead of reacting to stress with more resistance, the resulting stability will not interpret life as stressful.

Vata is the gross substance from which Yogis develop *prana* (life force). Similarly, the gross material for creating *tejas* (spiritual luminosity) is pitta, and from kapha we develop *ojas* (spiritual juices). These qualities, when refined, contribute to human evolution. In all these three systems—Ayurveda, Yoga, and Tantra—to advance is to sustain the experience of the all-pervasive prana, as its stability purifies our experience of the serene mind encountering its Lord, the inner Self. In a similar manner, we speak of refining the mind through the development of insight and discrimination, so that we can use the physical body more efficiently.

Tantra has two major forms; the primary form is for deepening the connection to your inner Self (White Tantra) with personal practice. The other forms build on that foundation of self-transformation. From a consistent personal practice, you can share your evolving spiritual and sexual energies with your spiritual partner to help bring you both into better relationship with your beloved via Red or Pink Tantra. Red Tantra encourages fulfillment of sexual energies with prolonged intercourse. In contrast, Pink Tantra promotes prolonged energy expression without intercourse. With grounding in the former (White Tantra), the latter (Red or Pink Tantra) becomes more accessible. These practices are appropriate only for people who are courageous and committed to enhancing their spiritually focused lives through developing meditation and intimacy skills.

## Seeking Energy with Yoni Mudra

The hallmark experience of Classical Yoga is slowing the mind, gradually bringing it to a still point. The key is the practice of *pranayama*, the literal meaning of which is "regulating the movements of prana." In the *Yoga Sutras*, third limb (or anga), asana is described as a means to "stilling the body" and being free of the disturbances the body has due to duality (II, 46–48). By becoming indifferent to moderate changes in temperature or not manifesting their desires quickly, Yoginis discover that subtle physical and psychological changes leave them serene (sattvic). This serenity evolves from balancing prana; when stabilized and consistent, a subtle form called *mudra* is generated. Pranayama evolves from prana into a more stable form of mind or mental energy. Similarly, as we deepen that stability to create a mudra, a durable form of prana awakens. This generates mudra, which are the techniques for the fifth anga, *pratyahara*. Pratyahara is the withdrawal of prana from the sensory objects so that the mind rests in the True Self.

I would like you to begin and end each Tantrik and yoga practice session with the yoni mudra, done by placing your palms downward, flat on your lower abdomen, so that your thumbs align straight across, with fingers together so that your forefingers touch, making a downward-pointing triangle in the space between your hands.

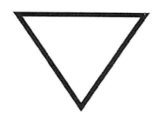

Yoni mudra

The pelvic bones resemble the physical shape of the yoni mudra. For self-healing and as a foundation for connecting with your prana, I recommend you deepen this energy pattern by placing your hands frequently in the yoni mudra. It is especially beneficial to do this after Hatha practice, as it evolves into Tantrik energetic bodywork. (In lesson 6, you will learn this technique to heal yourself and others.) Focus on directing your energies to come home from the extremities to this sacred shape (yoni, or Source) beneath your hands. This shape is the archetype of the feminine energy of receptivity. Follow your sense of the energy for some time, connecting to your energy until it feels steady. Then lower your hands to your four pelvic bones (the two iliac bones at the outer upper pelvis and the two pubic bones at the lower center) with a moderate pressure to receive the rejuvenated energy and store it into your pelvic bones and cavity. You may find that, in moving the hands lower, you need to support your elbows with pillows or a yoga block for comfort. Others find that bending their knees works best. Practice asking for guidance; it will surely awaken if you persist. Follow what comes and if you wish feedback from me as a spiritual mentor, you may email me with me the results of your experience.

The optimal time for this practice is at the beginning or end of your day, just on awakening or getting into bed. It can be done seated in bed or lying down. The morning practice will charge you up for an active day and the evening practice will help you dive into a deeper state of rest to rejuvenate you more thoroughly. It is especially beneficial at night if you are fatigued or have difficulty getting uninterrupted sleep.

# Yoni Mudra Practice

Do a body scan by sending your breath's wave throughout your torso (for details on this breath, see *Structural Yoga Therapy*, p. 53). Continue this for some time, then ask yourself to identify what are the strongest sensations that you notice. Place your hands there to feel the *"currents of sensation"* that may arise. Whatever you experience is your energy body. There may be an emotional, mental, or kinesthetic component to the sensations. Disregard analyzing it; just feel it and be with it.

If the current feels to be moving, identify the direction of the movement and encourage it to go the way that is most naturally arising. Follow the *"currents of sensation"* with your mind. Normally in yoga class, we end with *savasana*, hands and legs wide—a "posture of letting go." But now I encourage you to put your hands on the area of your body that you are breathing into and narrow or close your legs to assume a "posture of receptivity." As the sensations move, let your hands follow prana, the *"currents of sensation."* Continue as long as the energy pattern is moving. At first, do no more than five to ten minutes of this practice. Once you develop a consistent regular practice, it can be longer. Learn to both give and receive your pranic energy. This can be done from torso to hands, and vice versa.

If the sensation is not moving, identify how large an area it encompasses and get a three-dimensional perspective of its height, width, and breadth. Breathe with the intention of directing your attention throughout this area. Find out whether factors like pacing, volume, or intention of the wave-breathing pattern create a change in the sensation of this region. In doing this, let your whole body participate in the breathing, so that the subtle waves of sensation reach your inner skin. Open all you can without effort. Always remember to relax your effort until you find a naturally arising level, then you will be moving to deeper levels.

When the sensations feel complete, bring your hands to your heart while encouraging your heart to open and receive the currents of pranic sensation. When that calms and settles, place your hands in the yoni mudra where it feels most natural to conclude the session. Remain here until you feel a rejuvenation of your energy.

Remember to persist in your practice, yet stay detached from expecting specific outcomes. Tantra is a personal spiritual practice. When you feel complete with this lesson, read the Dialogue with Mukunda that follows before moving on to lesson 2.

**With Great Respect and Love, I Honor
My Heart, My Inner Teacher.**

## Dialogue with Mukunda

*Student:* I understand that we begin with our hands in yoni mudra placed on the lower abdomen. When the exercise states to drop the palms down to where the pelvic bones meet, do we keep our hands in the yoni mudra or overlap our palms so that the center of the palm is directly over the "actual yoni"? If so, is a certain palm better than the other energetically to have against the yoni? I find that keeping my hands in the mudra is more difficult than just doing the palms.

*Mukunda:* Yes, let your hands stay in yoni mudra in all placements if at all possible. There may be a need for a cushion under your elbows to help you maintain the hand position. In some cases, the hands just don't stay together when reaching for the lower placements. If you find it convenient to place your hands on top of each other, that is fine; just keep the intention of forming a yoni triangle shape with your hands or energy field. Best would be to keep your left hand on your body if they are overlapped.

*Student:* Is it correct just to be an observer and feel the energy flow and just follow it in lesson 1? I wonder how manufactured my experience is. Can experiencing just spaciousness, no tingling or surging, be considered part of the energy flow?

*Mukunda:* Mostly, I want you to feel the energy and follow it. Do not direct it. It will perform healing or spiritual awakening or whatever is most needed at this point in time. The prana is more intelligent than your conscious mind. It is the very source of thought.

*Student:* I found following the currents of sensation a bit difficult at first, but I have been practicing each evening and most mornings; with practice, it is coming. Do you have any advice?

**Mukunda:** Congratulations—just persisting is the major message here. Don't strive to achieve any specific goal; just do the lessons and, within a week or so, move on to the next one.

**Student:** May I have your help in understanding the following terms: *prana*—does this mean breath, or the energy affected by the breath? You used the terms *pranic energy* and *pranic body,* and I wasn't sure how these all fit together.

**Mukunda:** Prana is life energy, and it has a subtle body (the *prana maya kosha*). It is most easily trained through breathing exercises, but it is not the breath. Koshas are the sheaths or coverings that separate each of our five dimensions: body, prana, mind, intuition, spirit (amrita nectar), spontaneously arising bliss within.

**Student:** While studying lesson 1, I saw dreams about past years and felt quite depressed. Do you think that this relates to the Tantra lesson?

**Mukunda:** Tantra lessons as an energy practice can most definitely help you to open to your hidden abilities and find out what emotions have been unfulfilled or suppressed. It is natural that you move through these emotional states and past memories; consider them as a cleansing of your mind. The next two lessons will reveal more purification processing, what we call *kriyas.* They are invaluable for you to process so that you unfold spiritually.

**Student:** I've been reading your book *Structural Yoga Therapy,* and I'm finding it a wealth of information. I've been working with the Tantra lesson 1 and what I've experienced has been from my mind's eye. Upon forming the yoni mudra, I start to see images that I'm not bringing to my awareness and, in fact, the second I try to direct it at all, it stops. Any feedback would be appreciated.

**Mukunda:** Thanks for the praise of my book. I am glad to hear you enjoy and benefit from it. The opening of spiritual energies is a natural result of Tantrik practice. It is guided by my connection to Devi and the Divine Presence. The best attitude is to allow it to unfold you. As you are experiencing, it is spontaneous and does not respond to your mind. Namaste.

*Student:* I practiced for the first time last night. I noticed immediately my old conflict between being very frightened of feeling anything out of the ordinary and desperately wanting "something" to happen. Happily, I felt only the warmth of my hands on my heart and belly, and cool, slow breaths entering my lungs. Hooray, nothing to be afraid of there. Later that night, I dreamed that our beautiful earth was made up of rays of light and that these rays all came down to a tiny point that fit in the center of the yoni mudra made by my hands placed on my belly.

I'll continue this first lesson for increased intervals up to ten minutes for another week (unless you suggest otherwise), then write to you with further observations and the request for lesson 2. As always, I give thanks for the gift of your teaching.

*Mukunda:* All is going quite well. Keep it up. Good.

*Student:* For me, lesson 1 has produced a memory of freedom in my body. It takes a while to still my mind, or to be at peace with my wandering mind—it is very busy. But when it calms down, I see a vibrant blue behind my closed eyes. What I notice is that, as I return my hands to the yoni mudra, the light changes quickly, in an upward movement, turning bright white.

*Mukunda:* Great, you are doing well; just continue to let it evolve in its personal way.

*Student:* I have been working with lesson 1 for about two weeks pretty consistently. I find the yoni mudra to be very powerful in allowing me to feel energy concentration. I have been experiencing an upward flow to belly and heart, and then to jaw (where I hold lots of tension). The result of the energy flow there brings spaciousness to my jaw hinge. In the last few days, the energy has not been moving up to my jaw, but I still feel space there. I have not been able to retain the entire sequence in my head while I am doing the practice and see a bit more of the involvement every time I reread the instructions.

At times, I wonder how much of the sensation I feel is "real" and how much of it is made up. In other words, am I guiding the flow, or just allowing myself to feel it? And then I wonder what the difference is. I have been working with another practice of circulating prana, in which you are actually guiding the energy in a circuit—down my legs and back up, up my spine to the top of my head and down again, etc. I have been trying to focus on my jaw in general for some time now in daily life and asana practice, so the spacious feeling I naturally experienced in the first week of practice was a welcome relief.

The second week, I wondered how manufactured my experience was. Can experiencing just spaciousness, no tingling or surging, be considered part of the energy flow?

*Mukunda:* You are doing well.

*Student:* At first, I felt pain in a couple of areas of my body. I put my hands there and breathed into the areas. After a couple weeks, now I only feel the breath and a deep sense of relaxation. I do it before bed, but have done it at other times to see if I notice a difference. Yesterday, I received reconnective healing, a massage, and soaked in the hot springs; then my friend from Singapore brought a CD of toning healing sounds. We did healing work with one of us and then toned for about half an hour. Toward the end, I was lying down, and I used this lesson 1. It seemed to fit. At the end of the session, I felt complete. At the same time, the CD ended and said, "Namaste." I slept *soooo* well last night. I do not know what I am suppose to experience, but this is how I have integrated this lesson into my life and what I have felt. Am I ready for lesson 2?

*Mukunda:* Wonderful. You are doing fabulously well. Thanks for sending me such a detailed story of your experiences.

*Student:* I've noticed that my dreams have been very fearful as I continue the practices of lesson 1. In one, the sky opened with a thunderclap and a beam of light shone down. In another, I fell from a tree into a body of water, but didn't die. In a third, I could only see bright green light with no other shapes or colors. I've also noticed that my abdomen is more upset and distended, as if forming a taut shield. But I persevere with practice and know that, with consistency, things will right themselves. It's just a little disconcerting.

*Mukunda:* Thanks for your notes. Let me know when you are ready for the next step. Best is to move on and not concern yourself with the results of practicing lesson 1. If you stay there searching for stability, it will not come; that is not how Tantra works. It purposely seeks to uproot you where you are unstable and reveal that instability, so that you can seek elevation and true transformation—not merely superficial change.

*Student:* The first Tantra lesson has been interesting. It seems that it isn't so much developing a consciousness about the energy, as placing the focus on where the consciousness is already. It also seems to me that some people's connections between the physical body and subtle body are either more fixed or looser, just like physical joints. My purpose in my subtle-body practice is to know it and to organize it. I have a feeling your lessons are about doing just this very thing. So thank you again.

**Mukunda:** Good.

**Student:** When I place my hands in yoni mudra over the second chakra, I feel I must support my elbows on blankets so I can relax my hands and not have to exert effort to hold them there. So I do that; then when I breathe into the second chakra area, I have a feeling of strong resistance to receiving the breath here. I would describe the "feeling" as one of absence, nothingness, numbness. As I stay with it, I find myself getting anxious that I am not "feeling" something there—not feeling what I "should" be feeling, though I don't know what that feeling should be!

As I become more agitated about the numbness and absence of feeling in my second chakra, I become conscious of feeling heavy, blocked, and constricted around the heart and throat, as if something heavy and black were pressing down on my heart and two hands were wrapped around my throat trying to choke off the sadness and anxiety I feel there. This leads to feelings of panic and hopelessness, that I'm just not "getting it." This puts me in touch with a lifelong way of being and feeling—i.e., that there is something outside my perceptual abilities that other people understand and know and that I should be getting and am not.

If I stay with it longer, eventually the feelings subside, but I'm not clear if that's because I can't tolerate the distress I'm feeling, or if it's just a natural diffusion and relaxation of the feelings from staying there and experiencing them.

I had both my children by C-section, and the incision in my abdomen definitely numbed me to sensation there; I think that is a contributing factor to the "nothingness" or blockage I feel when I breathe into the second chakra area, but not the whole story. Do you have any insight or comments on what's going on in my practice here?

**Mukunda:** The sensations are natural, given your history. I encourage you to continue to do the practice and allow whatever comes up to come up. In Tantra, we conceive of what comes up as coming out. Blocked energies are being experienced as a way of finding their way to home. When that truly arises, there is a feeling of deeper connection to your yoni as the Source of your Goddess Tantrika energy. With C-sections, the numbness is natural, although with Tantrik practice, there can be consciousness increasing without sensations. In other words, sensation as neurology is different from perception as consciousness. We want the latter, even if the former is not hardwired. If you wish, we can do an individual session and help you open more. By the input of my energy into yours, you will have more to work with, thus clearing the pattern at a deeper level. It sounds to me as if there is some deeper, if not past-life, karma here too. *Getting* it is not the goal. The goal is *being* it— being the sensations and emotions until they release you from their grip. Once this is fully accepted, the goal is experienced.

**Student:** In continuing the practice with the first Tantra lesson, I do sense that I am "host" to something "not me"—an energy indigenous to my mother's side of the family, involving prohibitions against exuberance and fear of/resistance to wading into "dangerous" feeling. Whatever it is, I do hope it can be cleared. The persistent feeling/image I have is of being caged and fearful of emerging. I wrote down the images that came to me in my journal a couple of days ago, and felt that some small piece had cleared as a result of getting it down on paper.

I received counseling from a bioenergetic therapist over a period of about six years, and stopped eight years ago when we moved. The work I did with him helps me "get" your message that the goal is not to "get" it, but to "be" it. He helped me move in that direction up to a certain point, beyond which I was not yet ready to go. I'm hoping I am in a place now where I can let go of whatever this is and clear it out.

**Mukunda:** The issue is not for you to release it and clear it out. It is more about communicating with the entity and family history and telling it that you are now free, independent, and able to assume responsibilities that it was taking on for you due to your weakness. You are now stronger-willed and spiritually more capable of taking on the tasks assigned you by your previous karma. You are now consciously purifying yourself of your past limitation, from which this "veil" has protected you. By holding on to that positive and responsible role for yourself, the veil can be lifted from you. I have done some remote clearing for you this morning, and there is more for you to do by taking on a will to move ahead in your karmic spiritual life. When we meet, I can do and show you more. Blessings for wanting to be free.

**Student:** An automobile accident in 1994 left me with severe left-frontal-lobe brain damage and adult ADD with dyslexia, and brought on a rapid onset of full-body fibromyalgia syndrome and chronic fatigue. The good thing that came out of the accident is that it started me on a real search to find the Higher Source. Since that time, I have taken many detours trying to find my personal path. Luckily, you cannot fail as long as you are seeking Spirit!

I have been doing the *Flexible Strength/Joint Freeing Yoga* video every other day since the *Structural Yoga Therapy* intensive in Boulder, and it has helped a lot. However, I am in my second week of lesson 1 of the Tantra series and was starting to feel that I was either doing something wrong or on another detour.

This morning, for the first time, I could feel the energy starting to move, but randomly. I had a very symbolic "vision" upon exiting my meditation and felt energized! The best part of it all is that I feel calmer and more relaxed than I have felt in years. I can actually relax my shoulders and neck to some extent, and the pain is not nearly so uncomfortable. I have not been without pain since the accident and refuse to live on medication. Now, perhaps, there is light at the end of that tunnel. I keep blanketing myself in the soft blanket of the Lord's loving light and know somehow I will someday be able to reach a state of bliss. Thank you.

**Mukunda:** Wonderful of you to share of the power of my teachings. I am delighted to hear of a shift in your experience. I will be sharing this work in Atlanta this coming weekend and would like to read your story to them. In the meantime, I recommend that you linger on lesson 1, especially the Dialogue section. Then proceed to lesson 2. After a week or so, move on with lessons at your own pace. Clearly, you are doing well in your ranayama practice, as prana is making its presence so distinct. So let us just deepen your experience by mentored progression through all of the lessons

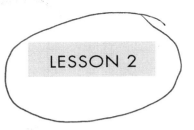

LESSON 2

# The Five Elements and Sensuality

With Great Respect and Love, I Honor
My Heart, My Inner Teacher.

Tantrik practice encourages a deep appreciation of the natural world. Through aromas, tastes, sights, and uplifting sounds and touch, the world of beauty found in art, literature, and the natural world is deeply enhanced. The Tantrik seeks to stay awakened to the senses, aroused by the sensuality of life and, through these sensations, comes to know the spiritual source of that beauty. Allow your mind to be captivated by sensual pleasures so that you will pause and enjoy the unexpected that God/dess is continually unveiling and veiling. Mother is a passionate dancer hidden behind the veils of a material life. When authentic beauty captivates us, we begin to see and know Her presence in life.

Each of the senses relates to the Tantrik and yogic view of subtle anatomy, called the elemental body. Earth, the grossest element, relates to smell; water to taste; fire to sight; air to touch; ether to sound and hearing. A beautiful practice is to observe your senses and encourage them to perceive the wonders of the world. In the more ancient philosophy of Samkhya upon which the *Yoga Sutras* is based, there are twenty-four evolutionary steps (*tattvas*) from unity awareness to the duality that we experience as the multi-faceted world. The five elements precede the senses. By acutely feeling the perceptions that the five senses give us, our energy will be elevated. We naturally feel more passionate as we perceive our sensual inputs with more uninhibited responses. This is especially deepened by practices given in lesson 5, which deal with moving from sensuality into prana. It is further enlivened in lesson 9, which deals with Tantrik love and natural expression.

We will develop an awareness of Self through the elements of the physical body as they correlate to the subtle-body chakras. Although the chakras are given an anatomical landmark for their location, they are not physical. They are affected, not by physical activity, but by the mind and senses. The elements and corresponding chakras are:

> Earth—first root chakra (*muladhara*), in the perineal pelvic-floor region

> Water—second chakra (*svadhisthana*), externally at the top of the pubic bone in men and internally at the cervix (opening of the uterus) in women

> Fire—third chakra (*manipura*), in the navel region

> Air—fourth chakra (*anahata*), in the center of the chest

> Ether—fifth chakra (*vishuddhi*), at the base of the throat

Two more chakras do not have a physical form as they are beyond the elements—the sixth or third eye (*ajna*) chakra and the seventh or crown (*sahasrara*) chakra.

While our physical health and vitality do not directly correspond to the subtle body, nonetheless Tantrik Yoga uses physical exercises for each chakra region as a doorway to finding the pranic energy hidden there in subtle spaces. Realize that, from the yogic view of anatomy, the chakras are in the second kosha, not in the physical body (first kosha).

One primary problem according to Rabbi Zalman Schacter-Shalomi, leader of the Jewish renewal movement, is that "the chakras do not talk to each other." They miscommunicate through the mind and body; clarity for them is non-verbal and non-physical—more intuitive. Their pattern must be known separately from their influence on the other koshas.

## Elements and Sensual Awareness—Nyasa Puja

This Tantrik exercise will unveil the elemental principles (known as the *tattvas*) that make up your organic body.

Sitting in your favorite spot, perhaps in front of an altar, each of the senses with something that is pleasantly stimulating exercise, offer each element in a ritual of worship (*puja*).

The purpose of worship is to cultivate higher consciousn and love of your True Self. Wave the offering three times vertic circle to the center of your altar, then bow to Spirit as you place the first sense (smell) offer an aroma that is particularly arousing; then move to offer a food that has a delicious taste. Next, offer a lit candle, symbolic of fire, then offer a cloth that is particularly soothing to touch. Finally, offer a prayer or mantra that is uplifting. Before making each offering, stimulate your senses with it—smell the flower; taste the fruit; look at the candle and contemplate the fire; feel the cloth; chant or sing the prayer or mantra. The offerings can be visualized or real, whatever is significant for you. The same offering can be used for more than one sense. For example, a flower can be used for both smell (earth, base chakra) and touch (air, heart chakra). In this exercise, you move through the gross senses toward the higher ones that are beyond your ordinary sensual perception—in essence, beyond the elements that comprise your body.

The second time you do this exercise, touch the physical location associated with each of the elements. By touching each location with the intention of imparting its element to the space, you are doing a Tantrik practice called *nyasa*. This technique empowers the gross elements that make up your physical body to seek their energetic connection to your subtle body's corresponding chakras via the sense organs. From this practice comes a thinning of the veils of the koshas that comprise the yogic five bodies. In the Tantrik model, the first five chakras relate to the senses. The base chakra's energy formed from the earth element is sensual in nature, thus its evolution will heighten your appreciation of pleasure and beauty.

I recommend that both of these exercises be performed at one sitting at the beginning of your morning. Practice the two exercises for the duration of this lesson and, if you enjoy them, they can become part of your daily practice. These lessons will expose you to many practices. Keep what is beneficial and let the rest go.

As touch controls the air element, it is the easiest of the senses to help you feel and regulate the pranas. Some Tantriks (specifically naga yogis and other wandering *sadhus*) do their practices free of clothing so that the perception of *vyana* prana, which flows through the skin and auric field via the air and ether elements respectively, is

19

ptible and thus more readily increased. Sunbathing is a wonderful way to
sitize the skin to the energies of nature and your own emotional body. As overdo-
ng this will imbalance pitta, it is best done before 11:00 a.m. and after 3:00 p.m. in
hot climates. For sadhus, sunbathing is a lifestyle, although, like others who practice
sunbathing for health, they use it with discretion.

When practices are revealed indiscriminately, their deeper meaning is lost. So
some of what I will share here is not meant for you to share with others, as the uninitiated may misinterpret its hidden spiritual meanings. If you are a yoga teacher, do
not consider what you learn as fodder to be shared with others. The intention of these
lessons is to give you a Tantrik *sadhana* or spiritual practice. This sequence of lessons
will first create emotional and mental health before going into the weaving of energy
practices that are the hallmark of Tantra.

> Tantrik Yoga proposes that we change our perspective on desire in
> order to improve our perceptions and our sense of taste. While drink-
> ing a glass of water, for example, if we believe that this water desires
> us, we will have an experience of consciousness; we will feel the water
> penetrate into us and cross through us. Everything we taste can then
> bring us the fundamental experience of union with the elements. The
> *Vijnana Bhairava Tantra*, 72 states: at the time of euphoria and
> expansion caused by delicate foods and drinks, be total in this delight,
> and through it, taste supreme bliss.[3]

As you make each offering to your elements, wait until you feel complete with the
process. Often this awakens a repressed emotion, so take your time and encourage
your senses to reveal their higher aesthetic sense. When sexual or emotional energy
is allowed to build, it becomes neutral energy. If you persist, it will be experienced as
spiritual energy. Know that these lessons are for the purpose of moving through yourself
to finding that deeper energy.

Make the offering first to yourself at each chakra location, then place the offerings lovingly on your altar as the symbol of your inner "sacred space." Offer the aroma
with your right hand, then touch with your left hand the outer part of the body associated with it—the root chakra at the base of your pelvis. Then offer the taste with your

---

3.  Daniel Odier, *Desire* (Rochester, VA: Inner Traditions, 1999), 44.

hand touching the pubic region. For the third offering of sight, touch the region of the navel. The fourth offering is made with contact to the center of your chest, the fourth chakra. The fifth offering is made while touching the base of your throat. As the sixth and seventh chakras are beyond the elements, there is no practice for them on this grosser dimension.

When you finish, place your right hand on your lower abdomen in the second-chakra region and your left hand at your heart. Then use the wave breath of *ujjaye* to connect all your energies into one stream. Allow it to be a natural process, and avoid the tendency to make something happen. Having the attitude of allowing whatever happens to be perfect will strengthen your detachment and encourage a serene (sattvic) attitude. For more details on this practice see *Tattva Shuddhi* by Swami Satyasangananda of the Bihar School of Yoga.

## Return to Your Source—Yoni Mudra

End your physical yoga practices with yoni mudra either sitting or lying. Repeat the sequence detailed in the previous lesson. As you seek to know where your energy is most predominant, that will help develop mental focus, which in turn will give your physical body more energy. Mind and body are coupled in this practice. As energy increases, it will tend to be healing and/or nurturing. Encourage whatever is a naturally arising experience by opening yourself to your own prana. Consider this practice as an energetic "self-hug." Later, you can share the same loving energetic hug with friends and/or a Tantrik partner to elevate both of you.

Sometimes the increased energy will tend to become polarized. In this case, you will find that there is not one place that grabs your attention, but two. When you perceive this, put your right hand on the lower energy spot and your left hand on the upper one. Encourage whatever is arising as an emotion, energy feeling, or a "current of sensation," and follow the energy wherever it leads you. This can result in a wide array of phenomenon—including deep stillness, physical motions, trembling, irregular breathing—or as suppressed emotions rising for expression. After the energy runs its course, it will naturally seek its Source. As it comes to completion, continue to follow its expression to a natural place of resolution. When the spontaneous component is over, slowly lower your hands to yoni mudra on your lower abdomen. You may be drawn to this placement as an indication of harmony.

Many students find that this technique is not really a technique, but the result of a feeling of pranic harmony. By lingering in this place, deeper insights into lifestyle changes that are wanted or spiritual insights will arise. This is the experience of moving through the koshas as you are uncovering the multi-dimensional experience of your energy bodies.

Although the essence of yoni mudra is to search for and locate the source of your energy, there are four specific positions that have unique benefits you can develop. From the practice of these four variations, you can develop your capacity to find the subtle elements that precede emotions.

> The first placement is with your thumbs meeting at the navel point. In this placement, you can locate a woman's internal organs. The forefingers will touch at the site of your uterus (shaped like a pear with its narrow end downward, about the size of a plum), and the little fingers will identify the ovaries. This placement is especially beneficial for healing your sex organs.

> The second placement is slightly higher, centered around your navel, the fire element. This placement can soothe intestinal inflammation or menstrual cramps.

> The third is with the bladder placed in the center of the triangle to locate your water element. In this position, your hands will rest on the bones of your pelvis. Your wrists will rest upon the upper outer-iliac pelvic bones, and your fingertips will rest on your pubic bones. This placement is especially beneficial in grounding your pranic energies. From this placement, you can learn to store prana in your bones, which may be of help with osteoporosis.

> The fourth placement is with your outer sex organs centered in the yoni mudra, with your fingertips reaching toward your pelvic floor, which is associated with the earth element. This position can be made easier by lying with your knees bent and pillows under the elbows, or sitting. This variation can be nurturing to your sexual expression or healing to unlock sexual events and blocked or judgmental patterns.

Do each of these placements for a minimum of five minutes or until your energy pattern stabilizes. Linger there, allowing your pranic energy to take you into yourself. Continue with this practice until you can both give and receive to each of your three elemental regions.

By deepening this training, you are forming the foundation for healing yourself and others as described in lesson 6 on Tantrik bodywork. I do not wish to tell you more of the effects of these four placements, but rather let you awaken to how varied the sensations are that move within your physical, emotional, and energetic bodies. Let this become a form of Bhakti Yoga, the yoga of love, surrendering to your feelings and the currents of sensation that generate them.

The subtler concept of yoni mudra is described in *Vasistha's Yoga:*

> The "I" enters into the triangle in its own conception; and because it is aware of itself, it believes itself to be a body, though this is unreal and only appears to be real. In that triangle which is the sheath of karma, the individual which is of the very essence of sperm and egg exists in that body just as fragrance exists in a flower. Even as the sun's rays spread throughout the earth, this individual which is in the sperm and egg has entered the triangle and spreads itself throughout the body.[4]

By placing your hands in the triangle symbol, you will reverse the process of energy spreading out to create your individuality as mudra generates the process of *pratyahara*, withdrawing prana back to its Source. With consistent practice of all the component parts of these Tantrik lessons, the secrets of Tantrik transformation will reveal themselves to you, naturally unfolding your innate spiritual nature.

You now have three ways to access and evolve your prana:

> Following the currents of energetic sensations from wherever they arise to their source

> Feeling the polarity of the currents and balancing their polar expression of lower and higher, tense and relaxed, stronger and subtler

> Directly perceiving your energy through yoni mudra

---

4.  Swami Venkatesananda (trans.), *Vasistha's Yoga* (Albany, NY: SUNY Press, 1993), 505.

Remember to persist in your practice, yet stay detached from expecting specific outcomes. Tantra is a personal spiritual practice. When you feel complete with this lesson, read the Dialogue section that follows prior to beginning lesson 3.

**With Great Respect and Love, I Honor
My Heart, My Inner Teacher.**

## Dialogue with Mukunda

*Student:* I am confused about the effect of unfinished *puja* practice. I experienced restlessness, anxiety, mind chattering, not balanced. I continued having heat waves at irregular times.

I started my morning with the puja. In the first chakra, I noticed a tremendous heat wave again originating from the center of my back spreading evenly through my whole body. I asked for a guide but did not hear any voice or spiritual input. After a couple of seconds, I felt comfortable with the heat sensation, and it eased smoothly. I was just in the process of the puja of the second chakra when the phone rang and I disrupted the practice and did not continue. I have done this before in a meditation session. So I didn't think it would be a problem.

During the entire day, I felt anxiety, restlessness, nervousness, and uneasiness with everything I did. My mind felt scattered. I felt angry deep inside. So I didn't do any other spiritual practice (meditation or chanting). When I was in town, I found other men attractive, but I have a boyfriend.

*Mukunda:* This is an effect of not completing the puja practice. It is important that, when you begin a spiritual practice, you not be interrupted by life. In this case, you considered the phone more important, so energy was lost and didn't know what to do, so it simply stayed in the second chakra stimulating latent sexuality. Tantra is more powerful than meditation. It is an awakening. In contrast, meditation is often a deeper form of the yoga pose of rejuvenation (savasana). Complete what you begin, but of course be practical.

*Student:* Could you please tell me if such practice can modify/reduce the flow of menstruation?

*Mukunda:* This practice definitely can modify menstrual experiences. Below, you will find the story of a woman who has not had a period in several years and she just had one from this lesson. So what I find is that which is suppressed becomes expressed, while that which is overly expressed becomes less so. Harmony is the natural result of deeper energy practice.

*Student:* The practice with yoni mudra is quite interesting to me. It is something that came to me spontaneously several years ago. I don't know exactly when, but at night when I go to bed, I lie on my stomach with my hands in this mudra. It's almost a ritual now. I don't seem to be able to get relaxed for sleep without it. Is that an attachment? I have never learned it from anyone; it just happened. When I received the first lesson from you, it was serendipitous. I knew it was something I like, almost need, to go to sleep. So I decided to try it sitting up. I realized how much I need to relax and how little movement is present, physical or energetic, in my abdominal region. When I do asana and formal pranayama practices, I release my belly, but otherwise it's pretty tight. What comments do you have about this? Is it fear or just a *samskara*? Should I try to wean myself from this nightly practice?

*Mukunda:* You are creating a natural response. Your subconscious past impression knew that energy needed to go there in order to create relaxation. If this is a samskara, it is a good one. I encourage you to learn from the response and continue to deepen your practice of the Tantrik lessons. In fact, this technique is what I give to those with difficulty sleeping. Even in the case of insomnia, it can be helpful when persistence is developed along with the capacity to follow the subtle currents of sensation that increase with its use. Persist. Don't discontinue.

*Student:* I have had physical pain in the second chakra pelvic area for many years. I realized by doing yoni mudra that it was related to my negative mental thoughts during sexual experiences. I consciously changed my thoughts to a more honoring, loving, positive pattern during my next sexual experience, and the pain was barely there. I still have, two weeks later, some tenderness, but not the intense pain where I have to guard against someone pressing on that area. No emotions came up; it was just in my mind, my thoughts. Does this make any sense? Could it be this easy?

I keep chasing the fear of it coming back by keeping focused on positive thoughts when making love (even to the point of saying "making love" instead of "having sex"). Nothing else comes up for me. Yet I do not feel complete, as it does not come naturally for me. I need to find another tool for this, and I haven't found one as effective. I am thinking Yoga Nidra by tape, but am not sure how to do it. My husband is not very open to that sort of thing. It is like an addiction I want to break. Was this lesson supposed to trigger this sort of thing? Should I move on to the third lesson while I continue working on this issue? Help. Thank you.

*Mukunda:* This is a natural response to the lesson of working with the yoni mudra. In some ways, you are ahead of the logical progression of the lessons, for they are written in a rational-mind sequence. And prana is not rational; it goes with the inner flow of what is needed. As a result, the healing that comes spontaneously is more profound and deeper. It tends to give each individual exactly what they need rather than what they think they need. Sounds to me as if this is perfect.

Yes, you can create a Yoga Nidra process to guide yourself.[5] I do not recommend using a cassette tape, as you mention your husband is not open to this, so respect his need for being as he is. Instead, do this tape by yourself prior to bed. This lesson often triggers such openings, as you will read from others in the Dialogue section of this lesson. Move on, by all means. The issue will be healed deeper as you progress through the lessons.

*Student:* I talk myself through a deep relaxation and then try to get a sense of the energy and place my hands in yoni mudra at the suggested places on my body. When I place my hands in the genital area, I feel a particular surge of energy all the way to my toes. It is not as if I have been totally ignoring the more sensual part of me, but I have not placed much emphasis on developing or nurturing that part of me either. I think it has, yet again, to do with boundary issues. I feel I need to be very clear about how I project myself as a massage therapist, yoga teacher, and mother—which is pretty down-to-earth, practical, and not particularly sensual.

*Mukunda:* Not uncommon. But the training in the Tantra lessons allows the energy to run its course without needing a sexual or sensual expression to someone else. Simply feel the "currents of sensation," rather than labeling them as sexual, since sexual energy tends to seek expression. Feeling feelings is a more powerful process. When you do this, you learn to hold on to your prana with more integrity and to express it consciously to elevate yourself and others.

---

5.  For those not knowing this deeply opening process, see tapes on this by Richard Miller at *www.nondual.com.*

*Student:* I find doing the mudra in these positions to be very grounding and calming. Sometimes I get surges of energy coming up through the muladhara center, which tends to make my legs shake and vibrate. Is this simply a release of prana moving through my body?

*Mukunda:* It is great that your body is having surges of energy. You are naturally moving on to the next lesson. As energy releases, it has a mind or higher intelligence of its own that redirects you to a more expanded and often detached point of view of your *vasanas* (latent emotional tendencies). Ultimately, this process leads us to a deeper experience of the naturally arising energy of yoga. Consider this one of many experiences you will walk through to a more integrated self.

*Student:* I have been working with yoni mudra for just over two weeks and have been experiencing a heightened sensitivity to things. I already, to an extent, had a sensitivity to energy, but with yoni mudra, my sensitivities seem to be heightened in a different way, in more of a psychic way. Don't get me wrong, I have not been able to experience a severe clarity, but do feel energy collecting in this place. What could this be?

*Mukunda:* Different dimensions of awareness (koshas) manifest different experiences of this yoni mudra. Heightened sensitivity showing in an increase in prana is a sign of nurturing the second kosha. Intuition or psychic sensitivity is due to an increase in fourth-kosha activity. That it is vague is natural, until it becomes more grounded. Grounding is a process that happens both in the physical body as well as in the subtler koshas. By grounding in the physical body, I mean the yoni mudra is felt in your tissues. Abdominal placement may connect to ovaries, intestines, or uterus. Placement of the hands on the pubic bones and iliac crests will ground the energy to your skeleton. Either of these placements can promote grounding. Explore lesson 2 and see which feels more settling for you. Over time, the vagueness moves in and out of clarity until, eventually, less fear is present—and that brings confidence in your psychic or intuitive perceptions. This, of course, is the subtle form of listening more to your Inner Teacher. Until that happens more consistently, it is important to follow your outer teacher more carefully.

*Student:* I have a question, but it does not relate to the lessons. I have found myself in the same difficult situation many times, but I have changed and I would like feedback on this situation. I have a son with cerebral palsy, and I am frequently asked the same question: "What is your son's prognosis?" Ten years ago, I would suffer a loss of energy. Today, I understand people have different belief systems and are unaware of other people's feelings. I was not drained, but rather wanted to act out of compassion. It was obvious the person was not ready for what I had to say. I answered by saying, "Who knows?" I want to make a healing connection with others, but I would like to know how you know when it is appropriate to give and when is it appropriate just to be blunt, as long as it is done with compassion. I believe I am ready for this lesson.

*Mukunda:* Your question does relate to the lessons. The Tantra lessons will help with this more personally than I can share here. But it is about feeling drained or charged as a result of how you share with others. By waiting and training yourself to observe energy, compassion and love will be emotional energies that build. We all lose prana in certain life situations, and these qualities seem far away. Learning to watch prana will tell you who to be with and how to share with them. Prana reacts instantly to all situations; it can be read in the pulse by Ayurvedic training or in the whole energy field. This training can give you some skill in these directions. Whether to be blunt is not the question; a better question is to see what raises or retains your energy. We seek to be sattvic (harmonious) in all situations.

*Student:* I have been meditating every Monday night for the last three years with the same group of four women. I mentioned to them last week that I was participating in your Tantrik lessons, and they are very interested in doing them together as a group. Would you mind if the five of us committed to doing the lessons on our own throughout the week, meeting every Monday to discuss how we are each doing?

*Mukunda:* Doing the lessons together is a great idea. I am delighted. I suggest you do practice for several days on your own, then read the Dialogue section and have discussions on your experience, as well as what others experience.

*Student:* I'm a yoga teacher. What do you say to my handing this yoni mudra exercise on to my class?

*Mukunda:* If you seek to be a guide to others, I offer training as a spiritual mentor for those wishing to use the elements of these Tantrik lessons. In order to share spiritual and subtle-body techniques, I recommend being trained for a minimum of two years. It is crucial to develop stability of the mind before training can be of benefit to others.

*Student:* I received from you lesson 2, and I found lots of power in the first part—making offerings to the chakras—but not so much in the second part. Should we be practicing the two parts together, one after another, when the lessons have multiple parts?

*Mukunda:* Do them sequentially, but you can also repeat some parts if they possess more captivating qualities for you.

*Student:* When I do the practice of the nyasa, do I experience/stimulate the senses with each offering or just offer it? For instance, smell the flower or taste the fruit? Is the sound offering in written form and/or spoken/sung?

*Mukunda:* You want to stimulate your sense with each offering before offering the object. Smell the flower, cut the fruit, taste a small portion and offer the rest. Sound can be chanted or sung.

*Student:* In nyasa, you make reference to touching the chakra points as you offer the second time. Is this how I should do it from then on—with the third, fourth, etc.? Should this become part of a daily practice? Is there a particular time of day that is recommended for this practice?

*Mukunda:* It is done for the period of this lesson. The best time is at the beginning of your morning practice. If you enjoy this, it can become part of daily practice. The lessons will expose you to many practices; keep what is beneficial, let the rest go.

*Student:* Does the offering have to be literal or may I offer an experience, like the scent of a ylang-ylang blossom after a storm or the taste of a childhood candy?

*Mukunda:* That is fine. You are free to do the offering that is the most significant to you.

*Student:* If the offering is real, does it have to be several different objects or may it be one, like a flower that has a beautiful scent, taste (if it is a rose), or touch?

*Mukunda:* You can use the same object for more than one sense.

*Student:* Does the offering have to be made during this practice or can I offer any sensations/experiences that I encounter during my waking moments? Now that I am re-awakening, I am more aware of the wonders around me.

*Mukunda:* It is ideal to do the practice at one sitting rather than throughout the day.

*Student:* As I'm reading the lesson, I'm first offering the element of a pleasing aroma to my root, taste to my second chakra, sight to my third. . . . Is this just a pleasing object to look at or a candle as in the previous lesson or does it matter?

*Mukunda:* It is up to your own naturally arising associations.

*Student:* Fourth chakra refers to an item in the second part, but in the first part it is something soothing to touch . . . yes? And the same for the fifth. Are we listening to a beautiful mantra as we just place our left hand to the base of the throat? I guess I'm not clear on what items correspond with which chakra; that's where I'm confused.

*Mukunda:* This is for searching for an association of a sense organ to a chakra. That is all.

*Student:* With regards to "returning to your source," I'm confused about the number of yoni mudra positions. On the last page, you refer to "three specific positions" and then say "the practice of these four variations," then describe four placements. You then mention practice until you can give and receive to each of your three elemental regions. Do only three of the four placements relate to elements? Could you clarify this?

*Mukunda:* There are four positions (a typo due to revising each lesson). The first around the navel; the second with your thumbs in the navel; the third with your hands touching your three pelvic bones; the fourth with your hands surrounding your sex. The first is covering the element of fire (third chakra); the third surrounds the bladder element of water (second chakra); the fourth places your fingertips at the root chakra (earth element).

*Student:* I have been practicing the yoni mudra in the four positions you describe, but have been having difficulty in doing the one where the triangle frames the genital area. I find it is an awkward reach to get the triangle down low enough so that it frames the center of this area. It is also difficult for me to relax in this position. I think one would have to have the arms of an orangutan to perform this mudra properly. Am I doing something wrong here? Do you have any suggestions?

*Mukunda:* A lovely image of you as an orangutan. They are blessed with convenience in such unusual yogic postures. For some people, this is more easily accomplished in a couple of ways—lying with your knees bent, which lifts the pubic angle, or sitting. The former is often more comfortable with pillows under the elbows to support the arms for a longer stay.

*Student:* Why do we place yoni mudra on the lower abdomen and not higher up? I thought the solar plexus area is where prana resides. (Don't remember specifically where I got that.)

*Mukunda:* It can go anywhere, but this is for helping vata to come home. Once vata is at home, the pranas can separate from it and go to their respective homes. Each of the five pranas has a different home. Samana prana's home is the abdomen. Others are throughout the body.

*Student:* At the moment, my progress is unfortunately very small.

*Mukunda:* Consistency is more important than progress. Just keep at it, and eventually you will be captivated by the energy. The fact that you are thinking of the pranas and their energy shows that they have your attention. Your mind is composed of prana; therefore, what has your attention has prana.

*Student:* I noticed that, when sitting quietly after making the puja offerings, there were sensations that moved from the bottom up through each of the chakras one at a time. I remember thinking, "Okay, this sensation is *energy*; this is one way that it can manifest." After that, there was a feeling as if a cool drop of something tingly had started at the crown of my head and was slowly making its way down the front of my face.

You said that it's important to develop serenity (sattva). I think of it as balance and indifference toward things that may happen. I am really enjoying the puja practice. I feel great reverence, love, and awe while making the offerings. I have to take a moment to calm down, it makes me so excited and happy. And, of course, I worry that it's not appropriate to have an emotion one way or the other (fear, angst, or anticipation).

*Mukunda:* Good to work with sattvic attitude, yes. That indeed is the evolution of yoga and Tantra. By becoming harmonious and detached from having a specific outcome to your efforts, the experience is, as you say, reverence, love, and awe. Lovely experiences.

*Student:* I'm finding that my awareness of energies is becoming more sensitive, especially in my lower spine. There seems to be no shortage of emotional energy to work with. I don't find it happens during the practice, but that situations or things people say suddenly open up awareness. My son was very upset at the prospect of going back to school and, on the way, asked me, "What do you hate most in the world?" The question completely floored me, and I haven't dared to answer it yet.

*Mukunda:* I find it is wonderful how family and intimate relations support the spiritual or inner work when one takes it seriously. I find that your son asking such questions is a sign of the depth of your inquiry. In such cases, you need not search for answers; being engaged in the search is the sadhana.

*Student:* Today, putting yoni mudra on my abdomen and feeling the sensations sent my hands to my solar plexus as the center (*bindu*) with fingertips on the navel. I noticed fear and emptiness there. I am elated to have this insight and am already practicing to reduce stress in several ways in my life. You originally gave me a practice to use yoni mudra with the heels of my hands on my ilium. That practice has been very helpful. It seems that layers are unraveling! I also oil my body every day now, mostly using sesame oil, and am eating mostly rice and beans as a cleansing temporary diet (*kechari*). I am grateful for the precious gift of your quiet presence in my life.

*Mukunda:* The oiling is also great as a deeper balancing of stress into the tissues. Both are working together, as you put it, to unravel the layers of your self.

*Student:* In August, I was stuck and in mental anesthesia. I became more sensitive than before, and I didn't have emotional and mental detachment at all. I feel the emotions and the thoughts of people. What I need, what I wish, is to perceive without going in the emotions and thoughts of others. To go in—empathy—is okay. To rest in, is not. It was worse than usual; that's why I didn't write to you. Deep unconscious fear was present. In August, I felt, for the first time in my life, the energetic power of jealousy and, at the same time, my energy was very low.

My goodness, Mukunda, such emotions are alive; this kind of presence has been strong to perceive and, at the same time, I could describe directly to my boyfriend what was going on in me. Fortunately, he knew the power of jealousy, so that I had the possibility to know it, to describe it, to live it in the body and transform this experience. Ouf! For a week, I've been in peace—I'm in total faith that all is becoming exactly as it has to be. No anger, no pain, no struggle, no confusion. Yoni mudra helps me a lot to bring vata more in the body. I would like to move on to the next lesson. One thing I realized in my body: fear is cold; heart energy is warm.

*Mukunda:* Wonderful, you are doing great. I am pleased to hear of your progress in working with such challenging emotions. Stay committed to doing all the lessons, and more blessings will come to you.

*Student:* I practiced today the puja you described and felt so connected to my physical and subtle body. There was a warmth that moved around and beyond my physical body. I need to delve more into the practice as I deepen my understanding of these sacred and hidden teachings you are passing on, for which I thank you. I will let you know how I am doing with the practices. It seems I was meant to meet you that day at the Tantra workshop. I would appreciate it if you let me know where I could find poems of Tantrik Yogis. I would like to include some in my *kirtans.*

*Mukunda:* That is very sweet. I am delighted at your insights. So many more blessings come from an open mind receiving insights into what was previously unavailable. Some poetry of Tantriks and mystics (for it is difficult to draw a line between them) include: *The Path of the Mystic Lover—Baul Songs of Passion and Ecstasy* by Bhaskar Bhattacharyya with Nik Douglas and Penny Slinger; *Love Song of the Dark Lord—Jayadeva's Gitagovinda* by Barbara Stoler Miller and Amritanubhav; *Nectar of the Awareness of the Self,* Jnaneshwar, trans. Swami Abhayananda (perhaps my all-time favorite). I have also written some Tantrik and yogic poetry in my book *The Yoga Poet,* which is available on my website at *www.yogatherapycenter.org.*

*Student:* My experience was changing while doing nyasa practice. At first, I had a great problem doing so, because it felt like sin. Please forgive me. I have to overcome a lot of conditioning. I disapproved of myself doing this worshipping of the senses. But I found trust and did the practice anyway, giving its result to God.

*Mukunda:* It is not really worshipping the senses, simply honoring them to see what they are trying to find that brings them contentment. This is a path to spirit. Giving its result to God shows a very good attitude.

*Student:* At first the offerings were, to my senses, on a different level, and I wanted to open up because I felt very tight and stiff in my fifth and fourth chakra areas. I knew that I was afraid of being who I am and of expressing myself. I had problems with receiving love and enjoying my life. I disapproved at first, but then thought it was alright to enjoy the good things of life that God created.

Then I became so grateful for all this beauty—flowers, tastes, smells, earth, and you. Then God *became* the smell, the taste. The chakras became the altar. I was a temple, an instrument. The taste adored me, loved me. It is not easy to describe what happened. It was almost like falling in love with the earth, the moon, the sun, and then God.

***Mukunda:*** Very lovely experience. So lovely that you share this with me.

# Yogic Anatomy and Sacred Space

With Great Respect and Love, I Honor
My Heart, My Inner Teacher.

Anatomy of the physical body is universal. In contrast, yogic subtle-body anatomy encompasses two additional bodies that are hidden by five veils. With spiritual practice, the veils get thinned and ultimately dissolve, revealing one true body called the Self. A more comprehensive view of these component parts is presented in chapter 6 of my book *Structural Yoga Therapy*.

We are multi-dimensional beings. The yogic anatomy of three bodies includes the physical body, but adds the subtle body as the mind and senses with three component veils, and a causal or bliss body with an additional veil. The five veils are:

1. Physical body (anna maya kosha)—literally "body of food that is an illusion"
2. Subtle-energy body (prana maya kosha)—"body of prana," emotions
3. Mind (mano maya kosha)—"body of thoughts"
4. Higher knowledge (vijnana maya kosha)—"wisdom body"
5. Bliss body (ananda maya kosha)"body of joy"

Each dimension is a servant of the higher one.

The soul is the vehicle of consciousness, ego sense is the vehicle of the soul, intelligence of ego sense, mind of intelligence, prana of the mind, the senses of prana, the body of the senses, and motion is the vehicle of the body.[6]

Such motion is karma. Because prana is the vehicle for the mind, where the prana takes it, the mind goes. But when the mind is merged in the spiritual heart, prana does not move. When prana does not move, the mind attains a quiescent state. Prana flows through subtle channels called *nadis* in the second kosha and is stored in the chakras there. Prana takes subtler forms in the third kosha (mental body) and fourth kosha (higher knowledge) and therefore any changes to it create the movement and stillness of the mind.

When the life force in the body stirs, the various organs of thought, word, and deed perform their functions. They flow towards the objects of perception in accordance with the deluded notions that prevail in the mind. But when the life force is not thus diverted by the mind and body, it remains rooted in peace within the heart. There is no movement of consciousness in the nerves of the body nor does life force activate the senses.[7]

It is like trying to answer the question of which came first, the chicken or the egg. When the prana becomes still, the mind also becomes still. As this stillness deepens, you move to a deeper place within yourself, to the fourth and fifth koshas and the presence of your innate wisdom and joy. For those who know meditation as detachment from cravings for worldly pleasures, the deepening of that state results in freedom from pain and suffering.

The *Yoga Sutras* II, 49 is a clear exposition of the progression arising from lifting the veils of progressively subtler bodies:

Pranayama naturally follows the perfection of yogasana with a cessation of the movements of inspiration and expiration.[8]

6. *Vasistha's Yoga*, 372.
7. *Vasistha's Yoga*, 161.
8. *Yoga Sutras of Patanjali*, 29.

Thus what is deeper, a more interior yoga, is very different from the yoga sadhana that incorporates only the third and/or fourth of the eight limbs, the physical discipline (asana) and breath awareness (pranayama). For those seeking spiritual life, it can only be found by experiencing the interior places, for the True Self transcends body awareness. It is an experiential knowledge that who you are is independent of the physical, energetic, or even mental functions.

Physical health is maintained by the quality of food we eat and the exercise we give to the body. The subtle body is fed by having positive emotions, encouraging natural expression, and self-control of the senses. The chakras feed the middle three bodies. The mind is maintained by positive attitudes, praise, uplifting thoughts, and an inward-directed consciousness. Wisdom is developed by reading the writings of wise people and cultivating a spiritual attitude about life. Bliss is encouraged by seeking the True Self veiled behind all experiences. From this, we allow ourselves to search for the source of pleasure when it arises.

By finding that each one serves a higher purpose, we begin to put into perspective the importance of the subtler forms of self. The True Self is not experienced as any of these bodies; yet it is constantly with us. It is best described as pure consciousness and remains the same in all states of body, emotion, and mind.

We have a lot to learn as we open the second body, for it is hidden from view due to the presence of prana. One of the major characteristics of prana is that it loves to hide. In its negative aspect, this is fear. We fear what we don't know. We don't know because the truth is veiled by the koshas that prohibit knowledge. In its positive aspect, this hidden prana governs all biological and subtle functions without requiring our mental attention. It allows the mind to function freely without interference. And yet, when prana helps the mind, the mind can function more clearly without fear.

## Tantrik and Ayurvedic Theory

In Tantrik Yoga anatomy, there are three levels to each of the chakras existing as the subtle body that comprises koshas two through four.

The first level of the chakras is the second kosha, made of prana. This is frequently represented in art forms such as *yantras* or mandalas with clear lines depicting the chakra boundaries. When in this level of awareness, physical pleasure is produced from the emotional biochemicals, endorphins and serotonin.

The second level of the chakras is the third kosha, composed of thoughts. It will take you to a deeper, more exquisite form of sensual pleasure. The vision of this level of the chakra is less definite—the lines or boundaries of the chakra field are unclear, as it corresponds to your emotional-body kosha. We often have to sit with our emotions until they become more physical before we know what to do about our feelings. This dimension is often characterized by a sense of losing yourself, or having unclear boundaries.

The third dimension of the chakras is the fourth kosha, made of wisdom. This level is even more subtle and hence will tend to spread out into a region that seems even less clear. The higher dimension of this chakra, when purified, will take you to the source of thought, the precursor to mind.

The ethereal/subtle body is composed of your materialized thought.[9]

The yogic science of health and medicine, Ayurveda, gives Yoginis another perspective on energy balance. The triple energies of this system are composed of five elements existing in the first kosha (physical body): vata (air and ether), pitta (fire and water), and kapha (water and earth). It is only when each of the qualities becomes balanced that they can be elevated to reveal their subtler nature within the second, third, and fourth koshas that collectively compose the subtle body. As they become balanced, the energies will move toward their home and, at that site, will be more readily recognized.

The home organ of vata in kosha one, the physical body, is the colon, especially in the region of the pelvic cavity. As vata becomes balanced, it will begin to increase prana, the energy that will return you to Source. This is the primary energy we are concerned with as Tantrik Yogis.

The home of pitta in the physical body is the small intestine, hence variation one of the yoni mudra, centered at the navel, will help balance pitta (fire). When balance is restored, pitta will become refined to its energetic component as *tejas* within the second kosha. Tejas is the spiritual light of discernment, and it reveals its true nature as discriminative wisdom.

The physical location of kapha is the heart. When it becomes balanced, it creates the quality called *ojas*, a spiritual liquid produced within secret cavities in the

---

9.  *Vasistha's Yoga*, 77.

body. Although difficult to discover, it is nectarian in taste (called *amrita, soma,* or *kechari*). In Ayurveda, these qualities are the inner experience of taste (*rasa*).

Lesson 3 is about balancing the physical elements in kosha one, which will transform them into their subtler substances as prana, tejas, and ojas. Thus the composition of the subtle body (koshas two through four) becomes stronger and self-centeredness lessens. Tantrik Yogis know these qualities by direct experience; they will not be satisfied with merely conceptual or theoretical understanding.

## Chakras in Theory and Experience

The chakras contain the grossest energy, as they are the first layer of the subtle body (kosha two), composed of prana. Physiological sensations tend to have emotional content, while purified prana is without emotions, save serenity (sattva). Each of the chakras described in lesson 2 are the gross material for the mind. But we must remember that we are in the second kosha here; the mind is the third kosha. It is the chakras and their pranic energy that generate positive and negative thoughts. They are the gross fuel for emotional expression. In the next lesson, we will focus on how to promote multi-dimensional healing by opening prana both to move more subtly and yet to remain grounded in the gross body. The overlapping of koshas two through four that comprise the subtle energy body makes for confusion in the mind, as it is looking at itself (kosha three). Therefore, it is common for people to misname what is happening when emotions, chakras, and prana are the field of experience.

In the same way, novices in Hatha Yoga cannot accurately tell if the sensations they feel during asana practice are stretch, strength, or release. They are different. Most are taught to focus on the stretch when doing yoga, but that is misleading, as often the sensation is one of muscle fibers contracting as they build strength.[10] In contrast, some experience tightness and wish to avoid it. So instead of building strength, they change their posture to eliminate that quality and their resultant negative feeling of tightness. In a similar vein, when your attention is upon the subtle body, you cannot tell if it is opening or closing your expression until you relate to someone else.

---

10.  See Mukunda Stiles, *Structural Yoga Therapy* (Boston: Weiser, 2001), 135 and *Structural Yoga Kinesiology*, 250.

The chakras open and close just like heliotropic flowers that follow the pathway of the sun. Only, for them, the sun is the mind and its emotional field. When the chakras are open, so is the mind, reaching outward to the external world. At this point, the chakras spin bigger and more rapidly in an outward fashion, giving energy to our senses. Spin is a relative term here. They seem to spin faster (thus the illusion of increased prana) when desire is blossoming. Conversely they rotate, subtly expanding as they blossom and spin inward, as they become detachment or the indifference of neutrality.

It also varies according to which kosha we are perceiving. The gross level of chakras is level-two prana maya kosha—the level of perception most commonly related to the desire for pleasure. When the mind is detached from desire, the chakras spin slower and awareness moves to the third kosha, where the chakras become more subtle and involute. With this, thoughts are clearer, and consciousness is perceived through its function of directing awareness. By continuing this inward awareness, one naturally moves through the cycle Patanjali describes as asana-pranayama-pratyahara (*Yoga Sutras* II, 46–55). The chakras become more like a column of light (*lingam*) in kosha four. As with the chakras, prana exists in koshas two through four and becomes more subtle as awareness moves from prana to mind and thought to wisdom. The latter feels as if it is given to you, not coming from you. That is what distinguishes the third from the fourth kosha.

The main motion of the chakras is like a flower closing at night and blossoming outward during the day. At night, they want to withdraw (pratyahara); during the day, they expand and reach outward through the senses. The opening of the chakras indicates sensual enjoyment. Those who take this to extremes, who focus on sensuality rather than the deeper opening toward spirituality, are called *bhogis*. This term means those who languish in pleasure. Yogis are not bhogis; their attention is focused on a sattvic state of consciousness, the attainment of contentment in all situations. In this procedure, the chakras are being trained to slow down. This training is described in the *Yoga Sutras* as leading to the stilling, not only of the body, but of the motions of the breath as well (II, 46–49).

The channels through which the prana flows into and from the chakras are called *nadis*. This term literally means a tube, through which consciousness can flow. When the nadis are blocked, there is a lowered awareness, a dullness—a *tamasic* state of mind. The nadis exist both as physical tubes—like the mouth, eyes, and the ten major openings of the head and pelvis—but also as subtler tubes without anatomical correlates. They form minor chakras at each of the joints of the body called *bindus*. The joint-freeing series (Pavanmuktasana) from my *Structural Yoga Therapy* book can open these energetic structures from subtlest to greater expression—that is from, nadis to bindus to chakras.

> Pleasure and painful experiences affect the nadis differently. The nadis
> expand and blossom in pleasure, not in pain.[11]

From this, we see that opening the chakras born from their nadis is the path of sensuality, enjoyment, and worldly fulfillment of "naturally arising" appropriate desires free of craving or lust. By the practice of careful observation, we can see the postural and energetic opposite when pain is experienced. It reveals not merely a posture of depression and sadness by a forward bend with rounded shoulders; it also shows us lowered vitality.

## Creating a Sacred Space—Puja

Up until now, our practice has concerned itself with the pranic body as the space for transformation. Let us consider making a container for the pranic energy that is bigger than the yoni mudra. In many ways, the physical body is a microcosm for the universal macrocosm. What is needed is a connection to a deeper truth than physical reality. For this, we need to create a sacred space, not only within ourselves, but also a space with which to surround ourselves—a space that contains us. Rabbi Zalman Schacter-Shalomi encourages everyone to have at least a "God corner"—a place where you can put your reverence, a space for sacred objects, a place that can both symbolize humility and embody Presence. With time, it will spread to the rest of your home, and indeed, to all your life.

Let us consider how the altar can be in your home. While it is ideal to devote a special room to your spiritual practice, with the altar being the central component, it may not be possible at this time of life. For myself, I never had a private room for spiritual practice until recently. I have a separate room for asana practice. They are

---

11. *Vasistha's Yoga*, 438.

different. The ideal is for the room or corner to be used only for your spiritual practices (sadhana)—chanting, devotional readings, and meditation.

The altar's central focus should be the teacher or teachings that are most inspiring to you. The proper placement is at your heart level when seated at the altar. To the right and left, place symbols of duality—a masculine and feminine statue, for example. Pictures of male and female influential teachers, or a lingam and a yoni will also do. Above the central image can be the source of that inspiration. Below, place whatever spiritual gifts you may have received from your practice or teacher. For elements, place a sacred stone for earth, a bowl of holy or blessed water, a candle for fire, incense for air, and a flower for ether.

The sacred space is a depiction of the elements and of the chakras. By your consciously placing an item that represents each element, it may feel more complete. Each of these can be offered in turn to your central image. By waving them clockwise in front of your chosen deity, you can surrender them and the elements that they represent to God/dess.

I learned puja, the art of worship, from my spiritual teacher, Swami Muktananda. He made it his practice to encircle the deity with the offering, and then follow that with a semicircle crescent below the deity. This crescent is the offering of humility. This was repeated three times, and then continued in multiples of nine, to cultivate devotion.

Children want to participate in all activities that are inspirational to us. They should be encouraged to do what is natural for them without being forced to participate. The same is true for your partner. When it is clear that your actions increase your capacity to be nurtured, others will want to join you. When children experience their parents meditating, they will want to do this too. We are models for all those in our lives. The mother is the most important model. The mother is the first guru or spiritual teacher. How a mother relates to life is carried, not only in her womb, but in all of her attitudes and interactions with others. Every woman is especially embodied to generate sacred space. The word *yoni* means not only source; it also means womb and sacred space. Every woman embodies that sacredness, as her womb is the source of life, which is innately both spirit and matter. By deepening these Tantrik lessons into generating spiritual experiences, you can know your body as a walking altar.

Recently, I went to India for the fifth time and rediscovered the power of the temple. It is essentially a home for you and your spiritual tradition, so that God, in one of Her or His forms, will come and live there. One of the most moving temples I have experienced is to the Goddess Bhadra Kali in the village of Ganeshpuri, forty miles north of Mumbai (Bombay). My guru, Swami Muktananda, had his ashram a half mile away from the village. In the village itself was his own guru's ashram. Nityananda, my guru's guru, was a huge Indian, well over six feet tall and deep dark in color, being from Kerala in south India. He claimed that, when he came from south India, Bhadra Kali had followed him. And, since he was respecting Her presence, he had his devotees make Her a temple. That temple is quite small, but has three rooms. The outer room is for the public to come and observe Her. The next outer room is for the priests to prepare the offerings that are given for donation to the Goddess. These outer rooms are always open. But the most interior room is often closed, for within this space is the Goddess Herself. She is treated as alive, not as a symbolic representation of the Divine Presence. The innermost room, the *sanctum sanctorum*, is where Bhadra Kali lives.

Similarly, in our bodies, we have an outer material body that receives guests. Then we have an inner body we call the subtle body that receives gifts and discerns what is beneficial—what is to be kept and what is to be tossed away. Then, within that, we have a secret heart that contains all that is precious. This is not to be shown to everyone who passes by, but is only shared with those who have a reverential attitude. Those who have discipline and regularity in their lives get to see what is hidden from public view. This is the way Yogis and Tantriks are. For those who persist in the lessons, who show regularity and discipline, lasting gifts are freely given. For others, a gentle encouragement is given. Transformation requires a bigger commitment than merely wanting your desires to be fulfilled.

Remember to persist in your practice, yet stay detached from expecting specific outcomes. Tantra is a personal spiritual practice. When you feel complete with this lesson, read the Dialogue section that follows prior to beginning lesson 4.

**With Great Respect and Love, I Honor
My Heart, My Inner Teacher.**

# Dialogue with Mukunda

*Student:* I feel, slowly, my perception of prana is increasing. I read in one of the Dialogue sections someone was talking about the difference between the physiological sensations in the body versus the perception of consciousness. Could you say anything more about this, please?

*Mukunda:* Physiological sensations tend to have both physical and emotional content, while refined prana is without emotions. Consciousness is the directing of awareness. This is done by thought; behind it is the third kosha of mind's prana. It is what directs thoughts and perceptions; it precedes all awareness of anything both inner and outer. Prana exists in koshas two through four, becoming more subtle as your awareness moves from prana to mind and thought to wisdom. The latter feels as if it is given to you, not coming from you. That is what distinguishes the third from the fourth kosha. Chakras in the second kosha spin (the literal meaning of chakra) when desire is increased; when the mind is detached from desire, then it spins more slowly and awareness moves to the third kosha. With this, thoughts are clearer and prana in the subtler chakras involutes (like a flower closing at night, then opening to desires later on). By continuing this inward awareness, one naturally moves through the cycle Patanjali describes as asana-pranayama-pratyahara (*Yogic Sutras,* II, 46–55).

*Student:* You said in one class that we should learn to recognize when we are in one kosha and how to move between them. How do we do this?

*Mukunda:* More is coming in lesson 6. The Tantra lessons can also help with this, but you will need to move beyond lesson 6 to know for sure. Keep looking for symptoms of physical vs. emotional or energetic experiences; by asking, answers that encourage discernment and clarity will come. Avoid asking "Why me?" or "How do I stop these feelings?"

*Student:* I find it easier to detect "feeling" states than energetic currents. Does that mean that this path is not suited to me or simply that it is early days and I just need to persevere and develop the skill without wanting to run before I can walk?

*Mukunda:* No, just substitute instructions that read "energy" with the word "feelings." Emotional feelings and energetic currents are the same.

**Student:** In your book *Structural Yoga Therapy,* you mention that emotions such as anger and fear are not negative, but that, when they are denied, they become toxic. What is the best way to deal with these emotions when they arise? Should we express them, or, if not, how can they be transformed?

**Mukunda:** Any emotion can be suppressed (tamasic) or overly expressed (rajasic). On the yogic path, we relieve this distortion with techniques that generate harmony and sattva, called kriyas. Some examples of kriyas are: prolonged breathing, tantrasana, and being in nature. These practices allow the pranas and emotions to find expression. Transformation of these qualities is an important step of these Tantrik lessons. Persist and, by lesson 6, a significant change can be made. You may even experience the beginnings of stability. That is necessary for sadhana to truly show its potential.


**Student:** I was reading in your book *Structural Yoga Therapy* that you should not practice yoga when you are angry or moody. Why? Isn't yoga to balance all the koshas and help with difficult emotions?

**Mukunda:** Yes, but it is best not to use yoga for psychotherapy, unless that is your profession. According to the main Ayurvedic text, "Exercise is contraindicated for persons in the grip of excessive sexual activity, traveling by foot, those who are in the grip of anger, grief, fear, exhaustion, children, old persons and those having the profession of speaking too much. Nor should one exercise when they are hungry and thirsty."[12]

Best is to do gentle practice no matter what state you are in. It is the commitment to regular practice that heals. Don't consider certain practices as healing for states of imbalance. Yes, it will always help to do sadhana, but stability does not come from merely managing emotions. As Patanjali tells us in the *Yoga Sutras:* "By sustained practice of all the component parts of yoga, the impurities dwindle away and wisdom's radiant light shines forth with discriminative knowledge."[13] Thus doing all the eight limbs results in lifting the veil from the fourth kosha so that wisdom comes regularly and, with it, a consistent experience of Spirit.

---

12. R. K. Sharma and Bhagwan Dash, translators. *Agnivesa's Charaka Samhita* (Varanasi: Chow Khamba Sanskrit Series, 1958), vol. 2. Sutrasthana, chapter 7, 31, 51.

13. *Yoga Sutras of Patanjali,* 23.

*Student:* Reading the Tantrik notes, I have become more curious about chakras. My gut feeling seems to tell me that, if I resolve the pain in my right hip (which happened recently), then my earlier knee injuries will heal better and my right shoulder pain, which seems to be recurring, may perhaps also resolve. Perhaps a latent muscle imbalance in the hips during my dance practice has caused these other problems. I have been reading that the sacroiliac is the center of the body (also mentioned in the sacroiliac exercise). May I ask, to which chakra do the hips correspond— the first or second?

*Mukunda:* The hip joints are actually between two chakras. The first chakra is in the central pelvic diaphragm, and the second chakra is at your cervix. For a man, it is where the penis attaches to the upper pubic bone.

*Student:* What are the underlying issues with the second and first chakras? In websites, some mention either, and I want to be sure.

*Mukunda:* It is not in a fixed location, as the subtle body is constantly moving, variable, more so than physical anatomy. Practice of the yoni mudra can lead you to finding the greatest source of energies and, with practice, you can feel how these two fluctuate. Tantra is not for emotional or psychological therapy. Its goal is to resolve all energies into the deeper koshas to know the impermanence of changing mental states. The sign of this success is serenity and being fully engaged in your proper life roles.

*Student:* This lesson was a real eye-opener for me. I have been doing chakra meditations for years and often lead my yoga students in visualizations and focus sessions regarding the chakras. I thought I was in touch with and experiencing the chakras directly and clearly all this time. However, the puja made me realize how overstimulating (rajasic) I was in my previous connection with my chakras. I was overpowering what I now perceive to be the sensitivity of my chakra system. My imagining and visualizing were actually a veil preventing me from seeing and feeling the chakras themselves.

Interestingly, differentiation is something that has been coming up in my life in other areas: between myself and my students, my husband, my daughters, and now my chakras. Making the offerings to the chakras had the effect of separating them from my ego. There was suddenly subject and object, where before there was only subject. You write in your description that the puja process has the effect of thinning the veils of the koshas, and that is what I feel. Since that night, I continue to experience the clear crisp spinning of the energy vortices. They are like diamond jewels with many facets, like snowflakes or crystals, sparkling. I have only had time to do one puja. I can do another tomorrow, but I am excited about moving to the next lesson.

*Mukunda:* Sounds very good for insights into perception rather than projection. I am delighted that you are spending such time on this sadhana. It evolves in a lovely way with time. As you have been blessed with such a powerful insight, do stabilize it by giving puja regularity before moving on.

*Student:* Over the last few weeks, I have been practicing lesson 3. The rush of energy has leveled off considerably; it seems much more balanced. There were a few days of feeling some aches and pains in unusual places, just during the practice—medial right knee, left elbow, etc. I just acknowledged the discomfort and, after a while, it went away. Am I right in thinking that was some kind of energy blockage in those locations? It has not come back.

Later on, there were times when I brought attention to the chakras. I started to shiver, even though my surroundings were very warm. That went away after two or three days. Over the whole time, I first felt a pulsing in my whole back that has become less intense over time. There was discomfort in what I figure is the kidney/adrenal area and what felt like constriction in the heart area. During the rest of the day, I am not aware of any discomfort in these areas. By now, the heart area feels fine, and I still am aware of something in the kidney area.

The emotions have been right on the surface. I have had several of those laughing/crying episodes like at the ashram, but not so intense. I have been moved to smiling tears many times. I guess there are all kinds of releases going on—and overall I have been feeling really well.

*Mukunda:* The variety of responses to opening to your own naturally arising spiritual energy is quite apparent here. For prana to awaken as it is unfolding by someone like yourself with many years of experience meditating is remarkable to those without a lengthy training. The experiences sometimes seem like fireworks and yet, once you persist through them, they become sattvic, as you point out. It is the variety of responses that clearly shows the difference between meditations done from self-centered practice and that which is given to you without your seeking anything except opening and trusting in the opening.

Harmony is the natural result of persisting, no matter what the Shakti prana needs to clear from your system.

*Student:* I'm not stuck on chakra locations, but I feel stuck or deadened just below my solar plexus. It is helped by the polarity technique, or continuous breathing. But it is right there every day I return to it. Should I be seeking progress in this area over time?

*Mukunda:* As you cite, the solar plexus, located well above the navel, is not the third chakra. Some mistake it to be, so let us be sure we are using the same references. Stuckness in the region of the navel is associated with the chakra, and it will definitely progress to flow over time. Try using all three locations for yoni mudra.

*Student:* I have been looking at a couple of Caroline Myss's tapes on the *Energetics of Healing.* I found where I was losing energy from several chakras. One important instance had to do with forgiveness. So, I went through my list of three people I needed to forgive that was linked to where I was losing the energy. I can see how I lose power from each chakra. The first one for me is about holding on to past negative experiences with my family. The second one is about how I fuel fears about making or losing money. That third chakra is really a bugger. That's where I didn't trust my intuition and gave up my power after that accident in the car and breaking commitments to myself. Then there's the fourth chakra, where past negative experiences limit my choices. The fifth is where I experience shame. The sixth chakra is where I hold on to old grief. And the seventh is when I am not living in the present moment.

So you can see why my spiritual development is so important to me and why the sutras have so much for me to learn from. And "every day, in every way, I am getting better and better."

*Mukunda:* I am glad that you are having such wonderful insights. Continue in every day and every way. Namaste.

*Student:* I feel that there is an integral part missing in my working with people, that I am unable to perceive their prana. Should I just be patient with this process? Can it be my fear holding me back from this perception?

*Mukunda:* Just be patient and persistent with yoni mudra, which reveals all the layering of the koshas. Move through these lessons without concern for mastery. Fear dissolves by learning how to experience the difference in the koshas.

*Student:* I have gone back to the first three Tantrik lessons to experience and learn more about energy. I think that I am able to discern the prana in me at times. This energy is subtle and flows more easily through the left side of my body than the right, where sometimes there is a block (pain) at my hips. I was reading Robert Svoboda's *Ayurveda for Women,* and he described pain as an imbalance in vata. I do tend to have a vata imbalance, and recently it was exacerbated by a lot of air travel. So I am taking balancing measures like drinking vata-pacifying tea infusions and reducing vata-promoting foods. I have also asked my body to guide me in working with this pain, and actually this seems to be helping. I am going to move on to lesson 4 to continue to work with this block. In addition to this energy, I also experience other types of energy. One type is vibrant, dynamic, and forceful; it occurs when I am meditating on someone and there is a "connection" and I feel as if we have melted. Is this also prana?

*Mukunda:* Yes.

*Student:* I am confused a little by all of these signs of vata imbalances I am having. I was very pitta-dominant for many years and feel as if that has shifted, but now I am having vata issues. Did I go too far? Or is it just going to be a constant back-and-forth?

*Mukunda:* These signs are normal for shifting prana. That shift occurs when working more deeply on yourself. Stability comes more from regularity in lifestyle and Tantrik sadhana, making it "same time, same place." That is the key to managing irregularity.

*Student:* Can you give me some tips on how I can develop more kapha?

*Mukunda:* Kapha is most often expressed as stability, strength, stamina, or a strong immune system. But, as when vata becomes elevated to prana, when kapha is balanced and elevated, it becomes ojas. That, for me, is more tangible than kapha. Ojas is mother's milk; when you were nursing your child, that energy, not just milk, was kapha's liquid form as ojas. It is also the feeling of love and devotion that is common in all situations where you feel loved or loving. To develop it, just be still, especially when you feel love opening your heart. In the stillness, kapha evolves to its higher level of ojas.

*Student:* I remember reading somewhere a statement you made about yoga and how it uses a different type of calorie burning. I can't remember where I read it. Can you point me in the right direction?

*Mukunda:* This statement about calories is a metaphor. Classical Yoga and Tantra burn karma; exercise burns only calories.

*Student:* I feel lost. In your introduction to Tantra, it said to finish each lesson within two weeks. Why? So I am discouraged about myself because I procrastinate so long. Actually, I feel guilty about taking so long with practicing the sessions.

*Mukunda:* It is best to move on, as the Tantrik lessons are designed to propel you to the next lesson. Getting all the benefits of each lesson as soon as it is done is not a goal to be encouraged. The Shakti or prana of the lessons propels you to states of consciousness not attained by lower lessons. Just move on.

*Student:* I didn't work with lesson 2 for too long, because I was more interested in lesson 3, the part about releasing emotional blocks. When I had my private session with you in New York last month, we worked on releasing holding in my liver, which brought up a host of stuff for me and cleared the discomfort I had had in my shoulder for some time. I can feel some energy in the pranic breathing exercise, but all I feel when I open suppressed energy is more of the same.

*Mukunda:* Just feeling it begins to release the suppression. Do not concern yourself too much with the idea of unwinding or changing, or even of being free of the suppression. By knowing that suppression is not what you support, your energy body must change toward the light and fullness of energy.

*Student:* I discovered during our private session that I need to take some action in my life, but I am unable to find the guidance as to what that is. Maybe I am checking out during practice so I don't get the guidance because I am too afraid to follow it. You say that these practices will give us clarity to see what the best course of action should be, so should I just continue to do them, or should I back-track to another practice that may be gentler? Before I started your training, I always took the more aggressive route to something. Is that what may be happening here, and so I am closing down around it?

***Mukunda:*** I recommend that you move on to the next lesson and yet continue to revisit lesson 3 a few times more, until you can see beyond it due to the influence of lesson 4. Clarity is an immediate response on the part of your energy body. Just by placing your hands in the mudra and asking for guidance, it will come immediately. Don't ask more than one question and be willing to follow the guidance that comes no matter what it says to do. This is a path of submission, surrender, and devotion to the Inner Teacher. She is always with you and can never leave. Just trust Her and allow yourself to be as you were before my training—more aggressive and immediate to your intuition. The course is to take you full circle back to yourself. So why not go there sooner rather than later? Blessings.

***Student:*** I have been receiving the Tantrik lessons, and I am ready for lesson 4. I do have a question, however, about a passage from the *Yoga Sutras* (which may be clarified by lesson 4, judging by the title of the lesson). It is passage II, 10, which describes how the "causes of suffering are to be reduced, then destroyed by the process of involution." I am unsure as to what is meant by involution, but it feels like something that I need to learn. I keep coming back to that passage and the ones preceding it.

***Mukunda:*** What this refers to is consciously reversing the stream of the mind from thought to feeling to action to result of action (karma). By reversing the flow in deep meditation, thoughts are returned to a subtler pattern and will be more sattvic in future expressions. What you're really doing is going to a thought-free state. To get there, you slow down the cycle of the mind; the impact of thought is lessened and, over time, eliminated. Future actions will no longer produce rajasic behaviors and their associated karma. The impact is lessened and, over time, eliminated. Meditation and finding the real Self is the key to eliminating all suffering and difficulty in karma. Tantra, like yoga, seeks to turn the energies back on themselves so their impact is negligible. Involution is attention going in, thus not being stimulated by the five senses, but rather by your intuitive sense.

***Student:*** With respect to creating a sacred space, when we moved into a new home at the beginning of this year, I decided to set it up in keeping with *vaastu*—the Indian version of *feng shui*—principles of placement, so that the north side of our rooms has a sacred space. Our home is small, so I practice in our living room. My altar is movable and, during my morning practice, I move the altar to the north corner of this space. This corner is also the entryway into the living room, but during my morning practice it is a sacred space. I think for the moment, this is the best that I can do.

*Mukunda:* That is fine. Spirit is omnipresent; mind isn't.

*Student:* I still love practicing puja, definitely a sacred moment. Following our last correspondence, I have followed your advice in order to be more aware and develop the connection with Divine Mother. Since I was a child, I have always felt a strong connection with Mother Mary. (I have a Catholic background, but don't consider myself as belonging to any religion anymore), I still consider Mother Mary as my protector, however, the spiritual mother of us all. So I was pleased when I read your definition of Goddess, as it made me realize that Mother Mary may well be a manifestation/connection with Her in my life. I feel grateful.

I would also like to share with you something that has manifested with the puja practice and lesson 3. I have been feeling some tension at work recently, notably with one particular colleague who has been rather sneaky and unfriendly. After a while there, I noticed some more compassionate thoughts arising and even recognized that it was all perfect the way it was (just for a few seconds). After the practice, I observe I still dislike the idea of her, but there was more detachment toward her attitude.

When I went to bed that night, I found myself crying and addressed a prayer to my guardian angel and Divine Mother. During the night, I dreamed that she was being verbally abusive to me and that I was answering back firmly and politely, asking her to be more respectful and to stay away from me. What a great surprise this morning when I walked into the office and she said hello to me with a big smile on her face and start chatting kindly to me, as if nothing had happened. I could not believe it! Usually, she does not reply when I say good morning. I can't help but feel grateful and to think that the power of puja, followed by my prayer, generated that shift.

*Mukunda:* So that is wonderful. You need to persist and see clearly how you want her to respond to you. The value in puja is one of offering the difficulty to a higher power. Let it rest outside of yourself in order to fix it. As you saw such a big smile, surely you cannot attribute that to your normal interactions. Subtler interactions with her that are soul-to-soul will change both your personalities. It is best to direct your mind to seeking praise of others rather than holding on to your lack of trust. Persist at your spiritual practice. Without sadhana, yoga is just exercise. Sadhana is what transforms us into what we were not. Yoga just moves material. Which do you want to support?

**Student:** Thank you for providing the sacred space for this. I long to be of service in the way you are, loving your name *Mukunda*, compassionate liberator, and to be able to really feel what is guiding me, and know when it is. I can feel myself retreat from these longings when I ask myself, "Why do I want this?" and then it switches to "What will I get out of it?" So I long to allow myself the space to just *long*.

**Mukunda:** Increase the longing. It is the longing that brings you close to your goal. *Yoga Sutras* I, 21 states the importance of a devotional attitude. "For those who have an intense urge for Spirit, it sits near them, waiting." For the most part, practicing humility, asking for guidance, and following what is given is the best. In this situation, I recommend more time listening to chanting tapes that move you deeply and having the intention to meditate deeply when you have time for a seated practice.

**Student:** Things have been so hectic with school and grad school applications that I have not had as much time as I would like for the Tantrik lessons. Even so, I am continuing on. I have been working with the fear and anxiety that come up as a result of that feeling of separation after connection. Because I am more aware of the strength of this fear, I have been able to talk to the part of me that gets afraid and kind of coach her to be okay.

The place where I experience fear and anxiety is mostly in my lower abdomen. I had been placing my hands there when this gassy pain arose, sometimes using yoni mudra. What I think triggered this was that, during savasana when you were teaching in New York, my head began turning from side to side, fairly vigorously and uncontrollably, a kriya releasing. And so much released after this. When I place my hands on my forehead (and I usually feel drawn to do so with a fair amount of force—like massaging the third eye, or pressing), the pains in my abdomen remit. It feels as if this is telling me that the origin of the pain in my lower abdomen is not actually an imbalance in the energy around my first/second chakra area. The root is not a gastrointestinal problem. It truly feels as if the anxiety is being created in my mind. It stems from fears and imbalances created in my mind, and then they come out as pain in my lower abdomen. Does this sound logical? The pattern for me, ever since I was a little girl, has always been: first I get anxious, and then I get a stomachache. So if the origin truly is in my mind, do you have any further suggestions on how to balance this energy?

**Mukunda:** The feelings of prana are not exactly where the sensations arise in the physical body. The challenge is that what you are feeling as pain is like the tip of the iceberg. By following the prana, it will lead to the source of the challenge. The mind is kosha three and prana is kosha two. Pranic imbalances make the mind unsettled. By settling the prana and returning it to its source via yoni mudra, the mind and pranic imbalances are resolved. They simply disappear. Seek the root not the flower, which seems to be in the body or as thoughts in your mind. Both have a common source.

It is most intriguing, although probably you are not unique in this pattern. I suggest two strategies: 1) place one hand over your lower abdomen or pubic bone, the other on your forehead—and encourage the excessive energy place to become balanced with the deficient space—and 2) start with both hands on your head where you experience anxiety arising and follow it with your hands, letting kriyas arise in both situations.

# Healing with Prana and Emotional Energy Expression

With Great Respect and Love, I Honor
My Heart, My Inner Teacher.

This lesson will encourage you to open at new levels of awareness, self-healing, and spiritual presence. All energy is healing when it is developed in a Classical Yoga context. Begin to label your experience to heighten your discernment of the signs of harmony or sattva as excessive, or rajas, and lethargic, or tamas. Sattva is the state of mind, body, and prana that we wish to promote in all our yogic practices. By using this context, you can see that tamasic energies need to be stimulated or expressed to be sattvic. Rajasic energies need to be somewhat sedated or neutralized to become balanced in the highest expression of sattva. When balanced, your energies will tend to be elevated to a higher kosha expression of the same chakra region. Ultimately, this will lead to finding Spirit in all your activities.

## Cultivating the Tantrik Mind

Tantra means "transformation of your energy." So what is meant by energy in this sense? From the yogic perspective, the subtle body is composed of prana. It is expressed as physical vitality and emotional health, and is the driving force of our thoughts. We often speak of negative or positive energy, implying the mental/emotional states of criticism or acceptance. Negative energy is experienced as stagnant, suppressed, blocked, or dark. Positive energy tends to flow, to create a feeling of openness, and is seen as light. Tantrik practice seeks to train you to find the precursors of both negative and positive energy so that you can be appropriate to both. By cultivating proper attitudes of openness to positivity and detachment or indifference to negative energy, you can gain self-mastery over your mind and emotional states.

Be courageous and look at how your blocked or suppressed patterns cause you and others to feel pain and suffering. The *Yoga Sutras* are very explicit on how pain arises from negative emotions and thoughts. Sutra II, 34 is the longest sutra of the book; hence it is the most important teaching to comprehend. These imbalanced emotional energies manifest from the more primal Ayurvedic elemental qualities of vata, pitta, and kapha. When they are left unchecked, they become a source of violence (*himsa*). This led Patanjali to a simple, yet profound, process of affirmation yogic style.

> Sutra 33. When one is disturbed by unwholesome negative thoughts or emotions cultivation of their opposites promotes self control and firmness in the principles of Yoga.

> Sutra 34. Negative thoughts and emotions are violent in that they cause injury to yourself and others regardless of whether they are performed by you, done by others, or you permit them to be done. They arise from greed (kapha imbalance), anger (pitta), or delusion (vata) and are indulged in with mild, moderate, or excessive emotional intensity. They result in endless misery and ignorance. By consistently cultivating the opposite thoughts and emotions, the unwholesome tendencies are gradually destroyed.[14]

This tendency to be disturbed by our unwholesome thoughts and emotions must be overcome for yoga and Tantrik practices to be successful. Otherwise, we are contributing to pain and suffering. As you learn to become detached from the mental tendency toward negativity, you are manifesting self-control. The state of detachment is not dispassion, for it is a mental quality of vata, while dispassion is an emotional quality of

---

14. *Yoga Sutras of Patanjali.* 25.

pitta. One of the most profound Tantrik Goddess texts states: "The state of dispassion only arises in one whose constant devotion is given to the heart as the Self."[15]

The Classical Yoga Ashtanga teachings describe the first two methods of self-discipline and restraints (the *yamas* and *niyamas;* see *Yoga Sutras* II, 30–44). From this core sadhana, we will naturally see that all we do creates our perception of the world. Transformation is just a thought away. When we admire the world and our most intimate friends, this takes the shape of yama and niyama into the form called admiration yoga. Similarly, when we seek to see higher consciousness, we will contribute to the evolution of all beings. This is the spiritual essence of these great practices. Exploring your naturally arising energy will free you from the tendency for these energies to become unwholesome thoughts or feelings. As you persist, this positivity will spill over to enhance all activities of your life. Detachment from what is negative will keep you free from leaking your own suffering to others.

What is detachment? My favorite comprehensive guide to self-realization is *Vasistha's Yoga,* a remarkable 12th-century text of Advaita Vedanta (non-dualism). It is considered a parallel teaching to the "mind-only" tradition of Yogacara Buddhism, as found in the *Lankavatara Sutra.* In his preface to *Vasistha's Yoga*, Swami Muktananda says: "[this text is] highly respected for its practical mysticism. The study of this great scripture alone can surely help one to attain God-consciousness. For aspirants of the highest beatitude, the *Yoga Vasistha* is like nectar. It is a storehouse of wisdom." Here is what the great sage Vasistha says about detachment.

> One who is detached is completely satisfied in their own self. They are not attached to anything or anybody; and they have no enmity in their heart. Attachment, on the other hand, causes the conditioning of the mind to become more and more dense, by repeatedly causing the experiences of pleasure and pain, thus confirming such associations as inevitable and thus bringing about an intense attachment to the objects of pleasure. If you have gained self-knowledge and you engage in spontaneous and appropriate action, you are unattached.[16]

---

15.  Swami Ramanda Saraswati, trans., *Tripura Rahasya: The Mystery beyond the Trinity* (Tiruvannamali, India: Sri Ramanasramam, 2006).
16.  *Vasistha's Yoga,* 321–22.

If, after doing these first four lessons, you have difficulty moving through any of your prior conditionings and emotional limitations, consult me. There are other energy-clearing techniques that I have to share that will be more effective at liberating deep-seated traumas. I am sharing those that you can readily learn on your own with a minimum of supervision. If possible, I offer my services to work directly on your energy body to free you from difficult karmic patterning. If you cannot see me in person, then consult me via phone or email.

## Pranic Breathing

Briefly repeat the elemental offering from lesson 2, then sit for some time in your sacred space and begin a deep wave-breathing pattern. Progressively open yourself from where the natural breath's wave is felt so that you are expanding it both higher and lower. Slowly move your breath to a full spectrum that extends the length of your torso. Then begin to connect the breath through the spectrum of your chakras. As you breathe inward, let your awareness move down; as you breathe outward, move your attention up. Do not concern yourself with finding the exact location of the chakras.

Detach yourself from needing to feel or see something that you have read about or been taught. Instead, focus on learning to heighten your own inner experience, regardless of what sensual awareness is predominant. As you continue with this pranic breathing, begin to slow down your breathing. Then let your breath pause on your perception of each chakra location as you continue to move awareness through the chakras. Cultivate an attitude of openness to feeling yourself at this subtler level as you continue. The objective in this practice is to heighten your pranic breath energy so that it is more sustainable in all activities. This will manifest as guidance to help you perceive what the best course of action is.

## Feeling the Five Pranas[17]

Start by sitting in a comfortable posture, either on the floor or on a chair. Then observe your natural breath. After a few moments, begin to slow your breath until its four

---

17.  Dr. David Frawley, *Ayurvedic Correspondence Course*. Edited by Mukunda Stiles, 2000.

components—in breath, pause, out breath, pause—reveal themselves. Do this for a couple of minutes.

To refine the pranas from the movements of breath, this next exercise will help you transform breath awareness into pranayama.

As you inhale, feel the *adhya* (in breath) prana moving the breath down from the head into the chest. As you pause, feel the *samana* prana in the abdomen; it moves in an outwardly spiraling motion. Then as you exhale, notice the main movement is upward, called *udana* prana. With sensitivity, you will notice a subtle prana move down through the pelvis relaxing the lower back. This prana is called *apana*. Pausing after exhaling unveils *vyana prana*, the subtlest prana. It may be felt as the aura or as an all-pervasive feeling of your subtle body.

Repeat as long as you can keep a relaxed awareness. Do not push against emotions or what feels to be an energy block. Instead, concentrate on opening what is naturally relaxing. Seek to open what is naturally spacious rather than seeking to change what is not ready to change. This is a profound practice and strikes at the core intention of Tantrik Yoga. Hatha Yoga is gained by control and self-discipline, while Tantra is given by surrender to a higher power. End the pranayama with yoni mudra—hands in a downward-pointing triangle on your lower abdomen or pelvis encouraging prana to come to its home (review lessons 1 through 3).

> Softly press yoni mudra during exhalations. Conceive of what you are doing as gently pressing your energy body into your physical body. Inhale, then soften your pressure.
>
> Repeat this six to ten times. Look for a lingering experience of the yoni mudra after your hands are removed.

## Seeking Prana's Openness

The intention of this practice is to become freer of your lethargic or tamasic quality, which can suppress insights and keep you from manifesting your fullest potential. Begin by focusing your attention on opening yourself, as in the first lesson of Tantrik energy balancing. If you have an intention to use prana, that intention will manifest and greatly assist in creating tangible results. Use your hands (touch is the expression of the element of air, of *vata dosha*) and direct your energetic attention with their assistance. Start with your left hand at your heart and your right hand on your abdomen, then begin your energy scan. In this practice, search for places where you sense your energy is suppressed or blocked. If they are not obvious, look for places where it is difficult to hold your attention. Place your closest hand on that spot and allow the other hand to remain as you began.

Begin to open your breathing pattern using the pranic breathing exercise previously described. As you increase your energy field, it will naturally move from the place of higher energy to the place of lower or suppressed energy. As it does this, you will begin to feel emotional changes. I encourage you to push firmly on the suppressed area, massaging or squeezing the area to encourage it to have more sensation. Allow your breathing to become stronger, occasionally breathing out through your mouth with vocal sounds. With persistent practice, you can feel yourself opening to more sensation and aliveness. Learning to release your energy comes naturally with persistence and clearer intentions. As you look at yourself, see what you do that causes you pain and suffering, and empower yourself with the decision to transform. When you feel complete, end with the variations of yoni mudra described in the previous lesson. If you feel strongly affected from the release, end by grounding yoni mudra, touching all three of your pelvic bones. Then lie prone on your belly (or sit up) and place the yoni mudra over your sacrum.

## Continuous Tantrik Pranayama

Pranayama are yogic exercises to feel, balance, and elevate the prana to higher dimensions (koshas). Unless this happens, pranayama is merely breathing exercises. You must feel the prana and know by direct experience its potential to heal and elevate your consciousness. Through pranayama, one gains true detachment and manifests natural appropriate actions.

When you feel a need and the courage necessary to break karmic patterns that are holding you back from living your full potential, a stronger intention must be made clear. For this to happen, you must tap into the source of your will. The act of intention (*sankalpa*) is to form a resolution that will manifest in lasting change.

This can only arise when you see the pain you are causing yourself and others and know there is no way back, only forward. By clarifying that intention, you can manifest a dramatic pranic energy that will propel your life force in a positive direction. The intention will be much more powerful if you find the most powerful, succinct words in which to frame it.

In continuous Tantrik pranayama, you will encourage a fullness and connectedness to the energetic component of your breath as a vehicle for transformation. In this way, we will be seeking an empowerment of your willful intention to remain conscious and elevate your awareness from its tendency to space out. There will be no pausing, only an immediate connection of the inhalation to the exhalation and back again. This can be done with my guidance, and using my words or hand I will point out areas in your body that are low-energy and not receiving your breath's pranic energy. I will also help you direct your breathing so that other areas that are excessively charged can be gently sedated.

If balance is not achieved, it is likely you may hyperventilate. This is not a dangerous situation; it merely means that your system has too much oxygen and, as a consequence, the muscles of your extremities may begin to cramp. This is most commonly experienced in the hands, by the fingers curling or becoming cold prior to a spasm. If this happens, just stop the technique, and the effects will pass within a few minutes of deliberate relaxation. As the continuous pranic breathing becomes more stable, there will be an increase in life force available to manifest your resolution. Along the way to that goal, any number of other experiences may manifest to distract you or reveal that more preparation is needed before manifesting your resolution.

Once again I encourage you to commit yourself to complete the entire eighteen-lesson course. Without persistence, the transformations achieved in the early lessons will not produce long-lasting, sustainable results. When you feel complete with this lesson, read the Dialogue section that follows prior to beginning lesson 5.

**With Great Respect and Love, I Honor
My Heart, My Inner Teacher.**

# Dialogue with Mukunda

This lesson generated the most questions, so I encourage you to read this section thoroughly before doing lesson 5 practices.

*Student:* While reading lesson 4, some new questions came up related to Yoga Sutra 33—"When one is disturbed by unwholesome negative thoughts or emotions, cultivation of their opposites promotes self-control and firmness in the principles of Yoga"—and Yoga Sutra 34—"By consistently cultivating the opposite thoughts and emotions, the unwholesome tendencies are gradually destroyed."

My question: If I try to eliminate negative thoughts, then I remain in the duality, because one side can never be realized without the other. If I want to differentiate, I always need both sides. So, if I invest a lot of power to obtain the good, there will always be the bad there as well, because they are just two sides of the same medal. The logical way would be to get rid of the bad by no longer differentiating. I can accept that both are parts of the ego and therefore not lasting. What is your opinion, Mukunda?

*Mukunda:* This is good insight. It goes to a deeper perspective than is meant by a superficial reading. The basic teaching is that violence comes from negative thoughts and emotions that are acted upon. Therefore, by turning thoughts to a positive direction like "How can I help?" or "Where can I open myself?" the difficulties with negative energies are gradually eliminated. This method is to help you wake up to how duality is operating and then direct yourself from doing harm or simply ignoring that which is unpleasant. First we have to wake up, then choose a path.

Patanjali states in *Yoga Sutras* II, 48 that "by perfecting asana duality ceases to be a disturbance." He does not say duality ceases. This is a very important distinction. Once you are firmly on the path, Grace may intervene and you can begin to have a non-dualistic point of view. To choose either will perpetuate the duality and the struggle. Thus one can pierce the veil of ego and see through it to the True Self, hidden behind the veil always there. "This only comes from submission to the Higher Presence of your inner teacher" (*Yoga Sutras* II, 26).

*Student:* If I share Ramana Maharshi's insight that everything that realizes, asks, or feels is the ego, why should I try then to get rid of good or bad? They do not remain; when

I die, they die too. So. . . ? Everything in me that feels happy after practicing something is my ego, because the Self doesn't feel happy or sad, the Self just is.

What is the aim of revealing all the veils if I know they are part of the ego and therefore not real. Isn't it so that the more I try to go into these veils, the more I get into the ego? Why should I do so?

Maybe there is a way to reveal the Self by pulling away one veil after the other. But don't you think that the awareness of Self is a sudden one? And when that happens, what is the motivation to care about veils?

*Mukunda:* Don't concern yourself with theory, just practice and the results of practice. Let duality and non-duality be resolved in the final eighteenth lesson. Some say the veils are slowly pulled off, one at a time, like lessening the density of the koshas. They say that self-realization comes slowly and gradually, and then there is the separate school of instant illumination, of self-realization without steps. I think both are true. In either case, when the veils are thinned or lifted during that period, there is no motivation except to do what is naturally arising and for the benefit of others. Selfishness and the ensuing desires are diminished gradually or totally.

*Student:* Regarding the balancing of energies (polarity) and your instructions to "put your right hand on your abdomen and your left hand on your upper torso to encourage a polarity flow of energy," here's what my experience is. As I place my hands in these positions, they tend to be on my heart center and on my abdomen, second and third chakra region. As I breathe into these two energy centers, I have two sensations. First, I feel as if each of these regions is expanding—the area becoming softer and wider. This is a very joyful feeling. Second, I feel the energies moving up and down repeatedly between the two energy centers. This feels energizing to me and also integrative somehow, as if these two centers are making peace with each other, communicating with each other, balancing their energies. This feels healing to me. Overall, I feel I am making "progress," if that's a word one can use here. I feel softer inside, more in the flow, more intuitive, since I have intensified these Tantrik practices. It's a "gentling" into my true nature—that's how it feels. I feel very very comfortable "being me."

*Mukunda:* You are experiencing the polarity to which I referred. Polarity will naturally tend to balance the opposites as they seek a harmonious relationship. By learning the sensations of this feeling, you will naturally tend to harmonize energetically within yourself when either extreme of polarity occurs within you. Over time, this balances Shiva to Shakti, masculine to feminine, receptiveness to giving, and the emotional polarities as well. Namaste.

**Student:** Would you discuss more about resolution (sankalpa) and how to get the correct one? How often does one's sankalpa change? I began (years ago) with a very lofty one and had to make the change to the simpler sankalpa that actually kept appearing in my mind!

**Mukunda:** For me, sankalpa (resolution or vow) is the force of the mind's determination to live an ethical life and have what is natural to manifest in that life. It aligns you with your inner nature, thus what is freely given will be given. What is not naturally yours or your role is taken away. When sankalpa is correct, then life is stress-free. It can change often as you align to your true nature.

**Student:** Unless I'm confused, I seem to feel some of my energies manifesting as thoughts. I guess it's useful that I can perceive this. The problem is that the thoughts don't seem to be the end of the line. I've taken to heart the sutra on cultivating its opposite. Will this eventually destroy these thoughts/energies? Am I missing something?

**Mukunda:** Thoughts can be perceived as arising from energies or vice versa. The goal is not to destroy thoughts that are unproductive. This is a major difference in Tantra practice to how most translators render *Yoga Sutras* I, 2—as control of your thoughts. Stopping or controlling the mind is not a good translation, as this produces suppression of emotions and pranic energies. My teacher, Swami Shyam, gave a better interpretation of this: "Yoga is experienced in that mind which has ceased to identify itself with its vacillating waves."[18] Detachment is the process that leads to yoga, and this is helped greatly by pranayama. Cultivate your capacity to hold or retain prana. By doing so, the mind will naturally attain a sattvic state, and peace will prevail.

**Student:** I am enjoying the process of studying the lessons. I came across the section on "Manifesting your intentions and continuous Tantrik Pranayama," and I feel the need to break karmic patterns that are holding me back from living life even more fully. I am talking about my love life and my relationship with men (and I am sure it's not the first time you've heard that one).

---

18. Swami Shyam, *Patanjali Yog Darshan* (Montreal: International Meditation Institute).

I will try to give you a brief background so that you get an idea. I grew up in a family rather split up and dissolved, where there was not much love and care shown. I have been attracting men who turned out to be unavailable physically, mentally, or emotionally, and who were sometimes unfaithful. I have been told by different sources (astrologer, psychic, and iridologist) that this was due to karmic knots I had to undo and that, in past lives, I had been mistreated as a woman and lost several children. Therefore, in this life, there was a lot of fear around men and becoming a mother. I was also told that this life was about finding liberation from this and opening myself to more love and compassion.

I have tried consistently to understand the lessons and to learn what was at stake, but I always seem to end up on my own. I have tried to feel detached from it by creating a nurturing living space around me, and I have some great great friends (and lots of hugs). In the last few years, I have focused a lot on yoga and my spiritual path, on bringing/giving love and care around me, and it has been very rewarding. However, I still feel a great deal of sadness inside me, and I have come to realize that, in order to fulfill my heart and accomplish my destiny, my deepest desire is to have a loving and caring partner at my side to share the journey, to make a home and family. When I read lesson 4, about the connection with clearing karmic pattern, I thought that maybe I could find help in your guidance. What do you reckon, Mukunda? Can you help me to help myself?

***Mukunda:*** Patanjali states that the way to success in yoga is by consistent effort over a long period of time and detachment from the results of those efforts (*Yoga Sutras* I, 12). So when you do the technique of looking for your energy, build it as fully as possible, especially in the lower three chakra regions. Any place that is difficult to fill, practice lingering on filling that area with prana, not letting it flow out. But stay within your body and/or hands. With persistence, you can feel your energy body sustaining the experience and feel it growing. Concentrate on the energy-body sensations and detach your mind from its tendency to make this into an experience of patterns of sensation that are memories. When memories come, think of them as prana and begin to deepen the sensations so that they stay in the lower chakras and don't move into your head. If they do, focus on interpreting them as prana that is displaced and needs to be returned to the lower chakras. Once you can build this, when memories come up, you will have detachment from the results, and being with attractive men will be experienced as sattvic. Sattvic states of mind are harmonious and reveal a stress-free state of body and mind that arise without effort.

A relationship can only come when you are sattvic—that is just natural. Building desire only increases the likelihood of you being rajasic—not true to your heart. If God/dess wants you to be in relationship, She will create that. But in my experience, it comes after building a relationship with Her and yourself. Blessings.

**Student:** I get confused about retaining prana. Wasting as little as possible? Retaining during pranayama exercise? I feel as if prana flows in and out of me. So how does retaining it help? Are we like fuel tanks, and the goal is to make our tanks bigger?

**Mukunda:** Your tank is sufficient for the vehicle. What is needed is to become more efficient with the fuel already there. What causes prana to go out is searching for pleasure outside—in any form of craving. By accepting what naturally comes to you, prana is retained. It is a subtle shift. Be yourself and do the tasks assigned by your roles in life; then prana increases. During all activities, just detach from the mind that craves results. The results are not for you.

**Student:** This week, I observed how my hormones are in control of me and how, try as I may, I was not able to detach from feelings of irritability for two days straight. I was aware that there was no reason for me to feel irritable—other than the changes in hormone levels—and, although I was trying to regain some kind of centeredness, I simply couldn't. I was able to control to a certain extent uncharitable thoughts that sometimes arose about other people and send them blessings instead, but I was not able to change the source of the feelings. Do you have any tips for many of us who go through this every month?

**Mukunda:** Just read the sutras again and again—especially those in chapter 2 (1–12 and 33–34). That is my suggestion.

**Student:** Perhaps this is a silly question, but when you say that "the objective in this practice is to heighten your pranic energy so that it is sustainable in all activities," do you mean simply that this practice will create more energy within you that you can use during your day? Or do you mean that you should be doing pranic breathing during all your activities to heighten energy? I think it would be the former, but the way it was worded was a bit confusing at first. Also, when is a likely time for this "guidance" that you speak of to manifest itself? Should I be asking questions after each practice to receive such guidance?

Any illuminations you may have of the above would be greatly appreciated. Thank you and many blessings to you for offering this service.

*Mukunda:* What I mean is that, by heightening prana, you will feel it during all activities. By learning to perceive it, you will begin to notice that some activities are characterized by less prana. This is a sign to detach or not do them. Other events increase your perception of prana, not necessarily increasing your energy. Prana is not the same as being excited. That is technically the Ayurvedic quality of pitta, not prana. Prana is the energy of guidance. It is sustained and elevated by pranayama and spiritual practices coming through the Tantra lessons.

*Student:* [The same student returned with the following question] I practiced it this week, and I am not sure if it is this lesson or if I am having stronger PMS symptoms this week. I have felt this week as if I am taking a colder, harder look at changes that I feel I need to make in my life and I wonder if this "eyes-open" practice could have this effect. I feel more intensely aware of where I am feeling "stuck" and, as I write this to you, am realizing this is just the effect we want some of these lessons to have … isn't it?

*Mukunda:* Indeed. Open-eyes practice is good at all times too.

*Student:* Thank you so much for your guidance and presence in my life. These past two weeks, I have been working on Tantrik lesson 4 and opening energy blocks now that I am aware of this energy. I observe that there is less energy on my right side compared to my left, and specifically at my right hip region, at which I have vacillating pain. This imbalance is somewhat balanced by the end of the practice, and during the process of balancing, I have fragments of memories (not mine from this life) or other images/situations that appear to me. They represent feelings of shame, arrogance, and envy. Are these negative feelings the cause of this energy block?

*Mukunda:* Indeed you are very accurate. This is often the case, as you interpret from emotional to energetic language. In my experience, these are all within the second kosha. Later on, in lesson 6, you will learn about energetic bodywork, which is a more specific way to release your own energy and emotional blocks. It can be done to you, so you can receive energy from other parts of yourself. By increasing that flow within you, from low to high, the blocked patterns will begin to dissolve. This can be done by me, or by my trained students, if you wish to have an individual session.

***Student:*** I am working through the eight limbs of the *Yoga Sutras* (II, 29 and on). At this point, I have enough detachment to examine my life and actions and can honestly say that I have a lot of work to do. Is it these actions and thoughts that also contribute to this energy block? The good thing is that I am able to recognize such actions and feelings, and I am grateful for your direction and blessings and introducing me to Swami Satchidananda and his translation of the *Yoga Sutras*. I still have work to do with my ego and its desire. But on the other hand, I surrender more and more each day to my heart's wisdom and guidance. Thank you for leading me to her.

***Mukunda:*** That is indeed a sign that you are seeing yourself as archetype II of the *Yoga Sutras'* second chapter, which contains all the major teachings you need to learn. Your thoughts are kosha three, and they will affect all other koshas, especially the next denser one, kosha two. Holding on to the teachings allows the mind to be purified and can lead to freedom from that kosha. I am glad to be of assistance in helping you find your way home. That is the duty my guru gave me when he named me Mukunda, which means "compassionate liberator." My job is to do this with myself well enough so that it spills over to others. Blessings.


***Student:*** I received Tantra lesson 4 two days ago and have not practiced the whole sequence yet. Yesterday, I got angry twice—something that hasn't occurred in a while. Then I remembered what you wrote about the "crust over the heart," and I felt anger at myself and then softened. Compassion comes then goes.

This morning, during joint freeing series #7, sunbird, I had sudden pain in the left sacrum area, which has been the site of most of my traumas since age seventeen (I'm now fifty-two). My immediate thought was for my structural body—"Too much effort when I start my period"—so I "backed off" and let go into the sacrum rather than resisting the grief, fear, doubt, anger. Spontaneously, I began growling loudly like a mad dog. Still protecting? Do I carry a layer of guarding to feel safe? I eventually transformed this into quiet affirmations of light and love with tears, with release of the pain. This would have gone on had I not been in a car and intentionally came to a place of stasis. You wrote that just reading the intentions for the lessons can be effective. Perhaps this is a quiet dawning of the multi-dimensional nature of chakra energy—pain appears as the messenger for my resistance area. Your words carry power, and I am again sensing the depth of the practices.

*Mukunda:* That is great. Now just remember to be gentle with yourself. These issues came over time, and yet they can leave in a minimum of time due to increased prana that comes from doing the lessons and asking for guidance.

*Student:* In the section on continuous Tantrik pranayama, I am unsure when or how we are meant to do this. I have used a sankalpa before with very positive results. Further direction would be appreciated. Thank you for your guidance

*Mukunda:* The pranayama is to be used while resting with a meditative intention. Meditation can follow this, but it should not be a method of meditation. The continuous pranayama should rather lead to a naturally arising meditation. Just be gentle with it. The intention, or sankalpa, is to find the naturally arising wave of pranayama that takes you to the distant shore of meditation. Eventually, the wave and shore meet without feeling any distance or time. Blessings.

*Student:* I have studied and practiced the exercises and techniques of lesson 4 and found them very useful in channeling vital energy and removing/reducing some of the tamasic thoughts limiting progress in sadhana (e.g., getting out of bed for morning practice). Now my tongue remains on the roof of my soft palate for prolonged periods during the scanning of pranic energy between my throat and heart chakra. My difficulty is that, after getting out of sadhana, this mudra takes place involuntarily while walking or at any time during work. Should I allow it to happen as it is or otherwise? Please guide me in this regard.

*Mukunda:* Although you are only at lesson 4, it is possible that spontaneous awakening has happened from your previous practices. When pranayama mudra and bandha arise spontaneously, that is a sign of Grace descending to help your elevation to a higher level of consciousness. In this case, when a breath pause (kumbhaka) occurs without instruction, it is the highest form of teaching. In addition, your tongue locked itself to the posterior upper palate without instruction. This is called kechari mudra, which means "seal of nectar." In this technique, the tongue is brought back and up past the uvula into a channel (nadi) that connects the throat chakra and the third-eye chakra. When this arises spontaneously, it leads to a breath retention that is effortless, and it produces a shift from pranayama to mudra. By this I mean that the prana is locked, sealed into a form that transmits effortless spiritual awakening. You should submit to what is naturally arising so that you can be in harmony with the awakened spontaneous motions of prana. Namaste.

**Student:** I have practiced the fourth Tantra lesson for about two weeks now upon waking up and just before falling asleep. I don't really work with the movement of the energy much; rather, the yoni mudra is so grounding and calming that I find myself focused there at my pelvis. It amazes me how much it activates the energy/heat in my palms, and sinks into my lower two chakras. Although this next insight is rather personal and embarrassing, I will share it. This practice has also reduced my compulsive desire to masturbate before falling asleep. Instead, when I practice the yoni mudra, all that boiling energy is soothed and quieted. Definitely *not* an anticipated impact! But somehow, I think it brings me more into the concept of *brahmacharya* to retain my vital pranic energy.

**Mukunda:** That is quite a lovely transformation. Thank you for confiding such an intimate truth to me. It is a natural result of prana becoming balanced that one's sexuality finds a natural and healthy responsiveness. Each person is different, so how one expresses that energy, especially its sexual component, is best found as what arises when prana returns to its sattvic pelvic home. In other words, it goes both ways. Natural sex expression results in a soothing yoni mudra feeling in both the general pelvic region and in the genitals. Brahmacharya (sexual harmony whether attained by restraint of over-expression or expression to balance one's suppression) is dealt with in lessons 8 and 9.

**Student:** I found finding the polarity of currents difficult and cannot say that I particularly felt areas where the energies were predominant. From time to time, I did get a little pain around my rib area, so I breathed into it and placed my hands below and above until it disappeared. I don't know whether you would term this energy.

**Mukunda:** Sometimes pain is energetic; sometimes it is physical. What you have done is a good test that has revealed, in this case, that this pain is energetic in nature.

**Student:** I didn't notice any energy movement in my body. But I was aware of different parts of my body being tighter than other areas. So I placed my hands in that area until I felt it relax, but I didn't feel the energy move anywhere else. At this point in my life, one of the things I'm working on is not being afraid of being afraid. I always feel that I need to be on guard to make sure I'm doing all I can do to prevent bad things from happening. I want to be free of that. During one of my sessions, I had a vision come to me that I could see that way of thinking starting to fall apart, as if it were a structure that was starting to crumble. But in that vision, I didn't know what to do with the pieces that were falling away from the structure. I didn't know how to get rid of them. I felt that they were going to stay in my body. Then, in another session, it became clear that I could just hand those pieces over to God and let Him do whatever needed to be done with them. I didn't need to figure it out; that was His job. That was very freeing for me.

*Mukunda:* You are doing great at these early lessons. Your attitude is commendable and will get you all you need in this course. Just persist and all the blocks get turned over into His hands. Persist and all will be well.

*Student:* While reading the Dialogue sections, I realized that I have not felt a positive energy flow. Mostly, I feel sensations of pain or discomfort in my pelvic area and lower back/sacrum. These were especially intense in the second week of this lesson. Since this coincided with the resurfacing of less-than-pleasant thoughts and memories from the past, I thought that this physical discomfort was a physical "memory"/response. Then, this Saturday, while practicing a sitting meditation on a blanket, I felt a release (both physical and spiritual), and the discomfort was gone. I have been so disconnected from this part of my body that simply experiencing the wave breath in my belly was a revelation and a celebration. It was the first time that I recall releasing my abdomen so fully and completely.

*Mukunda:* Great! I am so happy to hear that you are receiving such profound blessings.

# PART 11

# Tools for Tantra

# Transforming Sensuality into Prana

With Great Respect and Love, I Honor
My Heart, My Inner Teacher.

To the Yogi, natural urges are seeking a stress-free lifestyle both in outer and inner expressions. When this occurs, asana (the body) and prana (the life breath) become elevated to the forms called mudra (gesture) and bandha (lock) sequentially; this four-step process may not even be noticed. A sign that we are stress-free is that we don't observe the body and its subsequent pranic expression. Stress is so subtle that we don't even perceive it. In fact, from this, only natural urges arise. The experience of this is sensuality—sattvic sensuality. One retains energy through this natural four-step process.

Yogis with too much or not enough self-control lack harmony (sattva). Regardless of our attainment in yoga, we will not be stable until the gains are accompanied by a pervasive contentment arising from the field of omnipresent prana. Intitially, sensuality and prana are comingled, eliciting joy and comfort with the activity that we are engaged in. Often sensuality is blurred with sexuality, yet with yoga training, the consciousness of a Yogini will begin to shower fulfillment to all that she does as well as all those she meets. Thus, sensuality mixed with prana is a continuum flow that blesses the giver and the receiver. When neither seek to control it, it will continue to be elevated through bandhas that retain what was formerly lost—prana.

# Signs of Pranayama

"All the texts agree that pranayama is impossible until the nerve channels (nadis) are thoroughly cleansed," notes Theos Bernard in his Ph.D. dissertation.[19] Bernard points out that, by purifying the nadis, one gains natural health as the ability to experience prana. To the Yogini, natural urges are a way of feeding nourishment to the different dimensions (koshas). We must have freedom of expression of desires. Because our activities have not always been in harmony with our ideals, the yoga teachings recommend practices called *kriyas* to purify the subtle body for pranayama. The natural urges arise when there is freedom of the mind to generate emotional expressions, sleep, meditation, insight, appetites for food, sensual pleasure, and sexuality. Too much or too little self-discipline will generate stress, incomplete digestion, and loss of serenity.

To seek food is natural to all living beings. In performing one's natural functions, one need not be bad-tempered. Even selfish ends are gained by the wise through appropriate means and proper behavior, after they give up anger and mental agitation and resort to equanimity and clear mind. Give up your anger, and achieve your end by resorting to tranquility.[20] When this is done, a deeper hunger begins to reveal itself, and one can move to the higher dimensions of consciousness from the resulting increase in prana.

One way this hunger reveals itself is in your experience of giving/receiving hugs. If your hug partner welcomes your energy, you can do the practices in the previous lesson to find a polarity, gently remove stress-filled energy blocks, and even find the beautiful polarity of the heart-sacral connection. This is done by having one hand on your partner's sacrum and the other between his or her shoulder blades. When huggers relax, both will feel benefited. This is especially true in lesson 6, in which you will practice receiving Tantrik energy bodywork.

As energy increases, it will tend to polarize itself around activity and stillness, Shakti and Shiva. When these primal qualities are harmonious, we say that we are in the state of yoga. When prana increases further, it will shed light on the underlying three primal forces of desire, called the *gunas*. By diligently watching this play of consciousness, the Yogi develops discernment. Those lacking discernment will suffer.

---

19. Theos Bernard, *Hatha Yoga* (York Beach, ME: Samuel Weiser, 1972), 47. I highly recommend all four of his books.
20. *Vasistha's Yoga*, 99.

When desire is harmonious, the sattvic state is predominant. When desire is over-expressed, we are rajasic. When desire is suppressed or ignored, we are tamasic. When there is rejection of the natural urges, there will be a suppressed emotional quality, tamasic in nature. Tamas ignored results in energy blocks. Similarly, when there is over-expression of nature, we experience rajasic mental and emotional appetites. Rajas results in increased or inappropriate desires. Tantriks tend to work on subtler expressions of energy to restore the sattvic state. In Classical Yoga, there are physical methods of cleansing the gross channels (*strotras*) through which our physical, emotional, and sensory nutrition pass. The subtle can change the gross, and the reverse is also true. The gross purification can facilitate cleaning the subtle channels to sattva.

The six purifications were first described around the 14th century AD in a Classical Yoga text called the *Shatkarma Kriyas*. These practices cleanse the channels of higher consciousness (nadis) in the subtle body. The nadis are tubes through which prana, as consciousness, flows. The yoga texts describe ten major nadis that are the openings to the outside world. These channels end at the ten openings to the body—two eyes, two ears, two nostrils, the mouth, urethra, anus, and fontanel at the crown of the skull. The gross level of these purification practices changes internal pressures and heightens the capacity of the tubes to carry water, nutrients, waste products, and sensory impressions. This will improve digestion and the functioning of all the senses. When purification is achieved, pranayama will naturally result, and one can begin to perceive the prana directly. On a subtle level, kriyas create an inner-directed consciousness, free from the impulse given the mind by sensory stimulation. This process is called *pratyahara*. As this becomes stabilized by the arising of mudra and bandha, the natural flow of mind leads to meditation, called *samyama* in the *Yoga Sutras* III, 4.

# Fixed Gazing—Tratak

To prepare for deep meditation, fixed gazing (*tratak*) produces a most profound benefit for the short amount of time it takes to master. Its primary effect is upon the eyes and the lacteal glands (tear ducts). With regular practice, tratak also produces steadiness of the mind. Just as holding the body steady as a result of good asana practice enables one to more readily regulate the breath, so holding the gaze enables one to inwardly concentrate the mind.

To practice fixed gazing, begin by arranging your seat in a distraction-free area with a bare wall. Choose between sitting in a chair or on the floor. Of primary importance is keeping your sitting posture comfortable and supportive of your back, so you can remain stationary for fifteen minutes. Then place a focalizing object in front of your seat at the level of your heart. The ideal object is one to which you are neutral or attracted. It can be a flower, a candle flame, a scene from nature, or the picture of a respected friend or teacher. For this exercise, let us begin by using a candle.

Once your focal area is arranged, close your eyes and take several deep breaths as you release any superficial tensions. Then gently open your eyes and gaze at the candle flame. Allow your eyes to behold the flame without trying to focus on any details. Just look, without trying to see. Maintain an erect posture with natural breathing. Then just sit and watch yourself and the currents of sensation that move within you. Keep your eyes motionless for as long as possible. If they want to blink, close them for a moment, then release the tension from your temples, jaws, and eyes with full audible exhales. Then open your eyes and resume gazing.

Begin to separate your visual energy, which is used to perceive the object, from the object itself, from the underlying energy of consciousness. Conceive of the senses as an energetic flow from the sense organ to the object. In this case, the eyes have a field that goes to the flame and then returns with the impression, which is then projected onto your eyeball for mental perception. This back-and-forth flow of pranic energy can be subdivided any number of ways. One form is to observe the naturally arising beam of light that appears to be coming from the flame toward you. Follow this beam and begin to notice how your concentration will shorten or lessen it. Withdraw your awareness until you can feel a separation of your prana from the flame. Seek to make yourself separate from the flame and its energy, and your eyes and their energy. As you polish this practice, the senses separate the flame from its energy and your mind is free to choose its object. Continued persistence separates sensuality from pranayama. The objects are sensual, but the field that directs your attention is pranayama. By discernment of this distinction, sensuality, passion, sexuality, and lust are all seen as a comfortable spectrum for self-expression.

For the first few days, sit for as long as you are comfortable while holding your eyes open. During this process, there may be visual distractions—spots of colored light, memories, haze, changes in the candle flame, etc. There may also be hallucinations that produce distortions in the image. Just sit and allow these perceptions to arise without making any effort to alter them. Allow your eyes to remain soft, your lower jaw relaxed, with regular breathing. Tears may form, clouding your field of vision. Relax and close your eyes momentarily. With persistence and gentle sustained effort, your eyes can be held steady without blinking and tearing for the entire sitting period.

## Involuting the Chakras through Shambhavi Mudra

Tantrik Yoga can lead to the experience of emotional expression having an underlying energetic source—the chakras. The uncovering of the chakras reveals them as the field in which sensual expression occurs. When the chakras are open, we are responding to our perception of the world, and so we will be rajasic. When this is overstimulated, students need to withdraw from the world to find sattvic chakra energy and a corresponding sattvic harmonious mental state. Students with addictive responses need careful consistent guidance in finding their way to balance. In contrast to this, opening the chakras is the goal for those students who have suppressed their emotions and thus feel held back from living their potential. Once this tamasic quality is removed, we can begin to seek the sattvic expression of the chakras. When sexual or emotional energy is allowed to build, it becomes neutral energy. If you persist, it will be experienced as spiritual energy.

Let us consider asana bodily experience in this context. Patanjali describes the subjective experience of the yogic body awareness in his sutras on asana (II, 46–47), where he calls them "a steady and comfortable pose. It is mastered by relaxation of effort, lessening the tendency for restless breathing, and promoting an identification of oneself as living within the infinite breath of life." The goal of Classical Yoga asana practice is described in the next sutras (II, 48–49): "Duality ceases to be a disturbance. When this is acquired, pranayama naturally follows, with a cessation of the movements of inspiration and expiration."

These goals are secret, in that they do not often appear in contemporary yoga teachings. The *Yoga Vasistha* clarifies why this is true: "Pleasure and pain experiences affect the nadis (channels of prana) differently. The nadis expand and blossom in pleasure, not in pain" (p. 438). To be free of subconscious suffering and pain (tamas) and unfulfilling pleasure (rajas), we need to move in the sattvic direction.

All life seeks harmony with the inner and outer worlds. The harmonious state of sattva arises when the chakra energies begin to find the stillness of contentment, as is described in the *Yoga Sutras* on pranayama (II, 49–52). Following Patanjali's advice will produce a stillness of the prana, the energetic foundation of the mind.

The next step is for the chakras to involute, described in Patanjali's Classical Yoga system as pratyahara. This energetic movement leads the upward-rising (udana) prana to become spiritually awakened. This unveils the chakras as fields of consciousness, revealing the direct experience of our five dimensions, called the koshas or veils of the True Self. Each of the chakras is composed of three dimensions—energetic, emotional, and thoughts—that are the second, third, and fourth koshas. These five koshas are in three bodies—physical, subtle, and supreme.

The greatest example of this yogic anatomy is the three hearts. The physical organ is in the *anna maya kosha* to the left side of the chest. The heart chakra is in the *prana maya kosha*, centered in the chest. It is only accessed when prana is present. As the prana comes to a more sustainable balance, its energy moves inward to two more inner flowers, the first of which is the mind in the heart (*mano maya kosha*) and its higher function as wisdom (*vijnana maya kosha*). The third heart (*ananda maya kosha*) is initially experienced as uncontrollable rajasic bliss. The bliss transforms from rajasic to sattvic as the three hearts become united into one indivisible consciousness—pure consciousness. This third heart, ananda maya kosha, lacks form, and yet is experienced two finger-widths to the right of the breastbone, according to the sage Ramana Maharshi in chapter 5 of the *Ramana Gita*. Although it is initially experienced as the fifth kosha, as spontaneously arising bliss, others experience it is as the Divine Mother. She then takes the individuality and, in her own way, evolves the ego sense through the process of self-realization to show its true nature, beyond all the koshas, as the transcendental, the Divine, the True Self. (For more details, see *Structural Yoga Therapy*, chapter 6.)

A deeper form of practice will naturally arise when kriya purification nears completion. This takes the form of a mudra or "seal," which directs the flow of prana and seals it to a specific energetic pathway (nadi). The word *nadi* literally means, "that which makes happiness flow." Mudra is thus a way to direct the awakened prana Shakti consciously as an expression of higher emotional states. When one surrenders to the Shakti, she will produce spontaneous mudras that generate spiritual experiences as they help to sustain an open heart. This process of sense withdrawal is known in the *Yoga Sutras* as pratyahara (II, 51–53). All practices, when done in the flow of the guidelines set by Patanjali, tend to lead into the state of meditative absorption described in the sutras that follow. Tratak, taken to its completion, becomes a form of sensory meditation, called *shambhavi mudra*.

> With internalized one-pointed awareness and external gaze unblinking, that verily is Shambhavi Mudra, preserved in the Vedas. If the yogi remains with the citta and prana absorbed in the internal object and gaze motionless, though looking, he is not seeing, it is indeed Shambhavi Mudra.... That is the real state of Shiva consciousness.[21]

*Shambhavi* means "belonging to Shiva" and refers to the inherent power of Shiva (stillness) which captivates Shakti (motion). Thus the two are really one. When tratak is practiced consistently, it can lead to an awareness of a motionless state of mind called Shiva consciousness. Thus it is the training of the sense of sight that will culminate in the withdrawal of the sense to its source at the root of the mind. At that place, the mind has no thoughts. It is likened to the exploration of the source of a river. As one proceeds upstream, the quantity of water lessens, until, gradually, only a trickle can be found. But in the former case, something precedes thought arising, just as something precedes the stream becoming physical.

So it is in training with Classical Yoga. The study of the river of the body/mind reveals a smaller stream called consciousness, which in turn has its source in one-pointedness. In quantum physics, the basis of the universe is both a particle and a wave. In quantum psychology, the mind is neither thought nor matter, neither energy nor particle. The questions that are wisdom yoga (*jnana*) naturally arise as "What am I? Who am I?" Wisdom of the True Self remains as the silent answer to these questions.

Padmasambhava, the second Buddha, who brought Buddhism to Tibet in the 9th century, revealed "the secret of ultimate practice" to his consort Yeshe Tsogyal, princess of Karchen:

---

21. Swami Muktibodhananda Saraswati (trans.), *Hatha Yoga Pradipika* (Munger, Bihar, India: Bihar School of Yoga, 1985), IV, 36–37, 578.

Place your sight in space, straight in front of you, without moving the eyeballs, relax your awareness so that it will be sharp/keen, luminous, awakened, and embracing totality. May it be free from the fixation of observer and observed. Although there are many profound key points in the body, rest free and relaxed, as you feel comfortable. Everything is included in simply that.[22]

Note how singular these texts are. The steadiness of the Tantrik's Shiva becomes the same as the Yogi's asana. The standing steady pose, *samasthiti*, flows naturally into Krishnamacharya's tadasana vinyasa, palm tree, as described in my book *Ayurvedic Yoga Therapy*. Where motion ends, stillness begins. Where stillness ends, motion begins. There is no territory exclusive to Shiva, for He shares with Her his life of dynamic stillness/motion. Shambhavi mudra for the Devi Yogini is experienced as the same consciousness of maha mudra for the Tantrik Buddhist.

Remember to persist in your practice, yet stay detached from expecting specific outcomes. Tantra is a personal spiritual practice. When you feel complete with this lesson, read the Dialogue section that follows prior to beginning lesson 6.

### With Great Respect and Love, I Honor My Heart, My Inner Teacher.

# Dialogue with Mukunda

**Student:** In the *Yoga Philosophy* of Patanjali, translated by Swami Harihar Aranyananda, *Yoga Sutras* II, 12 (2), he says: "Attempts to derive pleasure by sensuous enjoyment sharpen the senses and intensify attachment, which in the long run cause great unhappiness." It seems to me that, in Tantra, we are trying to awaken the senses. Is the train moving in two directions?

**Mukunda:** This translation of the *Yoga Sutras* is highly regarded by my main teachers of physical yoga—Professor T. Krishnamacharya and Rama Jyoti Vernon. It is a good question indeed. There are two trains. Yoga and Tantra are going in opposite directions for the initial stages. However, I feel that they meet at the point where the student has developed

---

22. Daniel Odier, *Yoga Spandakarika* (Rochester, VT: Inner Traditions, 2005), 144–45.

detachment from the senses and their pull on the mind. Tantra encourages us to wake up all suppressed energies and emotions.

Sincere Yogis and Tantriks are seeking natural expression of desire and freedom from being controlled by the emotional tendency to make the mind rajasic or tamasic. It is really the mind we are seeking to discipline into a sattvic state of consciousness. By training the senses (pratyahara, step 5 of the 8 limbs), we can create, to some degree, a sattvic state in the mind. Yoga encourages pacifying the senses so that lust and attachment are removed from pleasures. It is neither pleasure nor pain that is the problem. It is that both tend to imbalance the mind so that attention cannot be focused to the underlying perpetual field of pure consciousness. I see Tantra and yoga meeting. It is, as Patanjali says in I, 12, that: "through persistent effort carried out over a longer period of time and detachment from the result of that sadhana that success in Yoga is achieved."

**Student:** I am feeling a definite resistance to going *in* when I am practicing the tratak. There is a point in the practice when I feel as if I am teetering on the brink of diving inward and something comes up to push me back out. The second part of the practice, the shambhavi mudra—is this something that will happen spontaneously?

There is also one more question that I have been struggling with. I have become overwhelmed with healing practices, and it is not practical/possible for me to do them all. I am pretty adept at tratak already. I don't know how to make a daily practice that is practical and possible for me at this point. I am referring to your joint-freeing series, yoni mudra meditation, chanting, puja, yoga nidra, and pranayama. I would like to take some of it on as a sadhana, but am not sure how to structure all of these into a daily practice. Once again, thanks for all your guidance on this healing journey.

**Mukunda:** Your first response is a sign of aggravated pitta. The mudra does naturally arise and can be deepened by practice. Basically, what you look for, once you know what it is, you will find.

To answer your second question, I do not want you to do too much. I recommend a practice that is shorter and more focused on your receiving prana. Learn to hold the energy within your yoni mudra placements. Do different positions until you find what allows you really to store prana. For some, it is the series of four placements; for others, it is only one that really works. Everyone's energetic body is different, just as our physical bodies are different. Chakras and nadis are in different positions too. My recommendation is for you to follow the sequence for practices that I give on the mantra card during all my workshops—that is, to do first the chants and puja worship, then do the joint-freeing series, yoni mudra, with the intention of three steps: feeling prana, following it where it directs your attention, and retaining prana. When that is consistent for a week or so, ask for the next lesson. Consistency and detachment from results give success in yoga, according to Patanjali's *Yoga Sutras* I, 12. This is a very important sutra to reflect on. Namaste.

**Student:** This has been an interesting practice. I generally find it difficult to make space for a practice later in the day; I usually do practice first thing. The need for a place with few visual distractions means that I do this in another room and leave the candle set up there. Although I haven't done the practice each day, I was interested to see that I could change my habit and practice in the afternoon, so that has been useful. Previously, when doing tratak with a candle, the flame was at eye level, and I was told to focus a soft gaze on the flame. Your guidance to look at the beam of light between the flame and my eyes created a different perception. I don't think I'd ever seen the beam before. After a few days, I found that I blinked less, but I still find it difficult to keep my eyes still. I was aware of a negative impression of the flame when I closed my eyes, but I didn't try to get involved with it. Also, as you said, when I reopened my eyes, I sometimes had a "hallucination," the negative of the flame also floating about among the light rays. I noticed, but again tried not to get too involved.

**Mukunda:** Good; that is going quite well then. The purpose of this lesson is to train detachment from the senses—pratyahara (see *Yoga Sutras* II, 53–55). Over time, it is extended to detachment and dispassion from the emotions. Namaste.

**Student:** During pranayama, specifically bhastrika, where is the inward gaze—third eye, heart, or somewhere else? Is an inward gaze also referred to as a *drishti*?

**Mukunda:** Inward gaze (shambhavi mudra) can go to either place—heart or third eye. It goes to the heart when you know or want to know your Inner Teacher; it goes to your third eye for seeking the outer teacher. *Drishti* means to gaze on an external object, usually done in still asana practice.

**Student:** Well, I did the yoni mudra along with tratak exercise last night before going to bed. Not entirely sure what I should expect to experience, but here it is. I felt fairly neutral throughout the yoni mudra. More energy seemed to be coming from my arms than my legs. I felt waves of energy descending from my shoulders down to the pelvic region, like a pool of concentration in that area. When I checked in with the clarity of color of my root chakra, it was a crystal-clear red. The clearest it's ever been! I also checked in with myself mentally and emotionally. Mentally, I was fatigued (mostly from the events of the day), but I was neutral energetically. Emotionally, I felt clear and centered. I will do the exercise again this evening. The interesting thing to me is that I am tightest in that area of my body—the hip flexors specifically. Yesterday in the Bikram class that I took, the teacher said that we carry a lot of emotional energy in our pelvic region and that can sometimes be the cause of physical tightness in that region. Hmmmm....

*Mukunda:* The pelvis is home to balanced vata, which is the source material from which prana is composed. Opening that on deeper levels brings about a potential for multi-dimensional healing.

*Student:* I had a very personal experience, but it's bothering me, so I still think I should tell you. After the practice, I felt a need to release sexually, but when I was trying to release myself, it was very hard. I'm blocked somehow. I feel that more often recently. Is that strange that I feel that need? Do you know what it is or how I can have a fulfilling expression? It feels as if I want to release very much, but am not able to.

*Mukunda:* It is not uncommon. The need is for being loving with yourself in a fashion that is soothing, nurturing, and connecting with the emotional or water quality of your second chakra. Be softer, gentler, and follow whatever you wish. Allow the energy to release without holding on to the idea that it must be sexual. It may be felt as an energetic orgasm, one that is without sexual climax. They are different. The energy that is love is seeking a higher expression than you may be familiar with. As a result, feeling blocked in your old pattern is showing you that a new direction is being asked for. The fact that you are reading this lesson shows you are seeking a spiritual experience of your sexuality. Sexual frustration is unbecoming to you; therefore prana blocks that to show you a new way. Seek instead to open what is naturally opening and disregard feelings of a block. There is always an opening near to a place of feeling blocked. All pranas are also emotions. All emotions are pranic expression. Prana seeks resolution by coming home to you as serenity. Be at peace as you unfold your beauty.

*Student:* Lesson 5 was actually the most challenging for me; I had the most resistance to it, where with the others, I looked forward to doing them. I am curious to read the Dialogue section for this chapter to see the challenges others faced and your suggestions. I practiced lesson 5 this week, and I am not sure if it is this lesson or if I am having stronger PMS symptoms this week. I have felt this week as if I were taking a colder, harder look at changes that I feel I need to make in my life, and I wonder if this "eyes-open" practice could have this effect. I feel more intensely aware of where I am feeling "stuck," and as I write this to you, I am realizing that this is just the effect we want some of these lessons to have—isn't it?

*Mukunda:* Indeed. An open-eyes practice is good during all times of the day and night. This is essentially a core practice that needs to be in place behind all the ones yet to come for you.

*Student:* Rather than the practice getting easier, I seemed to get more frustrated each day. The first day, I was more relaxed around it, and in the days after, I was frustrated with my inability to keep my eyes relaxed and not blink all the time. From the beginning, my candles had run out at home, so I have been using a wooden statue of Buddha. Should I also try with candles or stick with what I have been using?

*Mukunda:* You can use any object that allows you time and captivates your attention. Purification of the eyes will result in blinking a lot, and tearing is a natural side effect of a kriya (cleansing of the lacteal or tear ducts). It also purifies your tendency to project onto your perception of objects. Let it happen. If you do not wish to go through that process, just get more comfy and do the practice for shorter periods of time.

# Tantra Prana Bodywork

With Great Respect and Love, I Honor
My Heart, My Inner Teacher.

Tantra Prana Bodywork is a method I created to assist the release of subtle physical challenges—for instance, when a student is plagued with individual muscle-holding patterns or suppressed emotions that do not respond to asana practice. These students tend to be concerned about their blocked energy and find no satisfactory way of resolving it. In this process, we focus on opening what's already open and disregard what isn't ready to open. Those who have a spiritual practice find that this process connects them more deeply to their spiritual nature and forms a more durable connection to their teacher.

## Theory of Tantra Prana Bodywork

For a healer to be of true assistance in freeing you from the restrictions of your karma, he or she must have developed a degree of compassion in their empathetic responses to those in pain. This is developed over a long period of time from having a committed spiritual and energetic practice guided by a teacher. What protects both the healer and the client is two factors. First, the healer must be committed to his or her own spiritual practice, and second, he or she cannot react to the client's emotional or energetic responses during healing sessions, except to assist your liberation into a sattvic pattern. By encouraging both people to uphold these principles, prana will be elevated to its higher form as Shakti. In addition, healer and client cannot be sexual or romantic partners, as the intimate relationship will color your ability to be neutral and sattvic. With trust in your teacher's capacity to be focused on your healing, you can open yourself to levels of freedom that have been inaccessible until now. Your suppressed (tamasic) or overly expressed (rajasic) patterns can move toward harmony (sattvic) by the increased prana, enabling you to trust in a greater power than yourself. I offer trainings for Tantrik students to guide and transmit spiritual guidance. My method is cited by Joan Borysenko, PhD and Gordon Dveirin, PhD in *Your Soul's Compass – What is Spiritual Guidance?* (Hay House, Inc., 2008).

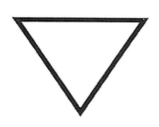

Yoni mudra

The Tantra Prana Bodywork process builds from the yoni mudra technique. Yoni mudra is the symbol of the Goddess or Devi ("being of light") as Her energy relates to descending Grace. The reverse is Shiva mudra, an upward-pointing triangle, which is our self-effort ascending toward God's Grace. Both forces are necessary for the fullest development of Tantrik Yoga. The meeting of these two forces creates the Star of David at the subtle heart center. In the harmony of these two primal forces—Shiva moving upward and Shakti moving downward—there must be upward striving self-effort to coax the descent of Grace. You must surrender to the full spiritual power of Grace to elevate your lesser emotions. Symbolically, the yoni mudra is the force of your karma coming back full force, seeking transcendence. Grace will naturally flow into the heart from above.

The three points of the yoni symbolically represent the three primary qualities (as Ayurvedic doshas) of our emotional energies. The upper left angle is vata in imbalance, manifesting as fear. The downward-pointing angle is pitta in imbalance, manifesting as desire. The upper right angle is kapha in imbalance, manifesting as attachment. In harmony, these angular forces are fearlessness, desire, and attachment to what is beneficial.

On a practical note, the three points of the yoni can be used to stimulate or suppress any one. This practice can be done alone or by a trained practitioner. As you do yoni mudra to balance vata, simply press the upper pelvic bone (*iliac crest*) on the left side. Do this practice rhythmically to your breath, pressing as you exhale, relaxing pressure at inhale. Allow your pressure to be firmer if you wish to stimulate and softer if you wish to sedate vata.

Similarly, to work with pitta, which is commonly rajasic, do the same procedure with emphasis upon sedating the pitta point at the pubic bone. For kapha, which is more commonly tamasic, your pressure may need to be firmer longer to elevate its prana. Gradually integrate use of both hands to bring out the kinesthetic insights into the three doshas within the pelvic bones.

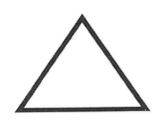

Shiva mudra

As we become more purified, we gain access to the higher koshas while appearing to be working on the gross body. Thus the prana maya kosha and the mano maya kosha are uplifted to fulfill a higher unforeseen destiny. This is the goal of Tantra Prana Bodywork—to make available forces that were previously unknown and surrender to those forces whose innate attributes lead to a higher level of evolution.

In the Shiva mudra, the three points of the mudra represent the forces of ascending self-effort. The effort to overcome our conditioning and past negative karma is enhanced by knowing that we can influence our destiny. From this place, the actions of a Yogini are able to overcome her past conditioning and sense of limitation. This is the symbol of the willful path of yoga. Yoga is self-effort directing your attention fully to the openings that manifest the divine presence. For many, Tantra emphasizes surrender to the Goddess in Her primal force as descending Grace.

The three points of the Shiva mudra represent the primary sadhanas Patanjali taught in chapter 2 of the *Yoga Sutras* to overcome karmic conditioning. This chapter is entitled "Sadhana Pada," the path of self-effort. Krishnamacharya taught that the teachings of the opening sutra of this chapter are the key to yoga therapy. The triple forces are self-effort toward purification (*tapah*), self-study aided by scriptural reflections (*svadhyaya*), and willingly following the guidance of your True Heart as your inner Self with devotion and humility (*Isvara pranidhanani*). This is the path that leads to total purification (Kriya Yoga). The upward angle is purification of the life force due to self-effort. The left base angle symbolizes scriptural self-study. The right base angle symbolizes devotion assisted by companions who are spiritual friends and seeking the company of holy beings (*satsang*).

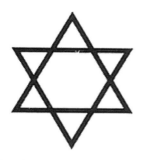

Shiva/Shakti mudra
(Deva/Devi mudra)

When the Yogini is in harmony with both her Shiva and Shakti natures, the naturally intertwining forces become the Star of David. On the mundane level, this is the symbol of man and woman in harmonious interactions. This ancient symbol is also the sign of the heart chakra in the second kosha. On kosha three, it signifies mind and body in harmony. The mind is Shakti descending with humility into the body, which is purified through discipline to ascend toward the Divine. In the fourth kosha (vijnana maya kosha), the field unknown to the mind attempts to be elevated (Shiva force) to know the Unknown (Shakti force). In the fifth kosha (ananda maya kosha), the Unknowable is encountered in one of its triple forms. It is the bliss of refined kapha being transformed into ojas, the root substance of love. It may also be revealed through vata being elevated into prana and taking tactile (air) or wisdom (ether) sensory experiences. Or it can come through the pitta dosha being transformed into tejas, resulting in real-life visions, like Moses's experience of YHWH as a "burning bush."

Let us move from theory to practice, for Yoginis will never be satisfied by mere understanding or even wisdom. Direct experience is the true hallmark of one who is a Tantrika or a Yogini. Without direct experience to guide you, all theory can be changed just upon the whim of what is popular to the culture. My hidden teacher, Yogi Hal, taught that "the true gains only come from your personal practice," not what happens in classes or in a weekend with a master teacher. Of what value are experiences in a class or given from an elevated teacher if they cannot be reproduced in your own Self.

Yoginis seek a sattvic state and its evolution. Yet they must guard against the quality of tamas, which tends to make us undisciplined, complacent, and unquestioning of our experiences of transcendence. Tantriks also seek this, but they realize that impurities are there; they are more willing to go through rajasic and tamasic experiences to root out the deeper impurities. One difference is that the Tantrika is not afraid to experiment with her pranic consciousness; the undisciplined Yogini will tend to follow only the cultural whims of contemporary teachings. By taking the best of both worlds, the Tantrik Yogini develops the discernment necessary for living an empowered spiritual life.

## Tantrik Bodywork Practice

Jacques Cousteau claimed: "We are organized as sea water." In commenting on this idea, André van Lysebeth says: "Our billions of cells are seawater at the same saline concentration as that of the tropical seas where life began."[23] This is a beautiful sensory guide for energetic bodywork. Consider that, when touching any body, you are touching a field of water. When we drop a stone in a small pond, we can see how the ripples move from larger to smaller as they wave to the edges, then, striking that edge, return toward the source, passing over the continuing initial waves.

From 1979 to 1981, I owned a holistic health institute that offered state-licensed professional yoga, health education, and massage programs in Sacramento, California. While there, I learned many forms of physical and energetic bodywork. In the spring of 1982, I was with Babaji Prakashananda near Mumbai, and when he learned of my background, he graciously encouraged me to give him massages daily. At first, I only did his lower legs as he lay on the floor of his meditation hut (*kutir*).

> One night while massaging his legs he encouraged me to continue and do his whole body. When I got to his belly questions began to burn inside my mind. Who is he? Who am I? While holding these questions, I gently pushed on his belly. The answer came that his body was like a waterbed. When I pushed on one side a ripple would go effortlessly through his entire body and then ripple back to me with the same force. I asked myself—What is he made of? What is this body? I closed my eyes and I saw a beautiful effulgent blue like the ocean shimmering in the morning light. As I continued to look the blue spread to the horizon and beyond to encompass the sky, I could not distinguish air from water. All the elements of his body and of my perception were the

---

23. André van Lysebeth, *Tantra* (York Beach, ME: Weiser, 1995), 20.

same glimmering blue. I had an image of a million tiny lights within the blue field all shining continuously.

My eyes began to water with warm tears of joy and great love as I felt his belly. Then I opened my eyes and looked at his body and he simply smiled at me. One of those all knowing smiles that allowed me to just be my Self. Just the joy that was his body while serving him through the act of giving a massage. There was no feeling of him giving me energy or vice versa. There was a natural acceptance of each other's role in life in this moment just being together. In that moment there was a grace that has never left me, that continues to live on and on evolving, vividly, as a connection to my spiritual Heart.[24]

As you reflect on this "body is water" contemplation, begin a process of Tantra Prana Bodywork. Focus your attention while doing a body scan to search out the greatest expression of prana, in the language of Master Krishnamacharya, as the "currents of sensation." Place your hands on that location. As you learned in lesson 2 on elemental practice, the sense of touch connects to the subtlest prana field related to the element ether, which manifests as vyana prana. The easiest way to perceive it is to lighten your touch, as vyana prana flows predominantly through the channel of your skin and the auric field. As ether, it also transcends the body and moves through the material world. For some, this sense is the strongest and will cultivate a profound connection to your prana as a healing force.

For those whose sense of sight is the strongest sense, you can visualize or imagine this next step with me energetically present to assist you. If you wish, you can do this Tantrik bodywork practice with me physically present, during a workshop, an individual session, a session over the phone, or via a Skype video connection.

Place your hands where you feel the "currents of sensation." Then visualize my hands where you feel your energy flowing or wanting to go. This step requires you to be open to feeling my presence and to allowing my presence to enhance your perception of prana. Move slowly as you become accustomed to my subtle presence and be sure that you are leading and I am following you. Once you experience this working

---

24. Titus Foster, *Agaram Bagaram Baba: Life Teachings and Parables of Prakashananda* (Berkeley: North Atlantic Books, 1999), 159.

for you, repeat the procedures in the introductory lesson until you become comfortable with another presence there. Focus your attention on fully perceiving your energy body. Do not concern yourself with depleting my energy. It is a foundational Tantrik concept that we are working, not to elevate or enhance your own individual energy, but rather to increase the collective energy field of all those we think of. Therefore, when we are connecting together, it will benefit your loved ones, family, and friends. The benefits can also be directed toward yourself when the intention is to be more effective to others. End the session with an energetic hug and open yourself to receiving and giving fully.

Place your hands on your second and fourth chakras (pelvis and heart) to encourage the polarity to become sattvic. Follow the currents until they nurture or awaken all areas that seem to want to open naturally during this session. Let your hands follow the currents of sensation, pacing your hands to follow just behind the change in sensation. Follow until a natural conclusion is experienced. Then conclude with the three yoni mudra variations described in lesson 2, taking your energies deeply into your first three chakras. Remember that Shakti energy moves downward and Shiva energy moves upward. You can flow up to connect to your Shiva's stillness by moving from the first to the third chakra, or flow downward to connect to more of Shakti's life force by moving from your navel to your pelvis.

For those who wish to direct their prana and come to be free of inappropriate fear, desire, or attachment, shift your intention for that benefit. As you place your hands on your abdomen, see whether the energy of the Divine is descending as Shakti energy or ascending as Shiva energy. Make a resolution (sankalpa) that you are going to be victorious and overcome your previous experiences. Remember that, previous to this, you were guided by a more powerful self-centeredness. Now you have strengthened your humility and devotional muscles, so a radically different outcome is due to arise. Have the intention of connecting to a greater power than yourself (pray to your chosen form of God/dess), one that allows you to overcome the limitations of conditioning. Become free of those thoughts, feelings, or pranas that have not manifested your victorious qualities through tantrasanas such as vira or vajrasana. Tantrasana will be presented thoroughly in the next lesson.

Place your hands with the intention of finding sensations of inappropriate fear (or anger as attachment). Now you have two choices: you can take the yogic path and involute the prana back to its source (yoni) or follow the Tantrik path and surrender to the prana's "currents of sensations." Both methods are equally effective. It is a matter of choice. In either method, understand that within the pranic flow is the energy you call emotions, thoughts, and conditioning. In either way, keep your resolution strong and have faith that you can be transformed into what you have never been before.

## Prana and Divine Mother

There are many yoga and Tantrik techniques whose benefits range to all the five dimensions of self (koshas), like pelvic-floor strengthening. These are different from childbirth-preparation Kegel exercises, as they are refined into a subtler form known as mula bandha—root lock. There are also breathing exercises elevated to energetic breathing (pranayama) to facilitate connecting to the life-force energies and initiations for sensual and spiritual awakening (Kundalini). These practices keep the Yogini awake to the beauty of the world as Mother's Grace descending into the visible world.

In Tantrik practices, the Divine Mother is principally known as the source of pleasure. In actuality, She is the threefold primal energy of creativity, nurturance, and transformation. In the human body, these energies have a source in the non-physical energy body, called the subtle body. They are located in dense fields called chakras, meaning spinning wheels, which are like vortices. The first chakra, responsible for creativity, is at the perineum. The second chakra, responsible for nurturance and pleasure, is located for women near the entrance to the uterus. For men, it is located at the base of the pubic bone. The third chakra, responsible for transformation, is located in the area of the navel. A strong energetic area above it called the solar plexus is located just below the breastbone. This is not the third chakra, but a grosser plexus formed by parasympathetic nerves.

It is possible that you may already be experiencing these specific energies building. They are the result of spiritual development and Divine Grace. When you connect to them, opening yourself when you feel your energy building, it can lead you to your higher power, source of wisdom, and if Grace is approving, to the experience of God/dess Presence. They can also come another way. While focusing on God in a church or religious service, the chakras may awaken and provide a physical experience of the Holy Spirit. When you feel spiritual or sexual, look closely at that experience and see where it is located, how it affects you emotionally, or whether there may be a vision or insight associated with it.

## On Divine Love and Kashmir Shaivism

Tantrik Yoga reverses the flow of outgoing pranic life currents and redirects them inward to your true Source, as was graphically shared in lesson 4 on shambhavi mudra. This can only come when you have a blend of knowledge combined with direct experience of your transformation. Remember that understanding yogic teachings alone is not spiritual practice or sadhana. If you have done these spiritual practices, your energy body will open naturally, culminating in the blossoming of your heart's flower. The ultimate experience for the Tantrika or Yogini is uncovering the inner source of love. No matter what we seek, that seeking has a desire for constancy that really comes from the formless. Along the way, we believe we will find that nectar in sensual worldly objects—and they may often give us joy, but not the illusive steadfast love we intuitively know exists. Our seeking is our finding. What we find is that the constancy of our search leads to the closeness of the One seeking us. Thus it is by seeking that the Dear One is felt in the intensity of that looking.

The text of Divine Love for the Yogi is Narada's *Bhakti Sutras*. It is a terse text of eighty-three aphorisms revealing the importance of cultivating the blossom of spiritual devotion for the flowering of love. This quality is crucial to protect the spiritual aspirant along the path of fulfillment that ultimately leads to self-realization. Here are some select sutras to reflect upon:

> Sutra 7. Spiritual devotion does not arise from desire. Its nature is a state of inner stillness.
> Sutra 8. The inner stillness consecrates the performance of worldly and traditional social duties.
> Sutra 9. Inner stillness, furthermore, requires a single-hearted intention, and disinterest in what is antagonist to spiritual devotion.

Sutra 10. When one is single-hearted, one relinquishes seeking security in anything other than the Divine Presence.[25]

As your energy opens from the practices we have been sharing, it is natural for your personal path to reveal its uniqueness. Hence you will be drawn to a unique path, teacher, and *sangha* (community) in which to share your spiritual evolution. I hope that my sharing of those influences that have been profound for me may also assist you in finding the profundity that leads you to know your own path. The safety and security that are needed for Tantrik Yoga to blossom are likely to become apparent to you now. A path that has greatly influenced me to uncover my spiritual devotion is the non-dual path of Kashmir Shaivism, as revealed by my spiritual teacher, Swami Muktananda, who teaches thus:

> The all-pervasive Lord
> manifests throughout the universe.
> The elixir of love pulsates through all things,
> radiates through every tree and branch.
> Welcome that bliss;
> get rid of fear and grief.
> O dear one, keep chanting God's name
> while sitting, or standing,
> or involved in the world.
> Never forget that One
> Unite your mind with the Self.

The most profound of the teachings of Tantrik Shaivism are in the 8th-century text, the *Vijnana Bhairava Tantra*.[26] My guru, Baba Muktananda, taught in the more contemporary Kashmir Shaivist tradition, which has its roots in this great work. In his Blessings to the first translation of this text, Baba said "among the ancient teachings of India the

---

25. Prem Prakash, *The Yoga of Spiritual Devotion* (Rochester, VT: Inner Traditions, 1998), 19–25.
26. The work is available in several translations, one in great detail with commentary by Tantrik Hatha Yogis as *Sri Vijnana Bhairava Tantra*, translated by Swami Satyasangananda Saraswati of the Bihar School of Yoga. Osho gave a series of lectures on these teachings that have been published as *The Book of Secrets: 112 Keys to the Mystery Within*. Two others with terse renditions and no commentary on the 112 meditations on Shiva are *Yoga Spandakarika: The Sacred Texts at the Origins of Tantra* by Daniel Odier and the classic *Zen Flesh, Zen Bones* by Paul Reps. Here, it is referred to as a pre-Zen text.

Tantra scriptures have the unique, in fact, the highest place. In them one finds not only the means for knowing the nature of highest reality, but also techniques to experiencing it."

In Jaideva's Foreword to the text he says, "The Vijnana Bhairava gathers up a treasure house of secret, yogic methods for experiencing the extraordinary and paradoxical reality of unbounded consciousness which is called Bhairava or Shiva. It is one of the bliss-saturated texts of Tantric Shaivism. True to its Tantric province, the text discovered the reality of Bhairava in unexpected and even apparently bizarre places."[27]

The work is written as a dialogue with Deva Shiva and his consort Devi Parvati. Deva and Devi refer to the masculine and feminine beings "who radiate light" to each other. Shiva refers to the primal consciousness experienced as stillness, steadiness, and commitment. His form is called a lingam, literally the "wand of light" as "his first form." Shakti Devi manifests as the yoni or "sacred space" that is the only container for his true form as stillness. Here is a beautiful series of sutras from the 112 meditations that Deva gives to Devi so that She can attain oneness with Her Beloved. Use this contemplation to move to a higher level of Tantra Prana Bodywork.

> Sutra 41. While being caressed, sweet princess,
> enter *the caressing* as everlasting life.
> Sutra 42. Stop the doors of the senses when feeling
> the creeping of an ant. *Then*.
> Sutra 43. At the start of sexual union, keep attentive
> on the fire *in the beginning,*
> and, so continuing,
> avoid the embers in the end.
> Sutra 44. When in such an embrace that your senses
> are shaken as leaves,
> *enter this shaking.*
> Sutra 45. Even when remembering communion,
> without the embrace,
> *the transformation.*[28]

27. Jaidev Singh, *The Yoga of Delight, Wonder, and Astonishment* (State University of New York Press, 1991).
28. Paul Reps and Nyogen Senzaki, *Zen Flesh, Zen Bones* (Boston: Tuttle Publishing, 1988), 199–200.

# Congratulations!

You have just completed the first third of the Tantra lessons. May you persist to the end of these eighteen lessons. Patanjali, in his *Yoga Sutras* I, 12, says the secret to success in yoga is "consistent earnest practice over a long period of time and detachment to the results of that practice" (*abhyasa* and *vairagya*). May you be blessed with both!

Remember to persist in your practice and stay detached from expecting specific outcomes. Tantra is a personal spiritual practice. When you feel complete with this lesson, read the Dialogue section that follows prior to beginning lesson 7.

**With Great Respect and Love, I Honor
My Heart, My Inner Teacher.**

# Dialogue with Mukunda

**Student:** I am still trying to develop more consistency in my Tantra practice, preferring to do it at night instead of during my a.m. practice, which I very rarely miss. Some of the lessons I have only practiced once or just a few times. I have tried to avoid being frustrated with myself about this, as I would have in the past, and just keep moving on. However, I recently went back and reread the previous lessons and feel that my understanding is improving. Also, I am noticing that I am beginning to process emotions more easily, moving through them without getting so stuck. I am working on living with more sensitivity and compassion toward myself. Thank you very much for your help and concern.

**Mukunda:** The major point I hear you saying is that you are learning to lighten up on how you take yourself. It is good that you are not too serious, but persist at the sadhana that you are given. This sadhana is one that is done over and over again. You need to learn the steps, then you can dance. Just as soon as you feel that you have some competency and are free from confusion and resistance to your emotions and triggers, move to the next lesson. It sounds as if you are doing that and it's going well. Namaste.

**Student:** I have spent the last few weeks engaged in self-examination. Upon reflection on the essays in Iyengar's *Tree of Yoga*, I realized that I was the cause of my back pains and all my other physical and emotional pains. That realization was a shock to me, because I did not know how disconnected I was to myself. I have been practicing energetic bodywork and giving myself the attention that my body and mind demand, so, of course, my back pain has been minimized. Reflecting on Rumi's poems revealed to me my dishonesty and hypocrisy, because I simply believed that, because I had a daily practice, I was spiritual, even though I left my spirituality behind at the end of my practice. This realization filled me with sadness, but I am trying to be more aware and engaged throughout the day. I have a long way to go. But then this constant practice/awareness has already begun to bear fruit. When faced with a situation with my husband in which I felt disappointment, I started on the familiar path of rebuilding a wall that I was working on disassembling, but then my heart reminded me of my intention to love him unconditionally and I began on a new path and left that wall behind. Such situations continue to be presented to me; I suppose they have always been presented, but that I am only just becoming aware of them.

I am so grateful for all that you have given me. With your guidance, my journey progresses.

**Mukunda:** Sounds to me as if you are doing beautifully on your path. I love hearing about reading Rumi. It is such a great inspiration to read from his work.

**Student:** It's been over a week since my Tantra Prana Bodywork session with you, and I am still experiencing lots of jerking and muscular contractions and releases while doing the yoni mudra exercise. Also, I have strong emotion and burning in the diaphragm. Tonight, I felt a complete void in the middle of the mudra for a few minutes and thought it was good (like a sattvic nothingness), but then it began to feel cold and heavy. During the past few sessions, my right shoulder has been jerking around a lot when my hand comes to my chest. I definitely have something stuck there. Should I just continue this way? Am I actually releasing something? What did you implant into my belly?

Also, can you tell me what the jerkings are? Are they energetic releases that are occurring spontaneously? It has now started to happen when I sit in satsang with my sadhana group here, when I am in meditation, and when I hear favorite chants. I had an emotional "vomiting" on my husband last week when I was challenged to touch upon a fear directly. This caused lots of the same kind of jerking around as when I was working with you. My husband was very supportive, told me I was safe and I should let it out. I did as much as I could, but he also said something that made me wonder. He asked me what was I fighting, and I thought, yes, from the motions of my body and the violence of it, it did seem as if there were a fight going on. So I have been wondering if that's what it is—that

I continue to try and suppress. It's mostly moved to my right arm now, not so much in the hips, which is where the pain is nesting. When you say you are awakening what is dormant and present in me, is it the physical and emotional desire for the release? Was it an awakening of the desire for union and non-separation? Or prana flow? Thanks.

*Mukunda:* When I work with you directly, physically using the Tantrik procedure, there can be many changes to your subtle-body energy. The jerking motions and irregular shifting are called kriyas. They are purifications of the first and second koshas—that is, they are both physical and pranic. You will be releasing physical tensions and suppressed emotion for some time. Just encourage it. Whatever is not beneficial will leave you. Whatever is beneficial will stay. I did not plant anything, only awakened what was dormant and always present within you. Continue with the lessons. The next two will help to stabilize you.

These motions and their emotional component are spontaneous as a sign of spiritual energy. When they pass quickly during the session, they are healthy pranic changes. They are likely to bring up suppressed emotions much more profoundly than the experiences that can arise from lesson 3. The pranic energy is seeking natural expression—physically, emotionally, and psychically. When that occurs, your pelvis especially will feel a deep release. The process varies from person to person; whatever fear or negative thought arises is what is being purified. If you desire union, that will come, until only beneficial actions and emotions remain. Be persistent and have faith in the process of your natural arising awakening. Namaste.

*Student:* You once suggested to me that, when I feel this energy while touching a client/student, it may be my own "stuff" I am feeling. Is it safe to say that, if I relax and it passes through me, then I am just a vehicle, and if it stays within me, my own "stuff" is being activated?

*Mukunda:* Yes to your first question. If it stays within you, your own vasana or karmic impressions are being purified.

*Student:* Will you be talking about kriya prana in the rest of the course or in your new book?

*Mukunda:* The term *kriya prana* implies that prana has a natural purification that comes to body prana and spiritual sensitivity. Experiences that arise and purify the mind are called kriya prana. As we become more serene in our sattva, we will also become sensitive to the prana as Shakti. Shakti prana is also called Kundalini. As such, Kundalini is a karmic housecleaner, and she is intensely desirous of a clean, clear house. Baba Muktananda used this analogy frequently in his talks. She clears out the energies latent in the central nadi (sushumna), analogous to the hole in the spinal cord through which cerebral spinal fluid travels. Details on this can be found in his spiritual autobiography *Play of Consciousness*, or in *Devatma Shakti (Kundalini) Divine Power* by Swami Vishnu Tirtha. More about this is given in lessons 11 and 12. Blessings.

**Student:** Experiencing the energy work with you at last week's session in New York helped to synthesize what I have been exploring on my own using the guidance of Tantrik lesson energy work. It was very clarifying on many levels. What are some of the other benefits of practicing mula bandha for the different koshas, besides the obvious pelvic-floor strengthening? Also, can you explain how the effect of Tantrik Yoga is to reverse the flow of outgoing pranic life currents?

**Mukunda:** The benefits of mula bandha are toning the pelvis to aid in all its functions, including sex, as well as heightening emotional sensitivity (second kosha), which increases prana and can be used to store prana in the lower chakras or lift it up to the third or fourth chakras. With detachment, one learns to allow sensory awareness and emotions, encouraging prana to flow into all experiences and not attach to them. This indifference and dispassion create the ability to retain prana and not lose so much. It is especially the case in the higher Tantrik lessons on sensual pleasure and attraction/aversions.

The person of discernment finds that the trouble is the uncontrolled mind. The five vrittis (instability of thought; see *Yoga Sutras* I, 5–16), especially memory, hold on to the past and cause the Divine Shakti to exert Her force of transformation. It is that force that manifests the prayer "May all the Beings in all the worlds be Happy." All are seeking to be free and loving. How we hold people is our way of trying to restrict the force of Grace. Grace happens to all, including those memories one holds as unworthy of Divine Grace. Grace persists in spite of our vrittis. No one remains as memory holds them to be. It is from opening to Shakti and persistent meditation that the mind becomes free of the instability that would limit its full capacity—that veil its true nature as the Self. The process of sadhana is the highest deity to hold on to, not to any living teacher. Opening to being free of restricted thinking is the true process of spiritual practice. Blessings for your life to be filled with Grace. Namaste.

**Student:** How can I better understand the process? With more guidance in pranic energetic bodywork? I understand to a degree what you mean when you say that the more effective way is to let it naturally arise, but I also appreciate the need to understand and feel more comfortable.

**Mukunda:** Mostly, it comes out of clearing your own energy field and making sure your doubts and hesitations are removed. Learning to follow the prana without hesitation and yet without investment in the outcome is a sign of success. It is definitely an opportunity for Karma Yoga or *Guru Seva* (service) according to your orientation. To understand is usually to reflect after the fact, not during the work. During the process, one should be so submitted to the Devi's energy that there are very few thoughts except how to feel and follow Her more clearly. As in the Quaker song: "O dear Lord, three things I pray—to see you more clearly, follow you more nearly, love you more dearly, day by day."

**Student:** My life has changed so much since beginning the Tantra lessons six months ago. I just wanted to let you know some of the impact it has had, since the holidays are upon us. When I began, my income was nearly a third of what it is now. I am teaching more classes, drawing more students, and prospering in many other exciting ways too. I am much more in touch with my energy, and know when to move into a situation and when to detach from questionable situations. I have taken over the care of two infants who needed a temporary foster mom and, being thirty-eight and single, this has really helped me examine my desire for children and family. The opportunity to open to the unexpected has been enormous. I am finding that, when I relax my tensions, my energy levels are increasing as I ask how I can be of service. I always heard that Karma Yoga was supposed to do that, but I am finding it directly now. Amazing!

My ability to connect to you is also profound. I feel a swirl of energy coming from my crown down into my body when I feel your presence. I rarely do this practice, because I am so exhausted at the end of the day. But I am surprised at how consistent your presence is with me when I look for it. It has also been the case in my expanded classes that I have occasion to ask my teachers to help me in situations that are arising with new challenged students. And guess what? They are there and give me tangible guidance and direction that is of benefit. Thank you for sharing.

**Mukunda:** What more can I say? All is unfolding as you learn to be free of your energy blocks and open to what is calling you. Continue to disregard the blocked patterns and just seek where opening is natural. It is always there, guiding and directing our lives. Trust your Inner Teacher regardless of her/his form. Truly, I feel that the time spent with my teachers is what keeps them connected to me, in spite of the fact that most of my teachers have passed on. We are blessed, and let us continue to open to what else seeks fulfillment. May your desires be fulfilled in the most gracious manner. Blessings.

**Student:** Thank you for sending me these questions and answers. It was helpful to read them and relate my own experiences to those of others. I am excited to move on with the process and definitely can relate to the precarious moving nature of Tantra. I feel as if the last couple of months have brought my deepest fears to the surface, along with pain in my physical body. I have wanted to contact you about this previously and felt stunted by my fears of not being accepted or not being ready for what I am doing. I have had multiple dreams in which I talked with you about whatever fear it was in that moment and you were so loving and so accepting in my dreams that I felt better the next day and the urgency to connect with you subsided. I just wanted to share this and say thanks.

**Mukunda:** Well that is great! Tantra and yoga are both aimed at purification, hence Kriya Yoga is the major issue in the first half of *Yoga Sutras* chapter 2. It is so different to walk through the experiences, as contrasted with just reading about them and sort of understanding them with your head. Thanks for sharing. Next time, share even when it feels resolved. Sooner is preferable, as it deepens your relationship with your outer and Inner Teacher. Blessings.

**Student:** Sunday, just one day after teaching my last Saturday class after reducing my schedule, ready for freedom to dive deeper into studies, I got a concussion/hematoma and am still feeling somewhat dazed. I was at the park with my dog. He ran under a jungle gym, and I rushed downward to grab his leash and slammed my head into a bar. My husband, John, saw a giant goose egg appear and rushed me to the emergency room. I'm doing okay, but feel pretty rattled in my head and spine. It's been difficult to concentrate much, but I'm better today. Have been taking it easy and doing lots of yoni mudra, your sacroiliac stabilization exercise, and lots of oiling. This morning, I returned to my structural yoga therapy practice in a more gentle form, minus the shoulderstand. Any other practice ideas to help me rebalance?

*Mukunda:* Do yoni mudra and bring its energy from your pelvis into your hands, then transfer it to the field above the wound. Gradually move down to physical contact. Going slowly will reveal pranic imbalances. Often, this will heal while in the field, not the body. Remember, injury mostly goes to vyana prana in such events. This prana flows through your skin and is the sheath of the aura. Increase your sensitivity to kinesthetic sensation, both subtle and gross. Though nasty, this injury is an excellent opportunity to learn deeper energetic Tantrik bodywork. The energy of both the injury and the healing will teach you.

*Student:* Thank you for this Tantra lesson. This was a difficult, painful one, but good, I think, because lots of challenges and clarity came with it. I visualized the healing laying-on-of-hands. My greatest sensation was in my left abdominal area. I had my hands in yoni mudra over my second chakra area, which felt like the right place to be. I visualized your hands and healing energy over mine, then a few other entities popped into the visu-alization/energy work! Amma then laid her hands in a yoni mudra over yours; Satchi-dananda laid his hands over Amma's; Sarasvati laid Her hands over Satchidananda's; Lakshmi laid hers over Sarasvati's; Durga laid her hands over Lakshmi's; and finally, Tara laid hers over Lakshmi's.

This happened spontaneously, without my really thinking about it. I feel close and nurtured by all these teachers and Goddesses, all of whom are on my altar. So, all of these divine hands were in yoni mudras over my hands in yoni mudra. I felt the healing energy toward my second chakra area. Then, out of the blue, the affirmation flashed into my head: "I Am Worthy of Divine Love." That phrase kept repeating in my consciousness like a mantra that has taken root in one's being. I would appreciate your thoughts, feelings, suggestions about all this.

*Mukunda:* How wonderful to be so deeply blessed in your healing. You are receiving blessings normally associated with those students who have completed the topics of lessons 10 and 17. For those who have done spiritual practices in other traditions, I find this Tantrik process cleans out the layers of the subtle body that create the belief and experience of sepa-ration and brings them into an integrated wholeness of self-acceptance.

All you need is the affirmation to be deeply accepted and received. Nothing more is needed. The blessings of many levels of your True Self are showing their healing of your history. As the Self becomes integrated into your personality, all the experiences of this oneness integrate with the multi-dimensional perspective, until the dimensions of your self become one Self. That is what I perceive to be Self Realization. It is the unconditional acceptance of Self, then living life with unconditional acceptance of all that you encounter. Blessings.

**Student:** I am not quite clear about energy flow when working with patients. My intention is there, but I cannot force or direct energy movement through my body. It seems to happen, or not, independent of what I hope to happen. It seems to depend on the receiver as well. In your opinion, should I be able to direct the energy more, in order to help the healing process; or is intention, and my own clarity, enough?

**Mukunda:** Sending energy to a client is like pouring water into a leaky bucket. It won't stay for long. Dependency is created, and the healer also becomes depleted. It is better to train yourself and your students how to move their own prana from places of rajasic excess to places of tamasic depletion. Over time, this training results in a capacity not to leak, but rather to restore and rejuvenate prana.

One who is competent at energy work can direct energy within others where it is needed without the use of their own energy. They can retain their energy regardless of how they are with others. The more adept can direct their own energy currents through their own bodies. That is what these lessons will provide, and more.

# Tools for Tantra

With Great Respect and Love, I Honor
My Heart, My Inner Teacher.

Tantrik teachings are empowered by your desire for prana and your capacity to imbibe the prana of your teachers and their lineage. Details of this process are given in lesson 11.

The tools for tantra include *mantra* (sound), *yantra* (form), *tantrasana* (body posture), *makara* (forbidden/hidden substances), and *svadhyaya* (self-study) aided by regular readings of the *Yoga Sutras* and/or the *Yoga Vasistha*. These first three words share a common suffix—*tra,* meaning "to transform." Mantras, or spiritually empowered words, transform the mind. The word comes from the root *man*, meaning "to think." Mantras take the mind to its root and allow your higher mind to receive from the True Self. Another meaning of the word is "the sound that protects you."

Patanjali defines violence as "negative thoughts and emotions as they cause injury to yourself and others. They arise from greed, anger, and delusion" (*Yoga Sutras* II, 34). Greed results from prolonged kapha imbalance, anger from pitta imbalance, and delusion or fear from vata instability. Yoga seeks to transform the mind into one that naturally produces a safe environment, both internally and externally.

## Mantras

There are two categories of mantras. The first includes mantras for material and health benefits (that is, for the first three koshas). These are called *jud* (dead) because their benefits produce serenity of mind and worldly contentment. Their effects depend on the intentions of the giver and receiver being aligned and a shared clarity about what is the natural desire to be fulfilled.

> Mantras for healing purposes as in Ayurvedic or Vedic astrology usage are not the same as mantras for spiritual (moksha) purposes. They can be used energetically and do not require being given by a spiritual teacher, though that is always better. What they do require is a proper understanding of their energetics and usage, just as do foods and herbs. In other words, one must have knowledge of Ayurveda and of the qualities and application of mantras.
>
> Such mantras, like certain homas and pujas (rituals), are prescribed for the ordinary goals of life of arogya (health), kama (sensual pleasure), artha (wealth) and dharma (righteous livelihood), including targeting specific diseases. Traditional Ayurvedic doctors in India have always used mantras as part of their health prescriptions, though modern Ayurveda, with its more scientific orientation, has generally not done this. Even many common people in India know the value of Mahamrityunjaya mantra for health problems, Ram mantra for calming children, or Sheetali Stotra for Pitta disorders. Or they simply use the mantras of their Ishta Devata (chosen deity) for this purpose.[29]

The second category is called *chaitanya* (alive) mantras. Ideally, this mantra is given by someone trained to impart, not merely the word and its meaning, but also an experience of the awakened energy that results from the mantra's practice. Mantras of this type are alive, in the sense that they impart a lasting connection to the master, the inner self, and in some cases, a feeling of the presence of the lineage with you, behind you, supporting you. These living mantras have the spiritual benefit of raising consciousness to experience the One Spirit.

Chaitanya mantras are the most popular mantras given and yet, without empowerment from the teacher, they don't produce the desired result. It is like having a lamp, but not plugging it into a circuit. The connection to the circuit comes as a result of the student doing the mantra according to the guidelines of the illumined teacher. That

---

29. See David Frawley's comments on mantras and Ayurveda in *Light on Ayurveda* magazine (*www.loa.com*).

illumination is noticeable by those who are seeking spirit. Mantras such as "so-ham" or "ham-sa" may be done for long periods of time without bringing about change in the mind. It is the commitment to sadhana, the study of the text on the mantra, and the devotion and submission to the Inner Teacher that plugs the mantra into its source.

An Indian disciple went to receive a mantra from my spiritual teacher, who was cordial in response to his request. He gave him the mantra "Om Namah Shivaya," which startled the disciple, because he had been given that mantra in childhood by his family's guru. Baba told him to go into his meditation cave. Meanwhile, outside, the devotees waited to see the results of this instruction. Since he had already been given the same mantra, there was controversy as to its effectiveness. Three hours later, the disciple came up from the basement cave and, with a startled look on his face, told Baba that he felt the mantra coming from the very walls of the cave. It was so captivating that he felt nothing but the pulsation and saw nothing but darkness filled with light. Baba told him to remember this experience, to talk about it frequently with devotees in order to enhance its blessing to his mind.

You can ask me for a mantra if you like; I have been authorized by my guru to give them to help you evolve your practice. It is best to receive a mantra personally, face to face, prana to prana, or Skype to Skype.

## Yantras

Yantras are rectangular geometrical symbols. They are captivating forms that take you to a higher level of consciousness. The root *yan* means a "vehicle" that takes you on a transformative journey. Another way of expressing it is through the derivation from the root *yan,* meaning "a vehicle" and *tra,* meaning "to transform." In this sense, the yantra contains the Goddess Devi's energies, making Her energetic presence condensed and accessible to the Tantrik practitioner. The lines of the yantra recreate the energy patterns preexisting in our bodies as the primal form of the Goddess. Those who honor the Divine Mother in this form use yantras to connect with Her energetic skeleton.

The highest of the yantras is Sri yantra, which depicts the fullness of consciousness as the manifesting of Devi. Her initial form is in the downward-pointing triangle. When one views the central downward-pointing triangle, one will count five below the bindu and four above. When reversed head to tail, the same yantra becomes Shiva yantra—with four yoni mudras below the bindu and five Shiva mudras above.

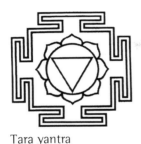

Tara yantra

Tara yantra is the form of the Devi associated with protecting the integrity and virtue of Classical Yoga teachings. Her central symbol is the downward-pointing triangle of yoni mudra. As the protectress of yoga, She maintains the integrity of those who seek Her assistance at staying connected to prana as Devi. The outer lines signify the lower states of consciousness and the inner the highest. In their center is a dot, or bindu, symbolizing the seed from which all life-forms spring. Commonly, they are composed of variants of three—and often having nine—downward-pointing triangles that "signify the primitive revelation of the Absolute as it differentiates into graduated polarities, the creative activity of the cosmic male and female energies on successive stages of evolution."[30] These are the most auspicious forms for the Tantrik.

For more on yantras, see *Yantra: The Tantric Symbol of Cosmic Unity*, by Madhu Khanna, and *Tools for Tantra*, by Harish Johari, which shows you how to create a yantra. If you would like a personal yantra painted for you, I recommend Michael Gilheany from New Jersey, as he painted a lovely Bhairava Shiva Yantra for me. In addition, I recommend yantra painter Nirlipta Tuli of London, who is creating large paintings of the ten wisdom Devis depicted in David Frawley's *Tantric Yoga and the Wisdom Goddesses*. I have also had them made into quilt-like silk wall hangings that you can see at my home/office.

## Tantrasanas

Tantrasanas are energetic asana placements that aid the prana to a higher level of expression, thus deepening meditation, pranayama, and even asana practice. These postures generally involve being seated with the spinal column upright. The best foundational sitting poses for floor practices such as puja, meditation, and Tantrik prana communion are samasana, swastikasana, siddhasana, padmasana, bhadrasana, and tarasana. True and empowered tantrasanas are given by a trained and empowered tantrasana teacher. These practices are the secret door underlying the transmission

---

30. Heinrich Zimmer, *Myths and Symbols in Indian Art and Civilization* (Princeton, NJ: Princeton University Press, 1992), 147.

of pranic Shakti through the combination of personal practice, later blossoming in partner tantrasanas as described in lesson 15.

## Bhadrasana

The word *bhadrasana* means literally "auspicious pose." This simple basic asana does not reveal its secret Tantrik nature without insights from the Tantrik texts *Hathayoga Pradipika* I, 53–54, the *Vasistha Samhita* I, 77, and *Gheranda Samhita* II, 9–10. In addition, as with all lessons, the texts in combination with consultation from your spiritual teacher will elevate your consciousness more than either one alone. Patanjali, in his *Yoga Sutras* II, 12, cites that consistent earnest practice and detachment from the result generate blessedness.

This posture often requires the aid of a wedge-shaped cushion to support the lumbar arch. This allows the skeletal posture and muscle levers to establish a minimum of effort in stabilizing the asana. Bring the soles of your feet together about eighteen inches in front of your pelvis so that the angle formed by your legs is a perfect diamond of 45 degrees at the knees. While pulling your knees down may, in the long run, promote steadfastness, seeking stability with a minimum of sattvic effort is ideal for all tantrasanas.

## Tarasana

One of my personal favorites is *tarasana*.[31] It begins from bhadrasana—seated with the soles of your feet together. Then move your feet forward enough so that, when you bend forward, your forehead rests on your inner heels. Interlace your fingers around your toes so that when the elbows are brought toward the floor, your forearms are straight across from your toes. This is a very vulnerable posture, for it affords access to deeper koshic realms and, as such, may manifest as Tara mudra. In this form, She is open to the space and air behind, as well as surrendered to the earth below. When this heaven-and-earth contrast is harmoniously experienced, the mind enters the realm of submission, and mudra results. In contrast, the primal Tara lives in the form of air and has no form save that of manifesting safety as *ahimsa*.

---

31. She is also called yoni mudra in *The Yoni: Sacred Symbol of Female Creative Power* by Rufus Camphausen (Rochester, VT: Inner Traditions, 1996), 30.

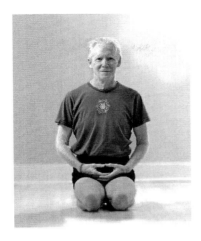

### Virasana

The word *virasana*, the hero, may be confusing to students of contemporary teachers, as this name and shape of the pose differ from the classical texts. The virasana of contemporary teachings is done by sitting on your heels or with your pelvis between your feet. However, the virasana of the texts is the half-lotus (*ardha padmasana*), as cited in *Vasistha Samhita* I, 70; *Hathayoga Pradipika* I, 21; and Vyasa's comment on the *Yoga Sutras* II, 46.

The contemporary pose is what I will describe in more detail. Virasana is done by sitting on your heels with your feet in a V shape, heels open, to bring your big toes together. Some teachers do the pose with the pelvis on the floor between the knees. A unique variation is *vajrasana*, the thunderbolt, which is done with the feet together at the heels and big toes to stimulate the *vajra* nadi (the urethra). It also is said to awaken Kundalini Shakti, sometimes bringing the lingam to an erect stature, hence the term thunderbolt. By the practice of these distinctions, one can discover the vajra nadi and enter the tantric realm of tantrasana.

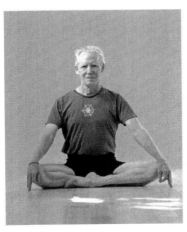

### Samasana

While not a classic pose, in that it is not cited by the medieval texts, samasana is a most naturally arising posture. The heels are placed one in front of the other, aligned with the pubic region. For men, the right heel is placed between the lingam and the anus, so that a mild pressure is applied to the perineum. The left heel follows, placed directly in front of the right with toes pointed. The legs are reversed for ladies. This pose is the posture of choice for the male partner in the Shiva/Shakti partner asana.

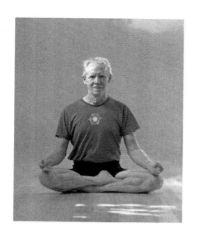

## Swastikasana

*Swastika* means "good luck or prosperous." This pose is the ancient symbol of the sun spinning out blessedness to all sadhus. The text references are found in *Hathayoga Pradipika* I, 19; *Siva Samhita* 113–115; *Gheranda Samhita* II, 12, and *Vasistha Samhita* I, 66. The lower leg placement is done as in samasana, then the upper foot is placed with the toes tucked between the calf and thigh. The upper heel can apply a mild pressure to the junction of the pubic bones, thus stimulating suppressed emotional prana.

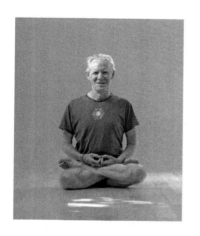

## Padmasana

Also called *kamalasana*, the lotus pose in the 9th century text the *Goraksasatakam* 7–9, this pose is found in *Vasistha Samhita* I, 69–70 as Bound Lotus, with the arms around the back, holding the same foot. It is also found in *Gheranda Samhita* II, 44–45 as yogasana, and in *Siva Samhita* III, 102–107, where one foot is placed on the upper thigh with the lateral ankle bone directly on the rectus femoris, the uppermost quadriceps muscle. If the ankle is placed into the deep groin where the femoral triangle of nerves and blood vessels are located, it will cut off circulation. Thus the higher the placement of the ankle, the safer the position and the longer it can be maintained. For some, externally rotating the lower medial musculature just above the knee helps to avoid inner-knee discomfort. Pulling the calf and lower inner-knee muscles also helps to maximize hip rotation. This adjustment is best learned from an Iyengar teacher familiar with the procedure. Once your lower leg is comfortable, place your upper leg in a similar posture, so the lower ends of your feet are beyond your thighs.

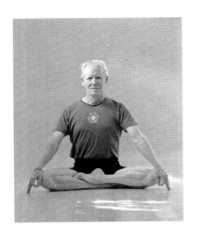

## Siddhasana

Siddhasana is considered the perfect pose, the posture of the *siddhas*—perfected masters. It is detailed in the *Goraksasatakam* 10–11, *Gheranda Samhita* II, 7, *Siva Samhita* III, 97–101, and *Hathayoga Pradipika* I, 34–43. In the *Vasistha Samhita* I, 79–80, it is called *muktasana*, the "liberated" posture. Most texts consider this the best posture for kriya and Tantrik pranayama and for practices to stabilize spiritual attainment and, ultimately, liberation.

The posture begins, as in samasana, by pulling the right heel to the perineum, adjusting the footpad or thighs so a moderate pressure is consistently felt at the physical site of the first chakra. By adjusting the male genitals, the left heel is placed above them, so that this heel applies an equal pressure to the central pubic bone. The lower heel goes to the lingam root, while the upper heel presses on the lingam's base. In his comments on this practice in his *Hatha Pradipika*, Swami Satyananda gives a different name to the pose for women—siddhayoniasana. This is done without clothes, so that the upper heel can be placed inside the vaginal canal (the physical yoni). With practice, the pressure is adjusted so that the first two chakras are calmed, thus generating sattva in worldly pleasures. The state of a siddha, an illumined master, is so sattvic that their activities swing naturally between the desire for worldly fulfillment and the desire for spiritual liberation. When these desires are balanced, worldly and spiritual fulfillment are not seen as different. (See Patanjali's answer to the question: What is the purpose of life? in his *Yoga Sutras* II, 18; 21 and IV, 24.)

## Tantrasana for Partners

Tantrasanas can be done as partner postures in which you mutually agree to share prana with your partner for spiritual evolution. Partner yoga books show a wide variety of poses that can be shared briefly by asana partners to promote a deeper stretch and to assist each other at doing a regular practice. Some variations include using these practices to enhance the spectrum of sensuality and sexuality. This is a mutually beneficial practice, whatever your desire may be—mild or strong. In the tantrasana practice, although any asana will do, the most beneficial are those that can be held for as brief a period as two minutes, or as long as half an hour. When practiced following the guidelines in lesson 15, these culminate in prana coming home.

The best tantrasanas are comfortable seated asanas where you can remain in a meditative state as you weave your energies into a harmonious communion. They are suitable to perform nyasa (energetic awakening and transmitting as described in lesson 2). They are described as *bandhura*, or "curved knot," in that they allow partners or individuals to be knotted into a pranic flow that suspends effort, space, and time. They are meant to be static to promote training toward *karezza*, prolonged intimacy. As you connect hand to chakra, or hand to bindu (minor chakras located at each joint space), you can learn to receive and send your elevated prana, thus increasing your capacity to assist each other to remove energy blocks and heal. Tantrasana reveals how delicate we are as humans, how easily we are touched, and how strongly we feel others. For we are not merely empathic; we are one. This practice gives that experience most tangibly.

The most famous of these practices is the *yab/yum,* or Father Mother Communion, frequently depicted in Tibetan Tantrik art. Notice, in the drawing below, that

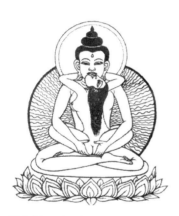

yab, or Father Deva's hands, are in an open yoni mudra over yum, or Mother Devi's sacrum—literally "sacred space"—deepening their energetic connection. In response, Mother Devi is arching Her spine to give Her heart more fully to embrace Her beloved. He is passive (Shiva), while She is active (Shakti). This can also be called Shiva/Shakti asana.

A delightful way of sharing a brief version of this tantrasana exchange comes when you share your heart's energy in a hug with a good person. Connecting chakra to chakra with hugasana, it is easy to feel the goodness of your partner. His or

Yab/Yum tantrasana
with yoni mudra

her goodness is felt as a natural communion that will make you both want to linger and, when you part, to do it very slowly. When this communion is enriched, it will become both a path to a deeper intimate coupling and a way to melt your individuality and merge into Spirit. For couples who have difficulty conceiving, these practices can encourage a soul to come through you, no matter what the obstacles.

Tantriks will see that Patanjali wrote not merely the Yoga Darshan (yogic worldview), but defined the progression of states of consciousness that culminate in self-realization and how to attain them. Thus the *Sutras* are a tool for knowing the experience of yoga. In the opening sutra to chapter II, Patanjali defines Kriya Yoga, the means to attaining a higher consciousness. The practical means for this have three aspects: self-discipline and purification (*tapah*), self-study (*svadhyaya*), and devotion (*Isvara pranidhanani*). The term for the first quality, tapah, derives from a root that means "to heat or to burn." It is often seen as an austerity to those who do not know it, but for serious students, it is done with a vow to attain the Truth and hold yourself to it regardless of the circumstances you face. For whatever can burn is not permanent. The serious student is not concerned about this type of loss. The second quality, self-study, consists of reflecting about yourself and the direction of your life. More important, this is done with the realization that you cannot do this on your own, that guidance is needed from those who can truly assist your evolution. This self-study is aided by the study of scriptures that are timeless, enabling you to perceive your destiny from a larger perspective. The third quality, devotion, is a process of gradually unveiling the form of the Divine that is of your choosing and that is attracted to you. In this manner, a personal relationship with the subtlest of forms begins. Over time, that One who is both formless and with the form of the entire world reveals Herself to you. Her omnipresence, omnipotence, and omniscience begin to comfort and guide you in all areas.

## Mukunda's Tantrik Yoga Practice

The practices of the eight limbs of Classical Ashtanga Yoga (described in the *Yoga Sutras* II, 29–55) can be utilized in a Tantrik context. The sutras on yama and niyama (II, 30–45), when given by your teacher and taken by you as a vow, will reveal how to uplift yourself and your companions to the attainments cited. The sutras on asana (II, 46–48) are not merely a guideline for how to practice, but also a path to clarify the state of higher consciousness that accompanies asana siddhi (attainments). In the same manner, the sutras that conclude the second chapter (49–55) reveal how to direct your practice to attain pranayama and pratyahara as a continually arising state, revealing your True Self. See my interpretation of the *Yoga Sutras of Patanjali* for details.

The first of my morning practices is mantra, which is the deepest for me and most profound for making transformation. The practice of mantra is charged from consistent use and opening yourself to feelings of devotion. Commitment and regular practice are the hallmarks for what empowers mantra literally to transform your mind. I have found that, as a result of thirty-five years of mantra practice, my mind functions less as a tool of my ego sense, and more as a receiver of guidance from a higher Source. As a result, I have regular access to the vijnana maya kosha, and insights into yoga sadhana and lifestyle arise on a daily basis.

I experience that mantra is truly a transformative process that gives me the greatest sense of transformation. For what I identify with most strongly is my mind, more so than my senses or body. By chanting the mantras and prayers I have been given with devotion and love, a wellspring opens up, connecting me to the deeper source of Life. I find that stress and pain dissolve completely through this practice. Yogasanas, in comparison, are much less effective for opening me. Yet they are a wonderful tool for maintaining physical health.

Devi puja, worship of the Goddess, is the second part of my morning practice. It essentially brings me out from an experience of formless meditation back into form. The four forms of the Devi yantras that I use are Tara, who is the space of the sky and lives in a higher realm of the fourth chakra, at the spiritual heart; Sarasvati, goddess of music, arts, and learning who manifests through the first chakra; Lakshmi, goddess of abundance, who comes through the second chakra; Bhadra Kali, goddess of removing what is not beneficial and restoring us to beneficence, who manifests through the third chakra. In the Devi puja, the combined practice of mantra and yantra allows you to connect to the cosmic energies within yourself.

I begin the puja by opening my heart to the Goddess Tara, who is said to be beyond the chakras and the elements. Tara is associated with the vastness of the heart as the sky and the vastness of the subtlest of the five elements—space, which is as near as the space in front of our faces. This same space exists within as our cavities, from large (digestive-tract tubes) to small (intercellular or subatomic space). Tara's yantra was shown in lesson 7. By placing your hands on Tara's home, your heart, in whatever mudra or gesture you wish, the inner Mother will begin to guide you in ways that, for this moment, will awaken you to the awareness of Her Presence. Affirm Her, as you acknowledge how She has already manifested in your life.

At first, you will experience your hands touching your heart or the center of your chest; thus awareness is of the first kosha (anna maya). As you continue to open yourself more deeply, you will experience the energy of Tara's prana, accompanied by a physical relaxation, signifying that you have moved to the second kosha (prana maya). Your mind will experience thoughts arising from yourself as the third kosha (mano maya). It does not matter whether you experience this inside or outside. Whatever comes when you are humble, that is Her Grace. As you continue to submit to the naturally arising experiences, you may slip into the fourth kosha (vijnana maya). In this state, uplifting awareness will be experienced as a gift, not arising from a self-centered consciousness. It is this kosha that marks the beginning of Spirit and the diminishing of self-centeredness. Should joy, the fifth kosha (ananda maya), arise then, allow your body to move, swaying, or even dancing in the Presence of the Divine Mother. This may come at any time.

The second Goddess to whom I direct attention is Sarasvati, who rules the earth element and the first chakra, situated in the subtle body of the pelvic floor. Sarasvati's Shakti creates artistic expression, literature, dance, poetry, and music. Affirm Her, as you acknowledge how She has already manifested in your life. Your hands can be placed here with the intention of encouraging your awareness, as in the practice of nyasa (lesson 2), or to feel how the Shakti wants to move in this region. If the latter, then direct your fingers to press in harmony with how you experience the Shakti prana moving. While awakening may begin here, it will naturally move throughout your body to any place that She feels is beneficial. So remember to continue to practice submission to Her creative energies. If She is dancing with Shiva, there is more stillness; if She is dancing by Herself, there will be more motion.

> Soaring on swan's
> Wings of Love and Light
> Weaving the web
> of ham' and sa'
> Embracing the worlds in
> Her ecstatic flight
> Bringing Her Yoni's sacred space
> to vanquish the enemy—fear

Her Grace knows no bounds
unconfined to body, space and time
She is shooting through sushumna's fire
Her blazing hair aflame
Love's de-Light
as She soars in Her ecstatic flight
The Soul's primal tunnel
holds Her not.

She is Tantrika Devi
weaving the web
on wings
of Love and Light.[32]

The third Goddess in this ritual is Lakshmi, who is the water element, the second chakra situated in the subtle body in the region of the pubic bone for men and the cervix for women. Lakshmi's Shakti, like Sarasvati's, is creative energy only. In this form, She creates life, sensual and sexual pleasure, prosperity, and spiritual abundance. Affirm Her, as you acknowledge how She has already manifested in your life.

During a physical hug, sexual energy will naturally flow due to the physical proximity of the sexual organs. Similarly, during a Tantrik hugasana, Shakti energy will naturally flow between partners as a sign of their energetic compatibility. This can be developed into a means of a shared Divine communion with the Devi by following the guidelines in lessons 13 through 15. During the sadhana, proceed as before by placing your hands on the lower abdomen or pelvis using yoni mudra. Again, proceed as before to sense your willingness and the natural desire of your prana for submission to Devi.

The fourth Goddess is Bhadra Kali, who is the fire element, the third chakra, in the region of the navel. Bhadra Kali's Shakti manifests as the energy of transformation to remove obstacles and old patterns of behavior and emotion that no longer serve you. Like Ganesh, She removes obstacles to your spiritual evolution. Sometimes, we misinterpret what is beneficial in life, and we hold on to what is not a blessing. Those

---

32. Yogi Mukunda. *The Yoga Poet* (Boulder, Yoga Therapy Center, 2000), 48.

who submit to Her energy see that whatever life gives or takes away is due to Her Presence. Affirm Her, as you acknowledge how She has already manifested in your life. To find this energy, use not only Her mantra name, but also gently stretch your chest up to elongate your abdomen. I find that, by doing this in asana, I can more easily experience Her Shakti enlivening my asana practice. When I finish offering myself to the Goddess in the form of Her mantra and yantra, then I spend some time reflecting on how all these forms are really One Being, One Omnipresence.

The final part of my morning practice consists of three *vinyasas* that balance the Ayurvedic doshas—vata, pitta and kapha sequentially. My first yoga teacher in the vinyasa lineage, Paul Copeland, was given individual sessions for nearly two years with Krishnamacharya, who gave him fifty choreographed yoga sequences for his research into their physiological and therapeutic benefits. After thirty-five years of practice of the vinyasas, he gave me permission to reveal them to the public. I recently wrote *Ayurvedic Yoga Therapy*, drawing from Krishnamacharya's posture flows and all of my Ayurvedic teachers. I have focused this curriculum into those vinyasas that balance the doshas in a manner that elicits their higher functions as prana, tejas, and ojas. These terms do not translate well, but correlate to the life force, vitality, and radiant spirituality. These energies need to be experienced to be understood. As Swami Satchidananda says, one must "stand under" the place that you are so that humility can reveal what your mind wants to limit. All of these tools are used in my daily sadhana.

In summary, the first hour of practice consists of devotional chants and meditation on the Inner Teacher; the second practice is Devi puja chants to the four yantra forms of the Divine Mother; the practice ends with an Ayurvedic Yoga program for balancing vata, pitta, and kapha doshas in that sequence.

The details of this sadhana are shared on 10-day retreats in India and other ashram-sponsored programs. The chants and mantras for this practice are available on CD. See my website *www.yogatherapycenter.org* to order. I encourage you to create a similar multi-dimensional Tantrik Yoga practice for yourself, or to ask for my guidance in creating a personal practice. Do also inform me via email or phone if you wish my assistance in your sadhana. More details will be shared in lesson 13.

Remember to persist in your practice, yet stay detached from expecting specific outcomes. Tantra is a personal spiritual practice. When you feel complete with this lesson, read the Dialogue section that follows prior to beginning lesson 8.

**With Great Respect and Love, I Honor
My Heart, My Inner Teacher.**

## Dialogue with Mukunda

**Student:** My morning sadhana usually shifts in such a way that sometimes I feel the need to do the joint-freeing series from your book right before meditation. My practice, based on my last private with you is:

Bija-seed sounds for the lower four chakras - *lam vam ram yam*
Bhastrika pranayama
Meditation
Four specific asanas
Yoni mudra

Lately, I have been reading a section of Swami Muktananda's *Where are you going?* and the joint-freeing series from your *Structural Yoga Therapy* book whenever I feel the need to do so. Am I too scattered in my sadhana? Should I keep it more consistent? Even though I feel your presence very strongly in my life, I'd like you to assist me energetically in my sadhana. When you are around New York, I would love to share your practice in person at your convenience.

**Mukunda:** It sounds to me as if your sadhana is going well. Just reading Baba's writings will help you to connect to the Shakti more. An energetic assist can come just by inviting Baba Muktananda or me into your practice as if we were sitting before you. Details are in lessons 11 and 14.

**Student:** You may already have solved this, but I feel that you need to explain a little on the rest of the chakras, the *bija* mantra, and moving Kundalini energy through all seven, and not just the lower three, chakras. A full set of yantra plates would be useful too, like the one's in John Selby's *Kundalini Awakening* and *The Kundalini Workbook*, which I found in a Massachusetts public library a while back. Thanks for everything. I am looking forward to your next book.

***Mukunda:*** Thanks for your feedback. I appreciate it. Let me remind you, however, that the chakras are most dense, somewhat physical, only through the fourth chakra, the heart. And the fourth chakra is the element air, so its form is the most subtle of all. Beyond that, the chakras transcend the elements that are perceptible with the mind. The fifth chakra is space and refers to consciousness. The chakra symbols appear as yantras and can be used for *dharana* reflections. They are tangible in kosha two and dissolve in the third and higher koshas. It is in these subtler dimensions that Devi and Deva yantras live. Beyond that is the transcendent realm. Hence there are no yantras or mantras for these dimensions. What can be given by spiritual teachers is not in the physical realm, but rather an empowerment or transmission of higher consciousness that appears to the student to be in the grosser chakras and koshas.

***Student:*** I just read an article in a Florida yoga magazine based on Russell Paul's mantra work. The author, Ramanada Das, says that most people do not differentiate between the various types of mantras—Vedic, Tantric, and devotional. He says that he uses Vedic chanting to gather strength and support for the day, the Tantric to get back into his body in the afternoon when the demands of the day's activities have moved him out of it, and the devotional in the evening when he wants to spend time with wife and family.

Are the chants that you taught us at our Structural Yoga Therapy intensive (Tara, Sarasvati, Lakshmi puja, and the Kali chant) classified as Vedic chants? He says the bija mantras are Tantric. I would guess that some of the Krishna Das chants are devotional, but they might be Vedic.

***Mukunda:*** Most intriguing ideas. All the Devi chants that I do in morning practice are Tantrik in nature, though they are devotional Tantrik. I would say that Ramananda Das is generalizing—nicely however. Tantrik chants are for transformation of energy, but when one does them in devotion to the Divine Mother, they become Bhakti Yoga, devotional. Other Tantrik chants, like the bija mantras he mentions, are focused on the purification of chakras and nadis, and for the awakening of Kundalini. Vedic chants are the mantras I use to open and close workshops. These are more for discipline of the mind; one could call them Classical Yoga practices. They are, like all mantras, to purify the mind and cultivate devotion.

*Student:* Could you expand on how to use yantras in practice? I feel drawn to Sri yantra. Thank you for being my teacher.

*Mukunda:* Yantras are symbols of Devi when the triangle is pointed down, and of Deva (masculine) when pointed up. Look for their energy lines in your body. In this way, the feeling of the yantras within your body will lead to sattvic meditation; these meditations will often arise outside the formal teaching. Energy points can occur at the knees and pubic bone, for example. Devi yantra may arise as the lower point at the navel or sex organs and as upper points at the shoulders or breasts. Deva yantra can also have variations—lower points at the hips and upper point at the third eye. Doing yoni mudra helps get it started, then these energetic sensations near the joints will captivate your mind into meditation. Your naturally arising desire for Shakti and its unfolding will promote positive emotional sensitivities. You are most welcome to benefit from my teachings. I only ask you to persist and be faithful to Spirit. Namaste.

*Student:* Are there people for whom the complete Tantra practice is inappropriate? If so, how is the situation managed?

*Mukunda:* That is a good question; no one has asked this before. Tantra is often considered appropriate for those who are brave enough to face their unknown feelings, courageous enough to see that their path is a path not a highway, and committed enough to their spiritual journey that they will seek advice of a competent teacher and be willing to follow that advice. It is not for those who are seeking pleasure or praise. Often, it brings about dispassionate introspection and the need for finding your own way. So it is not for the masses, as are the various popular forms of contemporary yoga. Namaste.

*Student:* I have begun my yantra meditation practice with Shodashi yantra. I have read Harish Johari's description of it in his book *Tools for Tantra* and it is beautiful; thank you for suggesting it to me. I need both Kali and Tara to help me negotiate this part of my journey. I would like to know of your understanding of Shodashi yantra if you would like to share it. Through yantra practice, I have become aware of how my ego keeps me from moving forward. I surrendered my ego to my heart, my Inner Teacher, and now turn to Her for guidance. Thank you for your spiritual guidance.

*Mukunda:* All yantras help the mind connect with the multi-dimensional three-kosha energy body within you. The outward worship can increase your love of Goddess in a form.

In this case, the Shodashi yantra, also called the tripura sundari yantra, relates to building the quality of communion of masculine and feminine within you and to helping you to see this harmony of Deva and Devi God/dess quality in others. The yantra depicts the merging of lingam and yoni triangles, forming the Star of David, symbol of heaven and earth in communion. Each part of the yantra has different qualities to experience and open to. Gradually, take in the entire image as you seek to understand its meanings. Blessings.

*Student:* Here is a poem that I scribbled down during a juicy asana practice one evening last week, inspired by the language of Invocation to Lord of Yoga (at the beginning of your *Yoga Sutra* book) and a new way of experiencing asana for me that I first experienced during practice one day at our last training:

> Tonight I honor my body as a sacred temple.
> With every shifting posture, I explore its secret contents.
> As Shakti dances gracefully, I come alive.
> My skin tastes the air around it,
> My spine takes pleasure in each wave of breath,
> My pranas slowly savor every undulation,
> My eyes and mouth water for the next move,
> My yoni welcomes each inhalation back to her sacred home,
> My mind lies quietly as my body makes love to my soul,
> My breath comes to rest and ojas begins to melt the coverings of my heart.
> Though I am not this body, in this moment, I relish in its delight.

*Mukunda:* Such a lovely, exquisite real experience of the power of tantrasana. I would recommend to all to reread that portion of lesson 7 with this poem in mind.

*Student:* Yesterday as I was meditating, I felt a very sensual energy arising from my first chakra. I almost felt my prostate vibrating and a warm sensation traveling along my back. I have no recollection of how long it lasted, but it was a strong and beautiful experience. What is it?

*Mukunda:* It is a natural arising of energy as it purifies the chakras. It can take a more physical or sensual expression, aiding you in having more enjoyment of life. It can occasionally arise as healing for an undiagnosed condition—perhaps an energy block which, if left alone, could become a prostate or urinary problem.

**Student:** My whole world has opened since our last meeting in person, when you liberated my heart! I feel the breath flow through my entire body—head to toe. I have had new encounters with energy. In the days after our last meeting, I could feel/see energy in my body and emanating through my fingertips. More recently, when meditating on my heart and offering thoughts of healing and love to certain friends, I feel that I have melted with their heart energy. This is a poor description, but I can't find the words to describe it exactly. Does this happen only with the people that are open?

**Mukunda:** Yes. It is common for sincere students to be in rapport with the Inner Teacher. The Inner Teacher's home in the body is the heart, so these feelings are often felt to be centered in that heart regardless of the feeling of its size.

**Student:** Will my offerings of love and healing reach those that I don't melt with? At the moment, I am specifically talking about my sister. She has dis-ease at many levels. After reading the *Anatomy of Spirit* by Carolyn Myss, I understand a little more about the possible causes of her state and also sadly understand my past actions that have contributed to her difficult condition. I am reaching out to her now, and I hope that I can provide enough love and compassion that she may choose a healing path.

**Mukunda:** My spiritual teacher used to say that whatever we do to help ourselves and others from our sadhana never goes to waste. It manifests as blessings in God's time, not ours.

**Student:** I am not clear about how to choose a yantra to work with or what to do with it. I am drawn to them, being a visual person. I attended a yantra-painting class in the spring where the teacher suggested starting with Ganesh, the half-human, half-elephant bestower of an obstacle-free life, so I have my own finished painting. Should I use this, or work with a goddess, or with more than one, as you do in your morning practice?

**Mukunda:** Ganesh yantra is a good idea to help with grounding your lifestyle and healing your root chakra. Once you have felt its effects in your energy body or devotion to the practice, then proceed to Sarasvati yantra. She has many forms. Any of the forms cited in

*Tools for Tantra* by Harish Johari, or *Tantric Yoga and the Wisdom Goddesses* by David Frawley would be valuable to contemplate.

**Student:** I started reading your spiritual teacher, Swami Prakashananda's, biography.[33] It is giving me more understanding of the photo you gave me of the two of you, and also your devotional energy. After waking at 4 a.m. and reading more, I returned to sleep and had a beautiful dream. I suddenly found myself in a mountainous region in India that was very crowded with small homes, rapid transit, street vendors—a noisy bustling area within the mountains. I went into a home and saw an older heavy-set woman. I could see that she needed comforting, and I felt inclined to hug her. As we embraced, she felt very soft and yielding, like a melting hug, and I could feel her lifetimes of suffering—but not in a tragic way, as a natural part of life. Quietly, a flood of tears poured down my face and formed small pools of water on the floor. As I looked down, I could see that the tears were magnifying small grains of sand and pebbles on the ground. Then I woke up knowing I had dreamed something very powerful. Just sharing. But as always, I welcome your thoughts.

**Mukunda:** Very lovely sharing. It is a natural sign of compassion growing in you and opening to all that is needed. The mountainous village you describe sounds very much like Suptashring, where Prakashananda lived to be near to his spiritual mother, Suptashring Devi. Undoubtedly, some out-of-body being was experiencing the power of your love. In dreams, all sorts of beings come to us for blessings. We are a great boon to them. Baba Muktananda spoke of this in his spiritual autobiography, *Play of Consciousness.*[34] This book explains the significance of many diverse spiritual experiences and the unfolding of Shakti from receiving Tantrik initiation. There are many dimensions of beings, including those of master siddhas who have left the body and remain in a world populated by other masters called *siddha loka*. From there, they are a blessing to all worlds. In the same way, we are also blessings to all beings in the worlds, known and unknown.

**Student:** I just wanted to share this experience with you. In my morning practice today, after intro chants and wave breath, I decided to try meditating using my mantra, which I had

---

33. Titus Foster, *Agaram Bagaram Baba—Life and Teachings of Swami Prakashananda* (Berkeley: North Atlantic Books, 1991).
34. Swami Muktananda, *Play of Consciousness* (South Fallsburg, NY: Siddha Yoga Publications, 2004).

let slip from my practice out of frustration almost a year ago. I now think I was not slowing it and my breath down enough, rushing and not allowing for the pause at the end of each breath. Anyway, it went really nicely, very peaceful, I think for about ten minutes. Then I did the palm tree vinyasa from your *Ayurvedic Yoga Therapy* book, very slowly with breath much steadier than I've ever been able to maintain before in asana! As I came back into standing centered pose, samasthiti, I spontaneously placed my hands on my upper chest just below the clavicles, maintaining the soft wave breath, ujjaye, in complete stillness without the desire to make any adjustments, just enjoying the interplay between gentle waves of energy and the stillness. Was I experiencing the dance between Shiva and Shakti? Samasthiti has always been a struggle for me, but this time I just wanted to linger there.

*Mukunda:* Your description of your insight into your practice is beautiful and clearly shows the Tantrik tandava dance. It is a delicate play of Shiva and Shakti. They are always dancing together, stillness beneath energy and motion. One must merely look and persist in the desire to experience them, and their dance creates a harmonious state in the mind. At first, either Shiva or Shakti may predominate, but as you did a vata balancing practice, as it sounds as if you did, then their harmony is felt as yours.

*Student:* This came as a surprise to me, since I've had an emotionally stressful week. My back has been hurting quite a bit and last night I had insomnia. But I think I am learning to respect my "delicate nature" and more often know when to be subtle and gentle with myself. One thing that I am trying to come to grips with is to know how a person with a mild sattvic imbalance can get anything done—full-time work, maybe having a child, etc. By continuing my practice, can I expect that I will have more stamina and be less easily thrown out of balance? Yet, one thing that I have learned is that doing the things that bring me joy gives me lots of energy. I guess I just need to keep moving in that direction. Thank you for your support and guidance.

*Mukunda:* The fact that you notice a subtle sattvic balance is a resolution that also changes rajasic and tamasic into more sattvic. Our goal is to promote sattva and by so doing lessen pain and heighten all functions of the body and mind. Initially, this shift will be colored with some lethargy of tamas because contemporary life is so stressful and rajasic. You expressed this concern clearly as "How does anything get done?" Over time, one becomes more productive and less stressed. "The more still and one-pointed the mind becomes, the more work it is able to do."[35] The unwinding of deep-seated tensions takes a long time. But there is always a movement toward a soul level of sattva, and given how we are in our culture, this appears as if nothing is getting done. But indeed, the mind itself is undergoing a radical transformation into sattva. Indeed over time, sattva becomes a well from which you not only draw, but with which you also have a continuous connection. What gives you joy is ojas; what gives you energy is tejas; what gives serenity is prana. When they are in harmony, these three qualities are naturally arising. Blessings.

*Student:* Although I have gone through this lesson, I have been unstable and irregular in Tantrik sadhana. In spite of this, I experience pranic energy often. With my new experiences with energy, I feel that I should return to the early Tantrik practices to begin to understand and experience this energy within me. Do you think that this is a right course of action? If so, may I have your approval to start all over at lesson 1? Also, can you recommend a text that can help me understand energy on an intellectual level? Or at any level?

*Mukunda:* Yes, a good idea. For books, there are quite a few possibilities listed at the end of this book. The main text I recommend is *Tantra* by André van Lysebeth, a very experienced Hatha Yogi who shares the subtleties of this practice. I suggest you also look at the Recommended Reading list on my website under Tantrik Yoga, as well as the Spiritual Life and Meditation subheadings. I update this list yearly, so go there to see in which direction your prana pulls you.

*Student:* When I was meditating on you and giving thanks for your guidance, I felt a sweet soft energy emanating from my head and flowing over my body. In Robert Svoboda's *Ayurveda for Women*, there is a description of ojas as a thick band of golden-yellow light that covers the whole body and radiates out into space. Is that what I experienced?

*Mukunda:* Yes. How lovely to have a unique personal experience of ojas, the subtlest taste of nectar.

*Student:* Lesson 7—that second look at energy awareness—has brought up a lot of anxiousness. I notice a stark difference between the warm centered feeling that comes from the practice of giving attention to energy in the body, and the way I normally move

---

35. Swami Muktananda, *Mystery of the Mind* (S. Fallsburg, NY: Siddha Yoga Publications, 1993), 24.

through the world, which feels very frantic at times. I wrote a note to myself in the margins of lesson 7, "non-acquisitiveness is one of the yamas." Just as soon as I'm not supposed to do something, it becomes *exactly* what I end up doing more than usual.

When I do the practices and meditate regularly the shift into living without awareness isn't as quick and can be diverted. I hope it makes sense when I say I can see myself making the choices that lead to anxiousness. It can feel as if I were watching a movie—I know, weird but true. At any rate, that's how it goes. I feel like quite the unworthy student, but I insist on persisting. Please send me lesson 8.

*Mukunda:* What makes a good student is not attainment or, as they say, the "fruits of your actions," but the doing of the actions with persistence and devotion. That is true Karma Yoga. What is given as the result of doing the Tantrik practices is not up to you. You are doing what is needed just by persisting. A spiritual revelation begins with seeking and not necessarily with finding. Blessings on your journey.

*Student:* I must say that I have never felt as blessed as I do at this moment. I am so thankful that you have led me to my heart, my inner guide. The more I rely on Her for guidance, the more at peace I am. And we have been showered with such blessings lately. My husband, who was out of work, has received three job offers. We have decided to take one—yet another opportunity to break free from attachments. Somehow, it is appropriate that I return to the region of my birth for a rebirth.

In my mind, I am "pregnant" with a new e-mail. Some questions and thoughts, things I found out in meditation. But it will take some time to "materialize" and write it down. By the way, I realize that I start to trust you. In my meditation, when you are with me, I feel very safe. I feel a warm embrace, being held without possession. I have the space to be myself and slowly develop other levels of the energy, going deeper without being forced to do something or to please. Thank you.

*Mukunda:* Congratulations. I am delighted to hear of help coming on both material and spiritual worlds. That is a sign of definitely good sadhana. Life should be easier from sadhana, not harder.

# PART III

# Healing Sexual Wounds

# Sexual Health Practices

With Great Respect and Love, I Honor
My Heart, My Inner Teacher.

Energy will naturally seek healthy expression. For many, the most challenging form of expression is when your prana, which is neutral by nature (colorless energy), becomes colored due to the presence of emotions that appear as sexual energy. In that form, it will seek healthy expression as well. When it is not freed, then it has no choice but to become either inappropriate (rajasic) or suppressed (tamasic). One without a partner may be comfortable in his or her choice of a temporarily celibate lifestyle, yet sexual energy will continue to seek emotional expression, including seeking extra attention from those to whom one reacts emotionally. Those without harmonious relationships with partners will also have challenges with this emotionally colored energy. In cases where healthy expression is denied, the organs associated with sexuality and pleasure will be subjected to a loss of vitality, function, and health. By health, I mean that expression that is free to move to all dimensions of the yogic kosha anatomy. A healthy mind creates healthy sexual expression and vice versa.

> Sexuality and anxiety present two opposite directions of excitation. The same excitation which appears in the genitals as pleasure, manifests itself as anxiety if it stimulates the cardiovascular system. That is, in the latter case it appears as the exact opposite of pleasure.[36]

36. Wilhelm Reich, *The Function of the Orgasm* (New York: Noonday Press, 1970), 110.

Tantrik sexuality is appropriate, regardless of your sexual preferences. Gay and lesbian partners can do the practices cited here in heterosexual terms. Celibates and those without a potential partner have the choice of visualizing the partner practices or simply skipping over them as they continue with the next lessons. The key is not your sexual orientation, but keeping these practices in the context of a spiritual sadhana. In so doing, all your activities can be a sacred event, as activities that purify your multi-dimensional humanity.

## Healing Life and Death

The yogic spectrum of health extends to all ages and dimensions. We are all dying. We are closer to death than we want to realize. Yet realization of Spirit also includes knowing it as omnipresent in life, birth, and death. Only when we know this can we truly accept death as life.

Regardless of how your sexuality is expressed, everyone is prone to fear when there is a diagnosis of cancer, especially in their sexual organs. This is not so much due to loss of function as to loss of the associated sensations they have experienced during sexual expression. The amount of pain or pleasure associated with sexual expression colors our attachment or aversion to these organs. Remember to focus on the practical guidelines in the quote from Reich above. When sexual or emotional energy is allowed to build, it becomes neutral energy, and if you persist, it will be experienced as spiritual energy. Know that these lessons are for the purpose of moving through your self to finding that deeper energy.

For those seeking not only health, but also pleasure, here are two techniques that can both increase sensual/sexual response and heighten lymphatic and cardiovascular circulation for improved health. Anyone with a family history of breast or prostate conditions is advised to receive these techniques on a regular basis as preventative sexual health care.

> Skin is our most sensitive organ, the one that "nourishes" us most. The health of a newborn who is not adequately touched, will rapidly decline. For Kashmir Shaivism masters a human being naturally recovers his unity when he is touched deeply—that is, when contact

is no longer a sexual strategy. When nothing is "wanted." To touch another in this way necessitates simply being the other, and to be the other necessitates living in a state of nonduality. To have been touched in this way restores to the body its sacred vibration and will sometimes render it intolerably sensitive to the unloving contact of unaware partners. From that moment on, the body will insist on being approached with veneration and true presence.[37]

## Prostate Massage—Ganesh Kriya

Hippocrates tells us that "the physician healer must be experienced in many things, but most assuredly in healing, soothing massages."[38] Although this massage can be adapted to free women's pelvic tensions, men need a different intention with these practices to reverse their naturally rajasic nature by directing the energy of the lingam downward and inward. In this shape, it will gain more Shiva energy, thus resembling the downward-pointing triangle of the Shiva mudra. Over time, this can heighten their self-control and stability.

A massage technique that benefits prostate health and also heightens sexual response is called Ganesh kriya. The name refers to the elephant-headed son of Shiva and Parvati who embodies the first chakra. This kriya is a perineal massage done with the area well lubricated with your choice of unscented massage oil—for instance, sesame or almond. I recommend that every man experience this. Once it is done, you can discover whether or not regular massage is appropriate. The massage can greatly increase the circulation of nutrients and the expulsion of toxic waste material (*ama*), helping to lessen the tendency for a tumor to form. In the case of hardening of tissue or excessive sensitivity, I recommend you receive the technique at least monthly and give it to yourself weekly. In all men over thirty-five, the gland will tend to become firm or even hard, so I recommend they should have the procedure as a preventative once a year.

Consult a good anatomy atlas to free the tissue of stress and pranic blocks for emotional release. See my website *www.yogatherapycenter.org* for recommended

---

37. Odier, *Desire*, 32–33.
38. Hippocrates, father of Western medicine, 400 BC.

anatomy readings. I especially recommend reading *The Female Pelvis* by Blandine Calais-Germain (Seattle, WA: Eastland Press). For women wishing to receive a pelvic-floor perineal massage similar to the Ganesh kriya, I have given instructions in the Dialogue section for this lesson.

Both partners can begin with yoni mudra positions, ending with the lowest place-ment, with the hands around the genitals. Gently press the yoni mudra into a smaller placement so that the thumbs press on the base of the lingam and the forefingers press on the perineal region. Relax and repeat this in a pulsing manner, while relaxing. The next portion is best given by your partner and received by a passive man. Later, you can give this to yourself.

Sit on the right side of the man and begin with a small clockwise circle massag-ing at the navel in gradually larger circles. Let your pressure be soothing, not erotic. Then extend the strokes to exploring the abdominal tissue around the lower rib cage, as low as the pubic bones. The diaphragmatic and intercostal motions of breathing are to be encouraged to promote emotional freedom. The massage points situated around the pubic bones promote an uninhibited breath, whose depth and slowness will permit the miracle of orgasm without ejaculation. In the beginning of training, however, your partner may need to use the ejaculatory inhibition pressure points located at the perineum, or two fingers above the right breast, to prolong arousal.

Have the man bend his knees, so that his feet are comfortably placed near his hips. Another position that often allows a deeper release is to have him in child pose, supported with pillows or bolsters, as in a restorative pose with the knees open. As you reach the pelvic floor muscles, give extra attention to the perineum before releasing the anal sphincter muscles. There are two areas to linger upon—the base and the root of the lingam. These two areas and the tissues connecting them are commonly sites of suppressed emotional and pranic energies. With loving attention, the primal male energies become freed for healthy expression.

The penetrating portion of the male organ is attached at the top of the pubic bone. But the lingam actually begins inside the body, below the pubic bone. As it moves externally from the pubic bone, this portion—called the root—is highly charged. The root of the lingam is held in place by the suspensory ligament that connects with the top of the lingam along the two-inch length of the pubic bone. The root is the lower surface of the lingam, where it enters the pelvis just in front of the perineum. In other words, two full inches of the lingam are hidden along the length of the pubic bone. When this tissue is freed from the pubic bone, it can be a source of greater pleasure for both partners. It is this manipulation that is achieved by tantrasana. Placing the heel at different spots along the lingam and surrounding tissue generates a softening of the male passions. As a result, sexual expression becomes more sattvic and prolongs into karezza.

This portion of the lingam between the root and the base is a site where suppressed prana and emotions are hidden. Regular massage (use sesame oil) from the root to the base can free up the primal fear men have of living up to their full vitality in all areas of life. Massage from top to bottom, external to internal, and with persistence and sensitivity to your partner's response. Often, massaging the belly or hips with your other hand will facilitate a deep relaxation reflex. Once this area softens, follow the root of the lingam interiorly along the anterior wall to the walnut-sized prostate. You will not find the organ until passing the two anal sphincters to a depth of a finger. The prostate should feel firm, but not hard. Your strokes should soften all the regional muscular tension, both internal and external. If it is hard and/or painful, your partner should have a pelvic exam by a medical doctor. With persistence, the prostate will soften and become more mobile—although, in it is the urethra, so it won't move very far. Let your strokes linger here, encouraging both of you to relax into a freer flow of prana. The ideal is a sixty-minute massage, with the first and last fifteen minutes spent in general soothing strokes over his abdomen and thighs.

Moving slowly and over a prolonged period is best, as, for many men, this region is highly charged with residual stress and traumatic memories. Sensitivity and gradual progression are imperative to release the pranic tension, so you may want to seek professional instruction in how to give and/or receive this procedure. When it is successful, the man will feel a tremendous surge of energy on all dimensions, without an ejaculation. With a less-effective massage, the result will be experienced as an overpowering sexual arousal. Although this may be intensely pleasurable, this form of release is not your goal, because this will result in the loss of energy rather than its increase. As a result, the tension released may make the man unconscious or cause him to fall asleep. This is similar to the common experience of yoga beginners, who fall asleep during savasana's relaxation effects. A good Tantrik practitioner and a good yoga teacher will allow students to enter any level of unconsciousness that is naturally arising, including sleep, until they learn to release their stress consciously, thus elevating their pranic field.

When the lingam is erect, it forms the shape of a Shiva mudra, an upward-pointing triangle with the testes at the base. When men gain control over their emotions, it will give them an ability to decide when or if to ejaculate. Until men gain control, firm finger pressure at the perineum will stop an ejaculation. By restraining this reflex through this process of *karezza* (prolonged arousal), you will retain your energy so that love-making truly creates love, taking both of you to higher dimensions of sexual and spiritual pleasure. This will lead to your capacity to open your hearts more fully. By knowing unconditional love, you can help your relationship get back to love more quickly when self-centered behavior arises.

## Breast Massage—Karuna Kriya

Just as men need special attention to the hidden gland that represents their virility, the prostate, so women need loving attention to the organs that are the symbol of their compassionate hearts, their breasts. The Divine Mother manifests as compassionate Grace in Her form as Karuna Devi. The chest is the home of kapha. In women, the sattvic expression of this energy is characterized by a strong immune system. Karuna kriya is a loving massage following the circulatory pattern of the lymphatic fluid. This liquid is normally mixed with the blood, except when it returns into the venous portion of the cardiovascular system. If you would like the details, see a good anatomy atlas that references lymphatic fluid circulation. If you have one, also refer to charts that can show you the difference between breast tissue and the underlying pectoral muscles.

This technique draws from my training in Esalen, Swedish, and Lymphatic Massage attained when I owned a massage and yoga school in Sacramento in the early 1980s. It is an easy-to-learn pattern consisting of only three basic motions. Sit above your partner's head as she lies below you on a massage table or on the floor. Begin by pouring some warmed oil onto your hands and spreading the oil over both sides of your hands up to your mid forearms. Place your palms on the tops of your partner's shoulders with your fingers toward the feet, and practice breathing in harmony. Linger in this posture until you feel a pranic connection between you, then do the first stroke of your massage moving down from the sides of the neck to the upper chest and outward to the shoulder joints. Then circle your hands as you move across your partner's upper back to come up the back of the neck. Repeat this ten to twenty times, gently modifying the pressure to suit your partner. Communicate, so she feels free to tell you if more or less pressure is wanted or if she wants you to linger or move on from specific places. Gradually, search for more anatomical detail, using mild pressure on the muscles and firmer pressure on the joints. Direct the flow in a manner that helps you feel circulatory fluids increasing in your partner's upper torso.

The second stroke is directed down the center of the chest, following the breast-bone with your fingers as you face each other. In this position, your fingertips will exert the greatest pressure to the body; let your palms be softer. Then let your hands form two circles, moving downward then outward to the lower side of the rib cage. Next, turn your fingers outward to come up the outer rib cage across the front of the shoulders and back to the top of the chest. Repeat this stroke several times, while directing your pressure toward the lungs to encourage a breath release. To facilitate this even more profoundly, hold your hands on the lower rib cage with your wrists to the sides and your fingers inward. Then press firmly with your palms (soft on your fingers), moving inward on every exhalation, relaxing your pressure on each inhalation. Continue this for some time, until you feel a sighing breath released. It is likely that this will also produce a mild emotional release if your partner has any suppressed emotions held in this region. This is called intercostal breathing (see *Structural Yoga Therapy*, p. 55).

Your touch will reach the outer perimeter of the breasts at this point. Do this pattern twenty to thirty times, or longer if your partner has breath or emotional releases. If this happens, do not break the process to give comfort, simply provide comfort with your words and loving presence. The pectoralis muscle that is underneath the entire chest region needs plenty of attention before you move to the breast tissue above it. As you continue these strokes, search out any signs of tension in the large muscle that ranges from the collarbone to the breastbone, then to the outer chest. Next, hold a steady pressure on the shoulder girdle, allowing your partner to take deep breaths and encouraging more stress to release. Continue to narrow the circular pattern slowly as you gently massage the breasts. Be creative yet sensitive with this delicate tissue. Whatever stroke you make, do it repeatedly so that your partner can become accustomed to your hands bringing attention to the body. If you find any delicate or firm tissue, be persistent yet warm and gentle to the area, so that the breasts begin to soften, thus melting to the consistency of the entire breast. Let your overall pattern resemble a spiral that reaches its center at the nipples. As you move toward the center of the breast, let your pressure become softer, more delicate, to encourage her feminine aspect. Feel that you are touching her heart, not merely her breasts.

For the third pattern of massage, reverse the procedure, returning to where your first strokes began. Although this third part will require only about a third of the total time for the massage, do linger and let prana direct you to where and how to touch. Your intuition will be much heightened at this point, as your partner's posture will shift along with her breath pattern, indicating how well she is releasing pranic tensions or suppressed emotions. Now is the time for you to practice sending your energy through your touch. Begin with feeling where your partner wants to be touched and connect with the direction her energy leads you. If you are not confident of your perception of prana, just ask what she would like, and where she wants more attention. Do not try to initiate energy connection; just stay open so that the energy itself will seek a naturally arising expression. If it is not there, just do a loving, nurturing massage. Not all partners have an intimate connection all the time.

Being humble increases the ability of all forms of touch to be healing. Occasionally, bow your head in reverence at being given the gift of trust and encourage yourself to release with some deep sighs too. Depending upon your partner and the nature of your relationship, massage can produce a wide array of sensations. By varying your pressure, you can create wonderful sensations that can run the spectrum from stress relieving, soothing, comforting, nurturing, healing, energizing, sensual, playful, or erotic, to arousing.

The intention of this lesson is to encourage you to develop your capacity for pleasure and experience the fullness of life by toning your pleasure muscles. By allowing this pleasuring to occur—during school, while out for a walk, while watching a movie, while enjoying dinner, while having intercourse—all of life spills over to an act of receiving and being deeply nurtured by a self-generated pleasure principle. Those who focus on sensual pleasure alone will be trapped, and the spiritual practice you have been developing will keep you alert to the hollowness of the *Kama Sutras* when considered alone, outside the context of lifestyle and spiritual evolution. The search for the Source of all experiences is the true nature of spiritual practice. It is called a practice, after all; practice gradually flows into spiritual realizations. Let the fountain of Spirit remain as constant as your determination to know your True Self, which is transcendent even within the heights of sexual pleasure.

# Self-Breast Massage—Karuna Kriya Variation[39]

The four-step procedure shown in this section will give you a simple massage technique that can be done by yourself, in the privacy of your own home. Although almost any gentle massage technique will have benefit, these four techniques should be a part of your personal regimen. The purpose of these techniques is to flush fluids from the breast (both venous and intercellular), bring nutrition to the tissues, and specifically remove toxins via the lymphatic system. Also, these techniques will enhance the health and elasticity of the support ligaments, which will in turn provide you with better breast support.

The purpose of the first step is a gentle motion designed to drain the breasts' lymphatic system; it is possibly the most important of the four steps. So take your time here and start with slow soft motions for several minutes before proceeding to adapt the depth and pace. Steps 2 and 4 are to assist in the movement of venous fluids. Feel free to experiment with these two movements and find what is comfortable for you. Step 3 is simply to help keep your support ligaments in good health and assist in the fight against gravity. This procedure should be done at least twice a week. It can be done on bare skin, but you may find that using sesame oil will be more comfortable. Stay away from mineral-based or scented oils.

> Step 1: This massage can be done in any posture; lying on the back is generally the most comfortable. Holding the breast with one hand, use the fingers of the other hand to gently smooth the tissue away from the nipple. These movements travel from the nipple and directly away, using no more pressure than what you would apply to your eyelid. Any more pressure will flatten the lymphatic vessel

---

39. For an excellent video tutorial of this practice, see *www.bodymechanics.net/subpages/ breast.htm*.

and stop the flow of circulatory fluids. Also, make this stroke slow, not fast, for it to be effective.

Step 2: Gently massage the breast with a kneading motion, using lifting and pressing movements.

Step 3: Slowly and carefully use your hands to twist the breast in a clockwise and counterclockwise direction, being careful not to put too much tension on the breast.

Step 4: Use both hands to apply several moderate compressions.

Remember to persist in your practice, yet stay detached from expecting specific outcomes. Tantra is a personal spiritual practice. When you feel complete with this lesson, read the Dialogue section that follows prior to beginning lesson 9.

**With Great Respect and Love, I Honor My Heart, My Inner Teacher.**

## Dialogue with Mukunda

**Student:** I have always gotten good advice from you. This time, I have a very intimate question that I hope will not offend you. I need advice for a man who is forty-five years old, with no medical problems he knows of (takes no medications at all), but who is not really fit. He has problems with erection; it is just about 50–70 percent. Is there anything you can suggest to help? I am sure he'll be very committed to trying what you offer. Thank you for getting back to me. Let me give you some details: This man is five to ten pounds overweight, healthy and active in his work and at home, and does a lot of physical work in his business and around the house too. He walks with his dogs, but has no fitness routine; his cholesterol is a little high. He does not eat junk food, and has a couple of glasses of wine with dinner. His stress level is pretty high, but he runs a good business and is a good father to two children, who live with him part-time. He has a girlfriend, with whom he is intimate two to three times a week. They are not living together. Their intimate times are very long, because it is stop and go. So that is the picture. What can you suggest? What do you usually recommend for men with this kind of problem? What could be the cause? Thank you again.

*Mukunda:* I need more information. Perhaps he should email his question to me instead of through you. This will take you out of the loop, unless you both want it this way. I am assuming many points—that his stress levels are normal and that he is fit, with no medical reasons for such complaints—but I will try to answer as best I can. I encourage him to approach sexual relations with a relaxed body and an open heart. Sometimes, this is due to many issues—not really making love, but having sex; constipation; incompletion with a former partner; pressure to perform; overly fantasizing about someone else; excessive media stimulation; inappropriate diet, etc. So let us consider that these are not the problem and address physical and pranic exercises that can stimulate virility and libido.

First of all, I would like to give a different attitude for sexual activity. In Tantrik Yoga, the penis is called the lingam, a word that means "wand of light"; the vagina is called yoni, meaning "Source or sacred space." Thus, spiritual intercourse returns the wand of light to its home in the sacred space within. The experience of being with his partner is the process of giving his light to her sacredness. The progressive series of eighteen Tantrik lessons that I have created are for opening your own spiritual energies. Use the lessons until you are prepared for sharing energies within a loving sexual (Red Tantra) or spiritual (White Tantra) partner. Anyone may receive them just by asking.

In Ayurvedic literature, there is an entire field of specialization in aphrodisiacs and related herbology for the promotion of natural sensuality and sexual expression. There are two herbs I am familiar with that help to enhance libido. Ashwaganda, "the strength of 100 horses," is for men; shatavari, "one who possesses 100 husbands," is for women. You can find details about their use are in *The Yoga of Herbs* by David Frawley and Vasant Lad. In addition, Ayurveda describes the massage of 122 vital points, or *marmas*, that can promote the flow of prana to debilitated regions when massaged. One point that may be helpful in this situation is *vitapa*, located a finger-width lateral to the pubic symphysis, where the spermatic cord passes. If there has been an injury to this site, it can cause impotence in men or women, according to *Ayurveda and Marma Therapy—Energy Points in Yogic Healing* by David Frawley, Subhash Ranade, and Avinash Lele.

Among the yoga poses that may help are those found in chapter 17 of *Structural Yoga Therapy* for optimizing mobility and strength. Do the whole series, but especially focus on the energetics and physical opening that come with the rolling bridge and the variations of the groin stretch. This series can open up many emotions, but especially those related to sensuality and sexuality. After doing the series, do yoni mudra, moving downward from the third chakra, centered at the navel, to the second chakra, centered at the bladder, to the first, in which the yoni mudra would envelope his genitals.

In each position, press the yoni mudra to the body with emphasis on the lower point of the first fingers. Once he has moved to the first chakra, this pressure will be applied to the perineum. At that point, work strongly on mula bandha by pulling up on the PC muscle group that lies in the pelvic floor. By building up the power of these muscles, his lingam will begin to lift up. By alternately tensing the muscles while pressing the perineum then relaxing these motions, his lingam will bob up and down, gradually growing into a stronger erection.

Once half a forceful erection is achieved, he should begin a massage from the base of the lingam to the root. The base is the uppermost attachment of the lingam to the body, located at the top of the pubic bone. From that base spot, the lingam is attached via a ligament to its root below the lower edge of the pubic bone, where it enters the pelvis. This two-inch length of lingam rarely receives attention and is filled with prana. By massaging the lingam away from the body at its two connective attachments along the length of the pubic bone, a greater energy will fill the lingam. This is best done by him alone. When he learns what pressures create arousal, it can be lovingly given him by his partner. Energy is light in its most pure pitta form; in vata's form, it is sensitivity and sensual arousal; in kapha, it becomes muscular stamina and love. All three expressions of Ayurvedic balance can be achieved when this is done with sensitivity, love, and detachment from needing a specific result. One of the three may happen; don't concern yourselves with having all three. Let me know if this is of benefit. Namaste.

**Student:** Lesson 8 has been very helpful in sensitizing me to my breasts. I don't have a partner, so I worked on the self-breast massage section. I can now identify ductwork, fatty tissue, and muscle. Although not much can be done about environmental factors that bring about breast cancer, at least now I'll be very familiar with my own terrain should any changes occur. Thanks, as always, for the gift of your teaching.

**Mukunda:** Thanks for the feedback. It is great to be able to distinguish such details in the breast. It is delicate tissue. Tissue of the heart, as I consider it.

**Student:** Thank you for your concern. These last couple of weeks, I haven't been able to continue, as I was moving and, with the holidays, it took a lot of my attention. So I was feeling that I was falling behind. My mind/ego was really getting in the way. I find the questions and answers help me. I feel that it's going to take me a while to really feel everything the way I think I should. I am going along and feel that my uneasiness is perhaps because I am in a transition stage, which is always a challenge. I am looking forward to being more mindful and having my practice back again.

I found the breathing a challenge, as I like to breathe into my lower abdomen first, then up to the chest. As I understand it, we breathe into the chest first, then lower it into the abdomen. The very first lesson, I felt a lot of energy, but as I continued, it felt dissipated. It's a journey, and I plan on staying with it. I know it's what can help me tremendously. I am single and have sexual issues about my past to work through.

While I was making my move into a new basement suite, I tried to take it easy but must have lifted something too heavy. Now I'm once again recovering from a lumbar 5 problem. My lower back is where I seem to hold my tension or pent-up energy. Any suggestions are greatly appreciated.

*Mukunda:* Best is just to continue to do the lessons at your own pace. They unfold very unpredictably. Each person has blocked energies or suppressed emotions; they are waves to be ridden. For your lower back, I suggest you try doing yoni mudra while lying on your belly with your hands over the part of your back that is stressed. Sometimes, you can also do this by placing them there while you're in a bridge pose, then lowering your back onto your hands. This mudra will build energy and help restore harmony, no matter what is disturbed in your pranic field.

*Student:* I have shared practice #8 with my husband. Can you tell me the modifications for massage of the pelvic area for women? I feel as if massage in the area of chakras one, two, and three would also be helpful for me. Thanks so much.

*Mukunda:* There are many methods for working with the female pelvic floor, externally as well as internally through the vaginal or rectal regions. These methods can be especially beneficial for heightening fertility, menstrual regulation, bladder function, coccyx manipulation, freeing sexual traumas, heightened sexual response, even for pelvic cancers. To me, the best is a progression similar to that done for men with the prostate, only centering the soothing touch on the yoni instead of the perineum. Release of the abdominal, hip, and perineal regions is the same as in massage for men.

Before touching your yoni, he can make the mukula mudra symbol of the yoni, in which the tips of the fingers and thumb are together to form the shape of a bud, signifying the yoni. This indicates an offering done with humility and reverence. Then I recommend lightly placing his hand on your yoni with fingers down, until you have a breath release. This should be as soft as necessary to cause your whole being to open to him—lingering there for some time is most beneficial. This can also be done over clothing as a way of making you feel confident that sexual pleasure is not to be denied regardless of what he is going through. This is called varada mudra. It is seen in many Indian statues and is the sign of bestowing blessings and serenity. In statues, it is usually done with the left hand and the right palm, with the outward-facing fingers upward in abhaya mudra, the gesture of protection.

After this invocation and soothing pause, bring the middle finger inward. If your yoni is not moist, then his other hand can massage your breasts to generate receptivity and cause ojas juices to flow. Once you are receptive, the middle finger will lightly massage the upper vaginal wall in search of the corduroy-like ridges of the G-spot. Yoginis call this the amrita-secreting gland. It is like the prostate in that stimulation to it can increase its secretions during arousal. But unlike the prostate, which can secrete only small amounts, it can release large volumes of clear liquid amrita or ambrosia.

Details of this are given in *The G Spot,* by Alice Ladas, Beverly Whipple, and John Perry; *Jewel in the Lotus,* by Sunyata Saraswati and Bodhi Avinasha; and an audio or videotape called *Freeing the Female Orgasm—Awakening the Goddess,* by Charles and Caroline Muir, available from *www.sourcetantra.com.* They offer workshops that train partners to experience this profound massage, often relieving traumatic sexual histories so that partners can be free of their karmic patterns.

Tender strokes should be made in varying patterns until your arousal is complete. Your energy body should be filled at this point and spreading Shakti to your husband. He can imbibe this with his other hand or just bask in the radiance of your glow as Tantrika Yogini. This can then be directed any way you wish—ending here or continuing to other forms of loving expression. As with other Tantrik methods, once you explore the basics of this, go with the feelings of what the woman wants; She is the embodiment of Shakti. Until that opening occurs, just do what feels most loving and follow your own Shakti.

***Student:*** I would like to ask your advice on the following: I have just heard from a dearly loved friend who lives in Cork (Ireland) and who has been diagnosed with psychotic depression. He has been taking some very strong medication that makes him feel drowsy and unable to hold his concentration much. He sounds quite helpless, and his mother has decided to give up work in order to look after him, as the doctors and psychiatrists were considering sending him into a hospital. Sean has had some suicidal thoughts before, and he made me understand that he could not bear going into an institution. I try not to empower negative thoughts; however, I have to admit that I feel really worried for him. He is a beautiful soul, a very bright young man of thirty, who has been doing lots of soul searching, with amazing abilities. Although I met him a year ago, I have often felt I knew him in previous lives. I feel very close to him, and there is a deep heart connection between us. I so much wish to help. I am sending him Reiki long-distance every day, but still I wish I can do more to help him. What is your insight, Mukunda? Can I dedicate my puja to him, asking the help of Divine Mother?

***Mukunda:*** In seeking help for someone at a distance, it is a good idea to share Reiki energy. Also, doing puja as a miniature version of the Yagna fire ceremony can help to lift the karma of someone who is a good person having unknown difficulties. Also, I suggest that you connect to Ananda Ashram in California. They are devotees of Paramahamsa Yogananda and offer a prayer council to help others. Their prayers have worked wonders, including for one of my dear long-term friends who was recovering from a horrendous motorcycle accident. Send basic information to *prayers@ananda.org*—name, age, location, and situation—and they will pass it along to a prayer group. They also offer instruction in how to pray effectively in order to send spiritual energy to others. Namaste.

***Student:*** As for the Tantrik lessons, I find that I go back and forth between the previous lessons. Is that okay? Does that mean I am not ready to move on to the next lesson?

***Mukunda:*** No. Moving back and forth means that you are reflecting on the previous lesson and seeing how it relates to your evolution and my sequencing of the teachings. These are not always what you may predict.

***Student:*** While I was in India, I spent much more time meditating than I do at home. There was one occasion there when I was focusing on the light, and after a while, it felt as if the light were in my heart and my heart was the light. I sat there for a long time afterward sort of wondering what had happened, savoring the feeling. It has not happened since.

Something really clicked for me last weekend at your training. I have been having a really good time with my own practice since then, exploring especially Surya Namaskar in different ways. I also love watching the flow of energy and the breath. I find that, when my mind goes in ways that are not beneficial and I get frustrated or otherwise out of balance, if I can remember to check the breath and prana, I can bring it back to where it needs to be. Remembering that I can do that is the biggest challenge. It is all so fascinating to me, how it keeps unfolding.

*Mukunda:* That is wonderful. Just by persisting, you find that you are ready for more. That is indeed positive. You are blessed from these experiences. Continue and you will find what you already know: that blessings happen.

*Student:* I think my husband has to do anal massage for his prostate. He mentioned something, but didn't talk about it properly and I did not ask.

*Mukunda:* Your question summarizes a commonly fatal attitude. Many people are like you, in that they would rather get cancer of the organs of sexuality than ask for a massage. This shows the fear of feeling the body and the fear of a possible arousal when what is being offered is a loving healing touch. Yoga is listening to your body's messages. Yoga therapy is taking action on the messages that come repeatedly. Yoni mudra is so powerful in keeping you healthy because of this simple principle of keeping you alert and actively responding to the body as your teacher. Stuck emotions and suppressed thoughts are tamasic. This is very common for men—when they say, "I don't want to talk about it," that is a sign of prostate or sexuality troubles.

*Student:* My husband and I worked with the practice #8, once with Ganesh kriya and once with Karuna kriya. Ganesh kriya produced extreme relaxation in him, and curiosity on his part as to why he didn't emote as suggested was possible in the instructions. He was also curious about what he has experienced me doing. I will let him address that with you directly if he is interested enough. For the partner Karuna kriya, I was very emotional, both in grief and joy, and very touched to know that my partner could be as gentle, loving, and caring as he was. At the end, it felt as if he were stroking my heart. I had not experienced him like that before. It was a very positive experience.

We have not had the opportunity to practice these kriyas again in almost a week, and I am frustrated by needing to have another person's cooperation in sadhana. I feel that he is resistant to try it again, because it turns into such a long ordeal and he hasn't been feeling well. He says he doesn't have the energy to go through it now. He has been rubbing my back instead, which has actually been quite amazing, because he triggers spots along my spine that send a very wonderful "something" up and down my spine, to the sacrum and to the top of my head. I also get a very spacious feeling in my "stuck" right shoulder under the blade. I find it curious that touch on the front of my body brings out feelings of grief, while on the back of my body, it causes very joyful pleasant experiences. I would like to begin the next practice and continue with #8 as we are able. Is that appropriate?

*Mukunda:* Wonderful responses. That is what this process is designed to produce. Deeper, fuller connection to your partner and to your hearts. I am delighted to hear this. Yes, by all means continue lesson 8 and move on to new lessons gradually when you are ready. Blessings.

*Student:* About Ganesh kriya: I have experienced the technique on myself twice and I find it extremely pleasurable. I have noticed that my awareness—control of mula bandha and energy level—has increased. However, lately I have been feeling aroused during meditation. It is really distracting. Do you have any suggestions? Do I get the same effects giving the technique to myself, in particular the second part? My male partner is not into it. Is lying on the side a good position? I am now near a forty-five-minute massage, so should I try to extend it or finish it whenever I feel the need?

*Mukunda:* For arousal, you can place the right heel at the perineum, just behind the root of the penis. This will dissipate the arousal, though it may initially increase it. Persistence in this will diminish that distraction. On the Ganesh kriya, I suggest you go slowly and not move too quickly to the second part. By lingering on releasing the external tissues, you can get much more benefit, resulting in more gradual pleasure, rather than rushing the energy to quicken. Just spend only a few moments on actual internal massage. Giving to yourself is not as complete as having your partner give to you, but it can be quite effective, nonetheless, if you move very slowly and imagine your beloved is pleasuring you. Curled up on your side is a very good position.

**Student:** In these past few weeks, I have given a lot of thought to the Tantrik practice exercises and have continued with my yoga and meditations (except when I was too sick to practice). To be honest, I feel very drawn to meditating and exercises that involve meditation. However, I find the Tantrik practices that focus on sex very challenging and, somehow, they don't feel right, as I lead a celibate life. What do you recommend for me? Is there another practice I could follow?

**Mukunda:** I recommend that you just skip over those practices that feel sexual to you and move to the next lesson. The practice is designed to bring you to a sattvic state. Some students of yoga are suppressed in this area. For them, it brings up those energies, emotions, and thoughts—that is, what has been tamasic. If it feels rajasic—overstimulating—to you, then move on. The last few lessons are both devotional and meditative in their nature. I encourage you just to complete the eighteen lessons and be detached from those lessons that are not appropriate to your celibate lifestyle. Blessings.

# Tantrik Love and Its Natural Sexual Expression

With Great Respect and Love, I Honor
My Heart, My Inner Teacher.

A fter we have mastered the wind, the waves, the tides, and gravity, we shall harness the energies of love," says Teilhard de Chardin. "Then, for the second time in the history of the world, man will have discovered fire."[40] The paradox exists that we love and yet fear love. Due to the arising of fear, judgment, and attachment to the past (vata, pitta, and kapha imbalances respectively), we miss out on loving fully. The challenge of human existence is to learn to be unconditional lovers.

## The Search for Love

I was given a beautiful new book that tells the story of a man's search for freedom from his oppressive, agnostic mind—*Agnostic Prayer* by Paul Sutherland. In the book, the agnostic finds relief from pain in this poem. The story ends well.

> Love
> Just Love
> Let Love guide you
> Love with joy
> Love when happy

---

40. Geralyn Gendreau, ed., *The Marriage of Sex and Spirit* (Santa Rosa: CA, Elite Books, 2006), 8.

Love when sad

Trust and let Love teach you how to express Love.[41]

The close proximity of the first two chakras makes it challenging to separate them into distinct feelings and understanding. What is the energy of sensual pleasure in the first chakra becomes sexual energy in the second chakra. It is natural for these feelings to flow one into the other.

> Spirituality and orgasm are different expressions of the same life force. There is a great similarity between an intense religious experience and a total body orgasm. Each is often called a "peak experience," a feeling of being at one with the universe for a brief moment. In orgasm, the experience of being swept out of the ego or mind is not uncommon. The giving of oneself to another with love, total surrender, loss of duality and merger describes the religious experience as well as it describes sexual union.[42]

The preliminary energy work of the first three lessons has prepared you for being able to sustain a fuller experience of all your emotional, sexual, and spiritual resources. As you persist with yoni mudra and energetic yoga bodywork, you can release your unconscious mind so that what has been suppressed is allowed to surface into awareness. From this, we can clarify which yogic practices are most appropriate for your deeper openings. The release of emotional energy is called *abreaction* in psychological terminology by Freud and others.

> Freud had discovered that remembering past dramas and memories was useless in the psychotherapeutic process unless emotional energy was released at the same time. This requires one to consciously relive the experience, thereby freeing one from dissipated and functional non-disintegrated energy that creates pain and suffering.[43]

Any yoga practice that is achieving this result is wonderful, provided the student has the resources to frame the experience and support its multi-dimensional unfolding.

---

41.  Paul Sutherland, *Agnostic Prayer* (Traverse City, MI: Karuna Press, 2004).
42.  Dr. Jack Lee Rosenberg, *Total Orgasm* (New York: Random House, 1973).
43.  Swami Buddhananda, *Moola Bandha* (Munger, Bihar: Bihar School of Yoga, 1998), 34.

How natural it is for us, when we experience someone who is being freed of their emotional suppression, to give them a hug. A beautiful expression of this was just sent to me by my mother. It was a photo of two prematurely born infants; unfortunately, I was unable to save the image for reproduction here. Nonetheless, here is the story, from an article called "The Rescuing Hug." The article details the first week of life of the set of twins.

> Each was in their respective incubators and one was not expected to
> live. A nurse fought against hospital rules and placed the babies in one
> incubator. When they were placed together, the healthier of the two
> threw an arm over the other in an endearing embrace. The smaller
> baby's heart rate stabilized and her temperature rose to normal. Let us
> remember to embrace those who we love.[44]

Yoga and Tantra encourage this natural expression of compassion and help you prolong it as a way of helping your friends stabilize all the emotions and their underlying energies seeking expression. From hugging, we discover the energetic goodness of their hearts and our own. There is an exchange of goodness in the quality of this experience that we who are within the spiritual community come to know. With sustained discretion, we can find our true spiritual place in life with our yogic and Tantrik partners.

Emotional releases are not due to technique, but to individuals feeling safe enough to open themselves to the unknown. The details of this opening are experienced as the nadis, which form subtle-body pathways to spiritual experience. Feeling safe is crucial for the Ayurvedic source for emotional stability, kapha, to be moist. As a prelude to emotional expression, kapha begins to water in the eyes, in the mouth, and in the sex organs. Yet, because of suppressed (tamasic) or overly expressed (rajasic) emotions and/or non-acceptance of these energies, it is natural for one to feel confusion. As a result, you may not know how to act appropriately when your feelings of sexuality and love arise. Yoginis seek to discern the difference and focus their attention on the development of love, rather than merely on self-centered hedonism or the suppression of their natural emotions.

---

44. This story was originally published in the *Worchester Telegram & Gazette* (November 18, 1995).

# Sexual Integrity—Brahmacharya

There are situations in which self-control of your sex drive is appropriate—when you have no partner, when you are grieving, and/or when you choose to reflect upon how to express your sexual self differently in the future. At those times, celibacy is the best option. For some Yogis, this becomes a lifestyle leading to vows of celibacy (*brahmacharya*) as a preliminary test of living a celibate life. Those who pass the test of foregoing attraction and sexual response, as confirmed by their teacher, can become monks by taking vows of *sannyas*. Orthodox Hindu-based yoga confers the title of Swami upon those who are ready for a lifetime commitment to serving others as they fulfill their sadhana.

Another definition of brahmacharya—one I feel is more appropriate for householders and non-celibates—is continence, in which men choose to engage in sexual relations without having a release of sexual fluids and climax. For spiritual partners, this practice can help you learn more about retaining your prana, while allowing natural functions to be fulfilled. This is particularly beneficial for those married partners who experience a difference in their sexual interests. It is natural for there to be periods of disparity in libido. But neither partner need suffer from this in a way that creates a loss of intimacy.

Tantrik Yoga also encourages chosen periods of celibacy to increase communication with yourself and your potential partner, to explore non-sexual relationships, to enrich your choice to be single, and to redirect yourself following times of transition. A beautiful book on this phase is called *Passions of Innocence,* by Stuart Sovatsky. This innovative, insightful book focuses on how to make choices, empowered with your sexual expression.

When one partner desires sexual intimacy and the other does not, they can still maintain intimacy and protect the more sexually desirous partner from entering inappropriate relations by having the less desirous partner practice selfless service. Thus, if the less desirous is the man, then his duty becomes to satisfy his partner sexually without seeking to be fully aroused himself. He will especially need to exercise caution that his lingam does not come into angles of penetration that arouse his fiery pitta, thus creating excessive friction, leading to loss of detachment. In general, this attitude is the most appropriate for a Tantrik male, as it will enhance the woman's fulfillment so she can then manifest herself as a Devi, literally "a being of light."

152

# Finding Your Own Natural Sexual Expression

In Kabala, the Babylonian Talmud of the Jewish tradition, we find these words:

> Lovemaking is far more than sex.
> It is the kiss of earth and sky, spirit and matter.
> For when you make love in earnest,
> know that you are unifying Creator with Creation,
> God transcendent with God immanent.

Sexuality and relationships have thus long been the most challenging facets of life. To sustain a relationship takes great skill and commitment. For many, the challenge is more than they can overcome, resulting in separation or divorce. The most common cause of divorce is an inability to deal with the problems of sex and money. From a yogic perspective, both issues are governed by the same chakra, the second. On the subtle level, these energies are governed by the energy of the goddess Lakshmi.

Goddesses are the primal energies latent within each woman. Yoginis can learn to connect to their energy within themselves through the practices of Devi puja cited in the last lesson. When they do, problems with abundance and sexuality tend to fade away. Lakshmi's energies are those of abundance, prosperity, and the fullness of sensual enjoyment. One does not need to study the *Kama Sutra*, the ancient Hindu text on love, to be skilled at loving life.[45] This Lakshmi energy manifests as Her abundant healing power. On a physical level, this healing will be of yourself and your relationships, and will result in a harmonious intimate expression. That energy will heal the wounds of two of the prime goals of life—*kama* (sensual pleasure) and *artha* (monetary prosperity). In America, the most prevalent Hindu temples are devoted to Lakshmi, for they realize the tremendous benefit that arises from finding Her qualities within family life.

And yet we have much to learn about love, in contrast with sexual attraction. That they are not the same is obvious.

> In youth, one is a slave to sexual attraction. In the body which is no
> more than the aggregate of flesh, blood, bone, hair and skin, one

---

45.  The *Kama Sutra* is focused on the pleasure of men. A wonderful contrast is *Kama Sutra for Women* by Vinod Verma. It is written by a Yogini for elevating women's intimate pleasure.

perceives beauty and charm. If this "beauty" were permanent, there would be some justification to the imagination; but, alas it does not last very long. Yet, while it lasts this sexual attraction consumes the heart and wisdom.[46]

From where does wisdom arise? Both the 10th-century *Vasistha's Yoga* (p. 496) and the 2nd-century BC text, Patanjali's *Yoga Sutras* (II, 1) agree that it arises from three factors: self-discipline and persistence in the pursuit of Spirit; knowledge of transcendence and how it has affected our living teachers, as well as the study of their writings in the case of deceased teachers; and devotion to Spirit as you understand your higher power to be.

The prevalence of sexual dysfunction is well-known, but greatly misunderstood. Women only tend to seek help when they cannot procreate. Men tend to not want to talk about their sexual lives unless they are bragging. This is commonly an expression of denial of their incompletion, which also relates to diminished kapha. A much deeper problem exists when we take into account the lack of true intimacy and communication that precedes the loss of sexual satisfaction and fertility. Robert Svoboda, an Ayurvedic physician and Aghora (Red) Tantrik practitioner, spoke bluntly about this problem.

> Unsatisfactory sex makes a woman frustrated, causing hormonal changes that imbalance and upset her system. As an Ayurvedic doctor I have occasion to consult with all sort of people on all sorts of conditions, and I have found that my Tantrik teacher, Vimalananda, was correct when he taught me that an unsatisfactory sex life is the root of many or most of the diseases that afflict women. When a woman's internal environment is disturbed by sexual misery, it impairs her creativity, and produces disharmony in the home and family, and in the nation and the world.
>
> A man's responsibility is to satisfy his woman, to direct her energy so that she can create or procreate. Sex forms an important part of this direction. He must make sure that she is satisfied, and no man who

---

46. *Vasistha's Yoga*, 14.

values his own happiness can afford to accept this responsibility lightly. According to Vimalananda, a good man knows how to help a woman produce the music of orgasmic delight. Most men are unaware of this and fail to fully satisfy their women. Many men are so concerned with their own gratification that they indulge in their own orgasms and deliberately neglect their partner's enjoyment. Whenever a man fails in his duty to his woman, her ability to create a happy home suffers, and life becomes hellish for them both.[47]

A woman needs to feel safe to make love. She needs to become a Devi with the encouragement of her beloved, thus finding empowerment to speak truthfully about her pleasures and what she longs for. Her beloved empowers her by expressing what gives him pleasure, such as how attractive her clothing is in arousing him. When she seeks to please him, he will reciprocate and show her the depth of his love. Lakshmi becomes/awakens Krishna. Together, they arouse the passion of each other.

When the underlying pranic energy that creates healthy emotional and sensual expression is freed, it is natural for the heart to open. So often, this takes the form of a transformation of the heart. The healthy heart is sattvic kapha, which manifests in a strong immune system. Its evolved expression is ojas, liquid love. When ojas is fully expressed, it manifests in several ways: in nursing women, as mother's milk; in sensual enjoyment, as an abundance of sexual fluids; in emotion, as tears that overflow the eyes. All these are signs of ojas, which I feel as liquid love; it makes your mouth salivate.

Sexual activity is natural and crucial for emotional and physical health. A recent article, "Is Sex Necessary?" by Alan Farnham (*Forbes*, October 2003), said:

> The risk of heart attack or stroke in men is cut in half by having sex three times a week. Vigorous intercourse burns about 200 calories, about the same as running on a treadmill for 20 minutes. Sex tones thighs, stomach muscles, buttocks and the production of testosterone results in stronger bones and muscles. Endorphins released immediately before orgasm alleviate everything from headaches to arthritis.

47. Robert Svoboda, "Sex, Self-identification, and the Aghora Tradition." Published in Georg Feuerstein, *Enlightened Sexuality* (Freedom, CA: The Crossing Press, 1989), 185–86.

In woman, sex produces estrogen that can reduce the pain of pre-menstrual syndrome. Post menopausal women who abstain from sex can suffer from depression and vaginal muscle atrophy. While women rarely have too much sex, it can be too much of a good thing for men. Penile tissues when overused can sustain permanent damage. Drugs such as Viagra can push men past healthy limits. Erectile dysfunction is typically a symptom of other health problems such as hypertension, diabetes or increased cholesterol. Men who exercise and have a good heart have firmer erections.

## Pelvic-Floor Tone—Mula Bandha

One means to a satisfying sexual life is to maintain the vitality of the muscles of love-making. While the gluteus maximus muscles (located at the back of the hips) are the short-term muscles controlling gross motions of intercourse, the subtler motions and those of sexual stamina originate at the sides and bottom of the pelvis. There is a group of muscles that makes up the whole of the pelvic floor in both men and women. They extend from the pubic bones in front to the tailbone (coccyx) in the back and from side to side. They are bounded on either side by the sitz bones (ischium). This diamond-shaped region has two segments: the front is called the urogenital triangle; the posterior segment is called the anal triangle. The common name for the group of muscles making up this region is the *pubococcygeal* (PC) muscles, or the pelvic diaphragm. Like the thoracic respiratory muscle, the diaphragm, they cover the entire breadth of the region, not unlike a trampoline or, more specifically, like a jellyfish. They are reversed in the thorax and the pelvis.

There is little difference in these muscles from women to men. They form the foundation from which genital muscle tone can be maintained. They are the primary muscles of sexual enjoyment. Studies have shown that, when these muscles are toned, both men and women have more pleasure during sexual expression. With a loss of tone, there can be pain, discomfort, or negative feelings prohibiting full sensual and sexual expression. Men who lose tone due to aging or impure diet will experience dribbles and/or a split stream when they urinate, causing accidental sprays. This is also due to the buildup of toxicity, *ama*, indicating not only a need to purify the urethra and prostate, but a cleansing diet to address the entire system's loss of health. Hence it is especially important to maintain this muscle tone throughout your life span and to eat a predominantly organic vegetarian diet.

Remember, before engaging in this more advanced lesson, that problems with the lower back, pelvic organ functions, and sexuality can come from the pelvic floor. These muscles, like all others, can suffer due to three potential problems: loss of tone (*hypotonus*), where mula bandha is needed; a subtle spasm, where external massage may provide relief; or excessive tension (*hypertonus*), where Tantra Prana Bodywork focused on the pelvic floor will generate not only relaxation, but emotional and energetic freedom. See the Dialogue section in lesson 8 for more details. For the general population, the most common problem is loss of tone. Personalized guidance may be necessary before proceeding with optimizing your sexual muscular tone.

To tone the muscles, sit in a chair (or lay on your back) with your feet flat on the floor. Tighten your buttocks and genital area firmly, as strongly as you can. Then gradually and totally relax. Continue this root lock (mula bandha) for ten to twelve times with full force. This initial level of training is for developing the outer gluteal and external hip rotator muscles' tone; it is not meant to extend to the smaller central pelvic floor. It is a start to help you differentiate the gluteals from the PC, or pubococcygeal, muscles that lie as a web between the four pelvic-floor bones (two ischium or sitz bones, the coccyx, and the pubic bones). Then focus on tightening just your pelvic floor—the vaginal or penile muscles (the ability to isolate these muscles is called vajroli mudra for men and sahajoli mudra for women) and rectal area (aswini mudra)—for an additional ten to twelve times.

Repeat this throughout the day, as you can secretly develop this tone during most activities. By being able to contract these muscles fully at will, you can prolong your capacity to retain energy in your Source center. With disciplined practice, these three muscular regions can be isolated and energy flows can be directed to and from these sites. Each of the three regions will produce different psychic and sexual attainments during sexual and spiritual practices. Once your body is responding more to the inner muscles, you can begin to shift attention to the multi-dimensional nature of the koshas and develop sensitivity to where you are and where you wish to go.

For women, mula bandha practice promotes health of the pelvic organs and increases libido and heightens pleasure. Adept women can direct their toned muscle control to the G-spot (a series of ultrasensitive corduroy-like ridges located on the upper vaginal wall an inch inward from the labia) or their clitoris and thus produce a stronger sexual-energy arousal. As was mentioned in lesson 2, the male site of the second chakra is external, at the pubic bone just above the base of the lingam. The female site is at the cervix. During energetic intercourse or physical penetration intercourse, these two points will come together, creating a strong energetic flow as the water chakras share energy. Often, it is this experience that can create a lot of emotional release in women during intercourse. The emotions can be of a known (memory) or an unknown nature—that is, not related to a specific memory, simply a release of pent-up feelings. Empathic witnesses to this opening often share their energetic reactions; even in a class where nurturing and safety are cultivated this can happen. By regularly encouraging a natural expression, more Shakti is created—that is, a natural expression of a fully empowered Tantrika. She no longer hides her feelings or thoughts. Every expression is in the open, because there is safety in being natural.

Physically, a woman whose muscular control is strong can grip her partner's lingam more strongly, giving her an ability both to regulate her own sensations and to control the pace of her arousal. This is particularly beneficial so that both can experience multiple orgasms, rather than be limited to how long the man can delay ejaculation. A trained man can learn to separate the two experiences, so that lovemaking can be prolonged for greater pleasure. This is the practice called *karezza*, prolonged caress—a beautiful way to flow the lines between the subtler bodies, as it is a cooler expression of love.[48] A woman's muscular control over her vaginal muscles will tone her partner's lingam, generating more ability for him to reciprocate pleasure. When men develop this practice to the variant called vajroli mudra, they can learn to withdraw or project their sexual energy through their lingam. The former helps them maintain arousal longer; the latter can sexually arouse a partner by producing energetic innercourse (Pink Tantra) without physical intercourse (Red Tantra). With patience and persistence, this practice can help couples regain their passion and help infertile women become pregnant. One benefit of Tantra Prana Bodywork is creating the fertility needed to become pregnant. A woman learns to become more receptive to the lingam's energy as her yoni expands its energy field. With practice, a tantrika can

---

48. André van Lysebeth, *Tantra* (York Beach, ME: Weiser, 1995). This book is highly recommended as the only Tantrik book by a committed Sivananda Yogi.

invite the lingam's energy into her body without taking the lingam physically. This is a practice that can be done in any posture and is very empowering.

Not all women have been able to regain vaginal muscle tone using Kegel exercises, especially when their tissues have been torn or damaged. This is why these more-detailed practices are given here and in lesson 14. They produce much more response, especially when coupled with energetic opening and the release of suppressed emotions. Persistence is often not enough to produce the desired results. I recommend an individual consultation with me to assist those who have not made satisfactory progress in developing this tone.

It is especially common for women who have had multiple children and an episiotomy (surgical enlargement of the vaginal opening to facilitate easier delivery for the doctors) to no longer enjoy sex due to the loss of tone in their internal muscles. Studies have shown that both men and women with strong PC and pelvic-floor muscles experience more pleasure than those lacking this tone. This pleasure extends to all avenues of life. Another option presented in lesson 14 is the use of a Shiva lingam stone to tone the internal muscles for women. This method provides some gentle downward pressure on the pelvic floor from above when the stone is inserted into the vaginal canal. This allows the internal muscles to release downward, thus regaining their natural range of motion by alleviating either hypotonus or hypertonus with regular practice.

While this practice is best done without clothing, a yogic loincloth called a *langouti* may be worn for the requisite seated poses. The langouti is easy to make and can be used by both sexes. It is described in detail at *www.derekosborn.accountsupport.com*. The key here is a special tantrasana foot placement that gives this sadhana the greatest benefit. To promote the optimal pranic response, sit in one of two tantrasanas: equal pose (samasana) or perfect pose (siddhasana). The first is done by placing your right heel (if you are a man; left for women) against the perineal root of the lingam and the opposite foot in front of it, so your heels are aligned, with both ankles on the floor. The second, an even stronger position, begins, for men, with the right heel placed as in equal pose, but the left foot placed above the lingam. In this position, pressure is applied to both the base and the root of the lingam—the sites of the first two chakras. With persistence, the pressures will bring sattvic qualities to these chakras, as it increases your root lock's power. An option is then to pull the right toes upward between the calf and thigh, and the left toes downward to lock the posture. The goal for men is to increase the upward flowing prana natural to the Shiva state.

For women, a Tantrik variation of the pose called siddhayoniasana is recommended by Swami Satyananda of the Bihar School in *Asana Pranayama Mudra Bandha* (p. 64). In this variation, the right heel is placed to press lightly on the yoni and the left heel placed directly above it, giving mild pressure to the pubic bone. For women, this pose promotes the downward flow of Shakti (apana), increasing the yoni mudra quality. Practice differentiating the various muscles of the pelvic and abdominal region until they can be isolated. (See *Hatha Yoga Pradipika* I, 37–43 for more details.)

Next, apply the four variants of yoni mudra introduced in lesson 2. In the first, the thumbs meet at the navel. In the second, the Devi triangle is centered on your navel, the fire element. In the third, the bladder is placed in the center of the triangle to locate your water element. In this position, your hands will rest on your pelvic bones. In the fourth placement, your outer sex organs are centered in the yoni mudra, with your fingertips reaching toward your pelvic floor. Practice feeling the detailed internal anatomy that follows with your practice of yoni mudra. Our goal here is to experience both energetic and physical awareness, and to observe how they blur the lines of distinction as you experience more Shakti and, with it, subtler awareness.

Find your uterus where the forefingers meet in the first yoni mudra. Just below that point is your vaginal canal, which is a collapsed organ until something is inserted into the cavity. The uterus is normally bent and tilted forward over the bladder. Reverse position is not uncommon, especially in women who have given birth. The latter position, tipped, may produce complaints ranging from painful menstruation (congestive dysmenorrhea) to pain in the labia, vagina or pelvis during or following intercourse (dyspareunia) to infertility.

Yoni mudra, Tantrasana practice, and receiving Tantrik bodywork from an adept (covered in the next lesson) can often free a woman of these symptoms. Where the cervix fits into the vagina, a circular moat is formed around it (fornix). In my experience, this area expands considerably during physical (or energetic) intercourse. The depth of the yoni as the vaginal cavity varies from woman to woman, just as the lingam varies in length from a tiny three inches, to an average six inches, to over twelve inches. Due to this range, the descriptions for locating your internal sex organs and the subtle-body chakras vary. What is given is for the average depth of yoni that is comfortable and satisfied by an average lingam. The *Kama Sutra* recommends finding your match for optimal physical love-making, so that romantic passions lead to fulfillment of your natural expression of pleasure.

## Congratulations!

You have just completed the first half of the Tantra lessons. May you persist to the end of these eighteen lessons. Patanjali, in his *Yoga Sutras* II, 1, defines three attributes that lead to attaining a stable elevated state of sadhana. These qualities are:

Tapah—self-discipline and a willingness to be purified

Svadhyaya—study of your self, aided by reflections on the scriptures

Isvara pranidhanani—devotion to the Lord/Goddess who attracts your love

May you be blessed with a deepening of these virtues!

Remember to persist in your practice, yet stay detached from expecting specific outcomes. Tantra is a personal spiritual practice. When you feel complete with this lesson, read the Dialogue section that follows prior to beginning lesson 10.

**With Great Respect and Love, I Honor
My Heart, My Inner Teacher.**

## Dialogue with Mukunda

**Student:** I have just realized that the openings that I have had in the past weeks, in which I have been flooded with love, are the results of lessons 8 and 9. Sometimes I'm dense! I was focused on the "sexual" term and forgot that love is the base. With these heart openings, I truly can love my husband and trust in him. We have been physically and emotionally distant in the last year because of all the barriers that had been built up. Now that my barriers have come down, his are coming down too. We are learning to love and trust each other as we once did in the very beginning. This is so very lovely.

*Mukunda:* Wonderful, and so sweet that you have moved to the foundation of the course. This is, of course, the foundation that gives meaning to all activities.

*Student:* I have also moved forward in my yantra practice. There was a release in the back of my chest, and I am able to breathe deeply into my chest as well as my belly. This helped to quiet my mind and allowed me to relax and be. And there she is again, removing those obstacles one by one.

With deepest gratitude for your guidance and love! A very big hug to you! Speaking of hugs, there was a woman at the vegetable stand who was asking for a hug from the shopkeeper. She had just lost her husband, and there was no one at home to hug her. I offered my hug, and she accepted.

*Mukunda:* Good for you that yantra sadhana is moving energy and the physical changes are so obvious. And you are so sweet to give yourself with compassion. Keep it up and blessings for your openings!

*Student:* Is one of the effects of Tantra also to keep the level of excitement high as long as possible, to postpone the moment of total discharge?

*Mukunda:* High, yes. But not outside of control for the man. For the Devi, yes. She gets to go outside of control. The man, Deva, is more responsible for what happens and should encourage the Devi to express herself fully. Yet she needs to feel safe so she will not cause emotional or physical harm. Therefore, she needs to be regulated gently in showing her that he will protect her. The total discharge is never fully a goal; the goal is spiritual orgasm, not physical ejaculation. They are quite different. Optimally, one reaches toward the former in their personal sadhana practice; through the closeness of Spirit comes also the closeness of the Devi.

*Student:* I guess meditation can be helpful, but after some time, you have to have someone to share. Meditation alone can hardly be satisfying for a longer time period without any contacts. Age-wise, I am now on top of feelings and sensuality. I am a red-moon woman now. Never before have I felt sensations so deeply and strongly, and never have

I wished more to get to know and explore my energies. I think I was never capable of enjoying more than I do at this age. I am very glad that I found the way to Tantra.

*Mukunda:* Wonderful that you can say that. Fulfillment from that energy is so different from fulfillment without it.

*Student:* I have already had many partners—some in relationships, most just for a short time. I tried out a lot. Most men are very simple regarding making love.

*Mukunda:* Men need to be educated, but they cannot or will not learn from each other when their egos are threatened. So a woman Tantrik teacher is best. As you are reading *Tantrik Quest* by Daniel Odier, you can see from that how powerful the Tantrika teacher is for Western men—powerful in the sense of truly transforming his ability to make love, and to let go of the wanting of sex.

*Student:* I realized today that I am not afraid to feel for you and that gives me great freedom! I can let my love flow. Thank you for that. More and more, I understand what a great gift sexuality can be, how much life power and transformation it can harbor! I always felt it, in a way, but it never seemed to be appropriate in society. I also never met someone who knew more and could teach me about all these secrets. Thanks to you, I learn to accept, love, and enjoy this present.

*Mukunda:* I am grateful to be so appreciated. Blessing also to you for unfolding completely and naturally.

*Student:* I have a woman in my class who has been trying to become pregnant for a long time. She asked me for help. I do not see her as a Tantric type of woman. She is very conservative. I've told her that I will contact you to ask for help and information. Is there something you can advise me to tell her? Thanks in advance.

*Mukunda:* I believe you can go to my website (*www.yogaforums.com*) and see some additional entries there for fertility and pregnancy that I have given previously. In general, if all that is possible has been done for both husband and wife in the medical realm, then yoga routine as sadhana can improve the fertility of both. If they are not doing sadhana, then a new program may not be so helpful. In other words, they need to consider yoga as a practice that takes them to the spiritual realm. From that place, they can visit souls who can potentially come into her body as her future child. If there is a match there, then the child will seek relationship with them. There are many practices for fertility, but this is a deeper question.

**Student:** I recently ran across something on the Internet that I wanted to ask you about. The website *www.makereallove.com* contains information about naturally arising tears during orgasm as a healing experience. This is the first time I have heard anything about this, other than my own experience. A few years ago (pre-yoga), this started happening to me occasionally when my husband and I made love. He found it confusing, but it felt beautiful to me, not at all sad. I think I may have started suppressing it for fear that he didn't feel comfortable with it. Tears can feel very cleansing to me, and I have recently started to allow myself to cry freely during my practice. I find that it can take me from a state of frustration to one of compassion. I'm just curious about the yogic perspective and your opinion on tears.

**Mukunda:** Tears are a natural expression of the Ayurvedic principle called kapha. When kapha evolves, it becomes the juice of love called ojas. So it is quite natural for tears to arise during true moments of love-making. When there is love being made, it naturally produces byproducts that are of the essence of kapha as juice: the salivary glands moisten the mouth, breasts swell to resemble those of a nursing mother, the sexual organs flow with a unique nectar called amrita, and the eyes flood with tears of pleasure, gratitude, and ecstasy.

Ojas is nectar that is found in these various ways. The Yogini also experiences this ojas as *kechari*, nectar that originates in a secret chakra behind the third eye and flows down the palate, eventually to be burned up in the solar chakra. Techniques like kechari mudra, in which the tongue goes upward, or viparita karani mudra (modified half shoulderstand) help the Yogini to retain the nectar so that it increases to become supreme love. When love evolves, it no longer is experienced as personal, but as Divine—that is, spreading equally to all that come into our consciousness. In truth, it is consciousness that is bliss, and it is natural to experience that as being filled with tears of love. I wrote several poems in my book *The Yoga Poet* on the eyes being filled with the black hole of love juice. There is no end to love, for the Yogi experiences that this is who we are.

**Student:** In this lesson, you say, "Emotional releases are not due to technique, but to the individual's safety to open themselves to subtle-body pathways." Does this mean that the person *feels* safe, or literally *is* safe and will come to no harm?

*Mukunda:* When people feel emotionally safe their energetic pathways are clear. As a result, the safety that comes is an opening to what would formerly have been unknown or unknowable. The mantra that protects you generates that safety because you are connected to the lineage that can give it.

*Student:* You say in the practice section that there are three muscular regions. Are these the buttocks, genital area, and pelvic floor? I remember once being told that intermittently stopping the flow of urine was a good PC-muscle exercise. If I occasionally stop and start urine flow, am I working the genital or pelvic-floor region?

*Mukunda:* The relevant muscles are the gluteals; the PC is the pelvic floor in its entirety, and in addition, the two sphincters surrounding the anus and genitals. These ring muscles are difficult to distinguish from the pelvic floor. As you mention, however, when you stop the flow of urine, you are contracting the sphincter, round-shaped muscles just an inch deep from your labia.

*Student:* I'm not able to distinguish between the two muscle groups. I don't know how I feel about paying attention to these parts of my body without being sexual. It's different. All the old stigmas I was brought up with—which amount to, "if you aren't washing it in the shower, you shouldn't be there"—come up. I thought I was past all of that. But I do look forward to being a little old lady who doesn't need to wear diapers. The work of distinguishing the sensual and the sexual is a challenge. It makes me feel undisciplined and childish when I don't keep sex out of the picture. (I don't fail all the time—just most of the time.)

*Mukunda:* It is natural, for very few can distinguish, which makes people uptight about their sexuality. The sequence of training from this ignorance of anatomy and emotions is very unique to yoga and Tantra. Yoginis make the distinction between the sensual, the sexual, and the spiritual. Tantrikas do not distinguish among these; for them, all is spiritual energy.

*Student:* I have been very committed to my practice lately, especially including energy work. When I received lesson 6 on sexuality and love, I really listened to this desire to try celibacy for a period of time—to renew myself and also to figure out what it is that I want to be creating in my next intimate relationship. So I am making the conscious choice to stay out of sexual relationships for the time being, maybe making a commitment of six months. I'm still thinking about that. But the thing that is confusing me is this force inside of me that doesn't want to generate sexual energy at all. So not only do I want to stay out of the physical contact of sexual arousal, I feel as if I do not want the energetic sensations of arousal or, in particular, of arousing feelings that then lead to a short-lived, vaginal orgasm that puts me right to sleep. I feel as if "What's the point?" Partner or no partner, I feel as if I'm through experiencing sexual pleasure the "old" way.

So I went back to lesson 3 and began to work on following the flow of prana, and really working with releasing suppressed emotions. This practice has been amazing. The only hard part is the time and place of the release—thank goodness I spend so much time driving (a good quiet place to cry). I have been able to feel and release the whole spectrum of emotions—so many of them. It's amazing. A lot is going on in my life, and I know I would be lost without these practices. I don't know what it is that I need to say, but I hope it's alright if I share with you my big news that is both wonderful and frightening.

When I think about this whole thing, I do not feel the deep sadness that I used to feel in my heart. It is more in the periphery of my heart that I feel it. And I feel a tremendous amount of acceptance around myself and the illness, too. But sometimes I just feel so exhausted. So tired of being physically tired. So tired of dragging this body along. So tired of being a body.

It's taken me so many years, almost twenty, to be okay being in a body and not wanting to leave. But I catch myself having those thoughts again, about how nice it will be not to be in a body anymore. In no way am I inferring suicidal ideation. I am just talking about looking up at the sky and just wanting to go home.

I am crying now and just beginning to get the release I really need. It is so hard being in this body, and I really feel as if all that is keeping me going is my practice. And I am so thankful for it and for the teachings and for all of the beautiful fruits of the practice. But it's just hard sometimes, being alive. And what's harder is hearing myself not being thankful for being alive. This is all so much. And the layers just continue shedding. And many days, I have no idea how I do this, how I have so many dreams and ambitions, and how I get out of bed every morning. And the only thing I can attribute it to is the Divine Grace that has been guiding me. Thank God. I think I released most of it.

**Mukunda:** Great in-depth sharing. Thanks for your confidence to share so intimately with me on your process. It is great that you wish to move from the "old way of being," to become transformed into something you obviously don't know what it will look like. I am happy to be supporting you. It is great that you realized a need to go back to lesson 3. That is a very powerful lesson, and I encourage you and others to do the same, frequently, as the more advanced sessions will bring out hidden blocks that lesson 3's basics can relieve. Continue with the next lesson; it will move you on more smoothly as a result of your persistent determination to be different.

**Student:** Tonight, after making my offerings on my altar, I started doing mantra repetition (*japa*) with Om Namah Shivaya and remembered an experience I had at one of your workshops. You led us through a Shiva meditation, having us sit in *baddha konasana* with hands in jnana mudra, palms facing shins and fingers touching the earth. I don't remember much more of your instructions, other than to make a pyramid with the third eye at the apex. I had a sense of Shiva coming into me, reaching his hands down through perhaps the top of my head and holding my heart in his two hands to try to crack it open. I can't believe I forgot about that experience when you recommended Om Namah Shivaya at first. I had a huge pimple at my third eye for a week after. So then tonight, when that image came back to me, I felt that experience when I worked with you last of something tangled around my heart and dry-heaving to loosen it.

One night last week, after making love with my husband, we both practiced yoni mudra, which sent me into an emotional spin centered at my belly and rising to my chest. With my husband supporting me, I pulled "the roots" out as you told me, coughed up a storm, and then couldn't stop laughing because all I could think of to say to my husband was "I bet you wished I just smoked after sex." (Okay, it still makes me laugh a bit.) It is wonderful to recognize this connection and then also to *know* it, at least during sadhana. Just as you wrote in the Ayurvedic chapters you sent us, students don't often know a stretch from a contraction. I am realizing more and more that I don't know how to differentiate the sensation of joy from sorrow or fear. But I am trying to take the time to sort it out before letting either consume me. My students are feeling your guidance in their dreams.

**Mukunda:** All is going very well indeed. I am delighted to hear of your memory of the Bhadra Shiva meditation that I shared. It has always been a particularly powerful, primal experience for me. It is performed with the body in the image of a four-sided (that is, three-dimensional) pyramid whose sides are lines connecting the arms, spine, and toes, so that all energetic lines lead to the third eye. The King's chamber is your heart; the Queen's chamber is hidden below that in the space occupied by yoni mudra. Continue to deepen your practice and especially encourage kriyas to be the way you let go of old patterns of your stuck emotions. Your capacity to love your husband freely, enhanced by this kriya practice will help release suppressed emotions. This can have a profound Tantrik effect, as it opens you to more safety to be free of your old ways. Allowing more energy to flow within you and around you is most natural, and your students will also feel some connection with your teacher. After a while, students energetically become, or at least channel, their true spiritual teacher. Blessings.

**Student:** My practice at the moment consists of daily japa mantra on *ham-sa*, although I find it difficult to sit still for thirty minutes right now, also feeling my mind very fidgety. I also practice Yoga Nidra and have started reading *I Am That*—on the hamsa mantra, by Swami Muktananda—and I like it very much. I now do yoni mudra first thing when I wake up (starting on heart center, then solar plexus, then belly button, then pubic bone and muladhara area) and in the evening, last thing before going to sleep, on the pubic bone area only.

I have been feeling very emotional, crying easily at times and very irritable at other times. I guess this is some link to the injury. I feel frustrated because I had to slow down my asana practice so much, because I can't teach as much as I would like, and don't seem to be moving on in my professional life and relationships. And at times, I feel very lonely. So, at the moment, I find myself in that space where I observe that life is not really going the way I hoped it would and that the only thing I can do is surrender to the Universe and see what comes up. I am not sure why it is going this way, but I can only guess this is part of the growth process and may be a slowdown before the breakthrough, preparing the ground, sowing seeds to insure a great harvest.

I hear your words when you advise me to keep moving and keep juicy, and I make sure I keep open to the world and what it has to offer. After all I have learned in the last few years, I very much realize that my practice is to apply it to daily life. This evening, I am planning to do a puja and connect with you for support and guidance.

**Mukunda:** With lesson 9, it is most important to keep a focus of yourself as the lover of the Beloved. The Beloved is your own Self. That Self is seeking nothing but your attention, with peace, love, and uplifting thoughts going its way. The Divine Couple is both an external manifestation and an internal one. As you love yourself more, in spite of the signs of success or failure, that love translates to deeper connection to the Beloved. No judgments; be free of them. Life is always giving to you. Being free of criticism and preferences is the path of yoga; the path of Tantra is to see that all is the Divine Couple sporting within all events. Keep looking for love; whatever you search for, you are bound to find.

**Student:** Mukunda, when I am close to my partner, I get lubricated very quickly and stay that way. In general, I am really working with understanding my energy and learning how to work with it most effectively. Even if all we do is kiss, this still happens. Now I am not complaining—it is a reflection of being interested and also feeling safe. But then, I am sometimes working with issues of feeling dry or achy in my body, and I wonder if getting so wet in that way drains ojas? Is there a way I can work with this to deepen a positive effect?

**Mukunda:** No, being wet is a clear sign of increasing ojas. It is different for women and men. Men need to retain fluids; women to express them. Just as it increases their energies, it depletes men's. When dry or achy, just assume you are not ready; allow for more caressing, loving compliments, foreplay of enjoyment. For more positive effects of ojas, there are many practices. See especially Tantra lessons 8 and 9, and their evolution into lessons 14 and 15.

**Student:** Last week, the week after you were here and speaking on much of Tantra to me and the other students, when I was close to my partner, I was completely absorbed and drawn in. But I felt no rush that anything had to be any particular way. I was very happy to stop and just rest, and even to do very little really. But I was getting lights, scenes from nature—even imagining smells, I think! I was more interested in keeping my attention focused on letting that unfold than I was on any physical sensations. To be honest, it was really quite ecstatic, and felt like some of the things that can happen in meditation. There was no sense of tension or playing either male or female roles. Just very natural. I have had experiences like this before, but not quite to that extent. It did feel as if the level of emotional intimacy and flow of the energies created the ability to enter into a really expanded space. Is that partly what Tantra is? The most outstanding thing, as I said to my partner, is the image I keep getting that there are no guideposts here. I have not been to this place before; it is really new ground. But then I begin to question whether one can become an ecstasy addict. This feeling is all very nice, but is it a place we can get stuck in, thus preventing deeper levels of opening and surrender? I would appreciate your guidance on how to work with my experiences. This is clearly a strong pull for me to be on this type of path, so I am grateful to have a Tantrik teacher who can help me weed out what is really happening here.

*Mukunda:* You are having an experience of lesson 15, without having gone that far systematically. The truth is the spiritual or Tantrik awakenings happen in God/dess sequence. And the explanation and training that I have set up is arbitrary and an attempt at being systematic so your mind can grasp what Divine Grace really is. The mind needs help understanding all this, and so we do need a spiritual mentor to move through the experience more gracefully. It is not the experiences of this world that are the problem; it is our response to them that needs to be corrected. The basic problem is *avidya,* as we know fully from reading over and over about the causes of suffering (*kleshas*) in *Yoga Sutras* II, 3–15. This ignorance of the Self manifests as doubt, confusion, and negative thoughts and emotions. They are not to be removed, only diminished by the cultivation of their opposites—that is, sattvic harmonious thoughts and emotions. Spending time with a Tantrik teacher is crucial; otherwise the mind develops many more confused vrittis.

*Student:* What you have said about the woman teaching the man is quite correct. I have indeed seen that in my own experience! And the more I realize the truth of your words and apply them, the better I get at not overextending myself and getting hurt in the ways I used to! So I am helping teach my partner how to learn more about himself, as I am also learning more about myself. Is that not yoga indeed?

*Mukunda:* Indeed, you must be his teacher when it comes to energy practice and evolution, and especially when working with these energies in a romantic or sexual expression.

*Student:* Since lesson 9, I've been trying to address repressed sexual energy with my partner—a conversation that took me six years to have—and I am very conscious of working with the lower chakras.

*Mukunda:* It is good that you are moving ahead and breaking down an old pattern. These lower chakras are often the major blocks to love. Sexual energy suppressed feels sexual, but when healthy expression is there, it is not experienced as sexual, rather purely as love.

*Student:* When I asked for my Inner Teacher, I instantly felt drawn to Ganesha and his mantra, although the mantra I was initiated into through the Sivananda was Siva. I feel this is very grounding.

*Mukunda:* This sounds like both natural and clear guidance. Since Ganesha rules the first chakra and his duty is to remove all obstacles, you are getting an increase in that blessing from following this guidance.

*Student:* In lesson 9, you said: "to tone the muscles, sit in a chair (or lie on your back) with your feet flat on the floor and tighten your buttocks and genital area firmly, as strongly as you can. Then gradually and totally relax. Continue this root lock (mula bandha) for ten to twelve times." Should I not do this with regular breathing then?

*Mukunda:* This is for outer muscle tone and not for the pelvic floor. It is a start to help you differentiate the process. Your body is responding more as if your inner muscles are reacting and your energy is moving inward. It is best to be gentler and use deeper sensitivity to tell where you are and where you wish to go.

# The Divine Couple

With Great Respect and Love, I Honor
My Heart, My Inner Teacher.

When matter united with spirit, when gods are with goddesses, the universe evolves, a new world comes into being. When they separate, the universe dissolves, the waters of doom engulf the world. Bhagavan and Bhagavati (God/dess), spirit and matter, support each other. When Brahma creates, Sarasvati is his knowledge; when Vishnu sustains, Lakshmi is his wealth; when Shiva destroys, Shakti is his strength.

Bhagavan and Bhagavati also oppose each other: While Brahma is beyond understanding, his consort Sarasvati is the personification of intellect, wisdom and cognition; Vishnu promotes detachment but his consort Lakshmi provides all that man desires—power, prosperity and pleasure; Shiva transcends worldly life while Shakti is the force of creation and destruction that rotates the wheel of the world. The tension and co-operation between Bhagavan and Bhagavati, between the soul and the flesh, the spirit and matter, is what gives life its vibrancy, power and momentum.[49]

These energies of the macrocosm are given different names when they appear as the microcosm of the human body. But they are the same primal forces. Again and again in Tantrik teachings, we are shown the

---

49. Devdutt Pattanaik, *Devi: The Mother-Goddess* (Mumbai: Vakils, Feffer and Simons Pvt., 2000), 120.

unique detail of personal transformation that reflects the highest teachings of the ancient Vedas in their summations known as the *Upanishads*.

> Whatever is here, that is there;
> What is there, the same is here.
> He who sees here as different, meets death after death.
> By mind alone this is to be realized,
> And there is no difference here.
> He who sees here as different, meets death after death.
> (Katha Upanishad)

Throughout the Eternal Teachings (*Sanatana Dharma*) of the Indian culture, there are archetypes of the God and Goddess living in harmony as symbols of living a sattvic yoga lifestyle. In the Tantrik teachings, this symbol of the Divine as both masculine and feminine is characterized by the polarity of opposites functioning in harmony. On the gross level, it means having the right and left brain both developed so that you can easily switch gears between artistic and analytical functions, learning to feel sensations in the body and interpret them correctly so that they arouse infinite consciousness. Ayurvedically, the vata dosha begins to be transformed into prana as a spiritual energy; pitta dosha is elevated into tejas as spiritual light; kapha dosha produces ojas, which is the moist elixir of Spirit. When disharmony predominates, there is rajas (excessive activity) or tamas (inertia).

On the subtler physical level, this is the balance of the right and left nostrils. In the subtle body, it is the harmony of the right, or pingala, nadi with the left, or ida, nadi. The balance of these subtle polarities creates a serene sattvic mind. When this is maintained, the Kundalini begins to awaken, purifying the central nadi (sushumna) that holds deeper karmic patterns of disharmony. As this awakening unfolds, you begin slowly to lift the veils that produce an illusion of separation and its accompanying emotional spiral of fear of the unknown, anger to protect yourself from the unknown, and attachment to the known. The spiritual process lifts this veil of avidya (meaning literally "without spiritual knowledge"). Without a veil, vidya manifests as spiritual wisdom, promoting safety, comfort, and enjoyment of life.

It is the dynamic energy of consciousness that is known as prakrti. That which is superior to this energy is consciousness itself which is the very self of consciousness, supreme peace. This dynamic energy functions and moves as long as there is the momentum of the Lord's wish. She dances as long as She does not see the Lord. Consciousness revels in duality till it sees its own Self. The energy of consciousness dances until it beholds the glory of illumination. When it beholds consciousness, it becomes pure consciousness.[50]

On the highest level, the experience of the harmony of duality becomes the union of opposites in which duality dissolves. It is symbolized in Tantrik Buddhism as the harmonic coupling of man and woman in the yab/yum posture, and in Indian Tantra as the primal couple of Shiva and Shakti, who are not two, but, as one, are the True Self. Shiva is characterized as masculine, but really represents the indrawn potential energy of the life force. Shakti is depicted as feminine, but really represents the activated energy of the life force. To experience Shiva is to be utterly still, silent, and immobile in a state of "peace that surpasses understanding," as described in the book of John from the Bible. To experience Shakti is to dance, sway, and be aroused in the delight of your inner being. The contrast between the two expressions is night and day. Yet, in harmony, they are the life force and all its manifestations. This harmony is the experience of the Self. When that awareness is sustained unbroken for the remainder of a life span, it is called Self Realization (see the last lesson).

## The Union of Shiva and Shakti

I offer my love to the God and Goddess,
The limitless primal parents of the universe.
The Lover, out of boundless love,
Has become the beloved.
Both are made of the same substance
And share the same food.
Out of love for each other, they merge.

---

50. *Vasistha's Yoga*, 575.

And again they separate for the pleasure of being two.
They are not entirely the same—
Nor are they not the same.
We cannot say what they really are.[51]

The sadhana to realize this union within yourself is Tantrik Yoga. That which is philosophical is of little interest to the Tantrika. What is of interest is the quest for the Divine and the removal of conditioned illusory obstacles that block you from sustaining that communion with the Divine Self. Sadhana arises from the desire to be fulfilled by your spiritual self. From that natural desire, natural activities are born to create communion. The sadhana is to see the Shakti as Shiva and Shiva as Shakti; to generate self-effort in sadhana is to see both the pain and the ecstasy as arising from these two apparently separated forces. By knowing the qualities of Shakti and Shiva, we can discern what to encourage and what to ignore.

The qualities of Shakti as the Divine Mother are worldliness and its illusory fulfillment of desires. The qualities of Shiva will naturally arise out of Shakti being fulfilled in Herself. The Tantrik sadhana is to know your energy, purify yourself of suppressed energy, and promote healthy energetic expressions that are beneficial to everyone.

The energies of Shakti as prana are to be expressed through the chakras when they blossom; but the energies of Shiva as prana are to be withdrawn, involuting the chakras, as mentioned in lesson 5. To allow Shiva's prana to withdraw without suppressing Shakti's prana expression requires surrender and submission to a will that comes from a power higher than your own consciousness.

At first, Shakti requires submission to be increased, so practice bowing with humility to the form that attracts you the most. Finding that form is a crucial practice of Tantrik Yoga. Persistence and humility are necessary for success. Humility comes from inwardly bowing, making the inner submission to your inner Self, your Inner Teacher, even when you are so imbalanced that you can't perceive that your efforts make a difference. The inner Self is omnipresent. Its qualities are consistency, reliability, persistence, and devotion. It is more devoted to us that we are to it. Grace is its nature. When we feel in touch with the Self, we will feel this consistency of love

---

51. Swami Abhayananda (trans.), *The Nectar of Self Awareness (Amritanubhav) of Jnaneshwar Maharaj* (Oakland: SYDA Foundation, 1979).

and devotion. It is outside of cause and effect, and yet our love for the Self seemingly manifests as freedom from burdens and an aura of profound serenity. Its Grace comes from you emptying your mind of a personal agenda. "May thy will not mine be done" is both the prayer and the experience of those who have submitted to the Divine. From this experience comes a lasting peace, no matter what life situations bring to you.

## Communing with the Divine Mother—Devi Puja

How are we to understand this concept of the Divine Mother? I suspect that most of my readers have not had the blessing of a devotional upbringing, let alone one focused on the Divine Mother figure. This is something organic and personal to everyone, and yet it is unknown without deep introspection aided by spiritual texts and a persistent spiritual teacher.

When Daniel Odier encountered his Tantrika Devi teacher, they had a most intriguing dialogue.

> "Tell me about your first experience of awakening."

> "If I am here, it is precisely because I haven't had any awakening experience."

> "If you haven't had any experience of awakening, I can't do anything for you. . . . Without prior experience of awakening, no asceticism, no practice, no meditation bears fruit. Without awakening experience there is no source, and since all Tantric sadhana consists of returning to the source, one wanders, not knowing where to go."[52]

The Divine Mother is the love expressed outside of selfish agendas. In a dialogue between two women, Lila (a queen, whose name symbolizes the play of consciousness unique to each one's search for their True Self) and Sarasvati Devi, Lila asks Sarasvati to grant her a boon to always be with her husband, even after his physical death. Sarasvati replies, in *Vasistha's Yoga* (p. 74):

---

52. Daniel Odier, *Tantric Quest* (Rochester, VT: Inner Traditions, 1997), 51.

I do not really do anything to anyone. Every soul earns its own state by its own deeds. I am merely the power of its consciousness and its life force. Whatever form the energy of the living being takes within itself that alone comes to fruition in course of time. In other words, whatever you long for will manifest due to your devotional persistence.

You never need fear God.

No human object ever had the power
to do anything against God's will.[53]

Remember to persist in your practice, yet stay detached from expecting specific outcomes. Tantra is a personal spiritual practice. When you feel complete with this lesson, read the Dialogue section that follows prior to beginning lesson 11.

**With Great Respect and Love, I Honor
My Heart, My Inner Teacher.**

## Dialogue with Mukunda

**Student:** There seems to be a synchronicity this week between what I am reading and hearing about the feminine deities. Yesterday, I was reading about the goddesses referred to in Tantra, and just a short while later a friend began speaking with me about Kali. I have started reading *At the Eleventh Hour* by Pandit Rajmani Tigunait and, in chapter 2, there is a reference to the goddess Chinnamasta, the goddess of Yogis. The author speaks of how Babaji followed her practice. When you refer to Goddess, are you referring to the Divine Mother, or to another deity?

**Mukunda:** My definition of Divine Mother is formless, but She takes the form of various Goddesses and Devis, and as every woman. From my persistent seeking of Grace, I have come to know Her as the true Divine Mother. In this fullness, She is the entire world—matter, energy, and pure consciousness. By getting to know Her forms, I lessen my vagueness, and Her Shakti comes to me more strongly. Nice to hear of your connection to Her. As

---

53. Ramesh Balsekar, public talk in Mumbai, India, January 12, 2002.

you described in your opening sentence, there is a huge synchronicity among those who seek Her. Namaste.

**Student:** I was reading over my Wichita, Oct. 2002 notes. As part of the complete vata program, you said: "Extend your prana through your wish to be of help with the emotion of empathy … clearing fear of being empathic, as in 'I am afraid to become like you,' absorbing others issues … and that you can stay protected by developing a relationship with a form of the Divine, not formless God." I discussed this idea with my friend, Annie, with whom I trade private yoga sessions for massage/energy healing (Barbara Brennan School). We are discovering many similarities between us. Both of us have a long history of being empathic and feeling responsible for others' feelings. She is very sensitive and, despite much training, has difficulty not absorbing her clients' issues, many of whom are very ill. She has experienced a great deal of pain, illness, and fatigue since beginning this type of work. She said the above-mentioned ideas on empathy "hit her right between the eyes." In myself, I have noticed improvement in lessening pain as I extend empathy through teaching (in your approach, not before), yet I can still get overwhelmed by the more intense/ill students.

We realized that we have both been reluctant to select just one form to focus on (Annie has studied many beliefs and forms and has a strong connection to Spirit from different traditions) and we both have preferred a formless God, the closest form being Nature.

Although I am feeling some beginnings of connection in Devi puja, Annie has asked me to find out more about empathy/Divine protection, and this is of great interest to me as well. Tantra lesson 10 seems relevant to this. Is this protection (from fear of empathy) a purpose of the Devi puja? Concentrating on and feeling the four forms of the Divine Mother? Developing a personal relationship with one in particular? Or with all four equally, and contemplating their Oneness? If I am on the right track here, would it be okay to share this lesson with her?

**Mukunda:** This is a very common problem of people doing energy work. One needs to keep clear of clients' energy. The safest training is to learn to use your energy, not to influence someone else, but only to perceive them. Otherwise, you cannot help but bring some "detrimental energy" back from working with them. This is due to avidya—that is, ignorance of the difference between the two of you. From that develops an unhealthy boundary, which, in turn, is not healthy technique. This, in turn, creates the illusion that you can give or receive energy from someone else. The primal form for energy work was covered earlier in lesson 6 as Tantra Prana Bodywork. The key is to understand the experience of your energy body as leaking, clogged, or sluggish, which, in turn, is detrimental to psychic, psychological, and physical health. My method is based on using my prana only to detect the situation and work with a client's field, not interact with it. Prana is omnipresent; therefore, to assume it can shift is avidya, according to the *Yoga Sutras* II, 3–5.

Since you have both preferred a formless God, it must be true that the formless one is all pervasive, affirming the bottom line of all traditions. Which is also to say that the details vary, but only the conclusion can be acceptable. Although God/dess is formless, it is only through sensory experience that we come to know and experience it—and thus it is through form.

The conditioned mind has preferences for different forms of God/dess, just as it may have preferences for the void, the formless form. As long as the conditioned mind predominates, there remains the sense of difference between your Self and the one you are seeking. (See *Yoga Sutras* I, 21: "For those who have an intense urge for Spirit and Spirit's wisdom, it sits near them waiting.")

With reference to the Devi puja, its purpose is to get to know the forms of the Devi that Divine Mother assumes both externally and internally. By this practice, one will naturally feel comfortable with some and unfamiliar or uncomfortable with others. Through persisting in this Tantrik sadhana, devotion becomes awakened because of the inherent feelings of oneness with that toward which you direct your awareness. For me, Tantrik Yoga without devotion leads to self-centeredness and perhaps even to arrogance. Devotion is the quality that purifies us and allows us really to know the Oneness. It is fine to share my response with your friend. If she wishes to do the lesson, it is open to all who ask. Spiritual practices are given freely. Blessings.

**Student:** I had an understanding so deep today that my inner body is still vibrating, my heart beating in happiness at such a deep level. Simple, but for me very profound: The connection between living and speaking the truth and Shakti. Since Shakti manifests Herself as the alphabet, if you do not speak the truth, you are going against the Self. So, in that way, you almost cancel out your Self, who you are, why you are here. I'm having problems putting it into words, but the depth of my understanding of the importance of this is incredible! I do now understand the power of one's words at such a deeper level.

*Mukunda:* Indeed, when you fall in love with yourself, the truth must manifest. The Truth and Shakti are the same. Until that experience predominates, they are both veiled, covered by the koshas, the perception of difference. When the veils are lifted, there is nothing but Shakti. All sounds are that One. In fact, She is called Matrika Shakti—the Mother of Sound. She creates and embodies all sound of all creatures and all movement is Her expression. Whatever moves, moves in Her and makes a joyful sound crying out to Her. This is a profound Tantrik science—the science of pulsation described in the *Spandakarika* text and expounded in the Devi Mahatmyam, the Gayatri Mantra, and so many other Devi texts and teachings. Blessings.

*Student:* I can't remember exactly what I saw, but I felt an energy around the second chakra area, though something told me it was really more about the first chakra. The energy was very strong and noticeable. The context in which I typically feel this energy is one that confuses me. It is usually with a male teacher, and I feel sexual energy. It's as if I feel drawn to the person, or to their energy, and it is pure and harmless and loving, but then I start thinking it is sexual. I know it's not, but the only sensations I have ever known in that region and in that way have been sexual. So, in the visualization, I felt this strong, intense, potent, red heat or energy. It was easier to identify in that state of consciousness, but I am wondering if you can explain this energy a little more.

*Mukunda:* Indeed, it is sexual energy, which is difficult for most of us to distinguish from emotional energy, moods, and sensuality. After all, the home of these energies is the first two chakras, barely two inches apart. It is compounded by the fact that prana, as emotional energy, is highly mobile. So what is felt in the genitals feels clearly sexual, but the same pranic energy in the heart is translated as love or compassion. A subtler level of the same prana is experienced as a mental energy fluctuation called a vasana—a subtle memory from which you associate this particular energetic pattern as being sexual. All energy, when followed, fully leads to higher consciousness—both higher subtler koshas and higher chakras. The challenge is not to hold it back by your initial impressions. As you allow the sexual energy to be what it feels like—that is, sexual—it will transform to spiritual energy with persistence. Sexual energy opens all others above it to become elevated. You are doing well to maintain your curiosity with caution and not to act on these impulses with your teachers. Instead, keep this reflection to yourself or share it with your female yogic friends.

*Student:* With the practice of lesson 10, I was able to feel a physical opening of my upper body; I am able now to breathe fully into my open chest and can fully appreciate the wave breath. During that evening's practice of opening suppressed energy, I felt a burning sensation in my left hand and arm that was placed over my heart; then, for a moment, my physical body disappeared. With this opening, I have been able to trust in my relationship with my husband further and let go of my fear of his possible rejection and the pain that would follow. I also realized that I had become invested in his spiritual development, so I have now fully entrusted that task to him—only he knows what is best for him. And then I was able to release the pain of fear and rejection that resided in my right hip. I also am now able to nurture myself. I had not been able to cook for the longest time, and now I am in the kitchen enjoying the preparation of foods again. I am once again able to savor the tastes and flavors of love and life!

*Mukunda:* Wonderful. A great example of what I shared previously—that if you are not getting lessons, just move on. The energy is there, awakening within you, and you will get what you can handle in time. I created a list of attainments from each lesson and placed them at the back of the book so you can see how you are being transformed.

*Student:* Tonight, I experienced stillness with Tara and Saraswati. As I moved to honoring Lakshmi, an upward motion took hold, drawing my diaphragm up into my rib cage and holding it there for some time. In the back of my mind, I wondered if I would need to breathe sometime soon. When the mind took over, I released the pause (*kumbhaka*), and it happened again. Afterward, I logically thought this was Lakshmi taking my understanding of abundance from a lower realm to a higher one. Then, on to Kali—immediate flame engulfing my heart, again strong stomach lock (uddiyana bandha), and a strong breath retention, this time focused in my chest, which resulted in my feeling my chest was being sucked into itself. Retention was not as long. Then I practiced tratak (fixed gazing) on the Bhadra Kali picture you sent from your trip to Ganeshpuri. My intention was, as with the flame, to feel the connection between myself and the object, then remove that visual connection and feel the inner presence, detaching from the form. The form, very blurry by now, kept pulling me forward toward her, physically, over and over again. Finally, I closed my eyes and felt how She called to me. I bowed to that calling, asking for continued guidance toward making me a worthy vessel for Her Grace to come through. The night before, during the tratak practice, there was fear. I do not know if, in this practice, I am feeling a spiritual communion. I feel as if I am taking much and not coming from a place of devotion. It feels very self-centered, selfish.

***Mukunda:*** The spontaneous and frequent arousal of purification (kriyas) over a long period shows that Shakti Kundalini Devi is awakened. Grace is given you as perfected techniques arise spontaneously. When kriyas like uddiyana bandha and kumbhaka arise with more intimacy than those learned from an outer teacher, this is a sign of blessings.

Practice is called practice for a good reason. Patanjali, in *Yoga Sutras* I, 12, says that practice does not bear consistent benefits unless it is carried out over a longer period of time with persistent devotion and detachment from the results. Often, one is doing good practice and what is given is a dharana not a samadhi. Dharana is feeling the presence; dhyana is communing with that presence; samadhi is merging oneself and losing that self into the Divine. Sometimes, they flow together into what Patanjali calls samyama (see *Yoga Sutras* III), sometimes not. Practice requires persistence and patience. Remember that work is not done until God/dess is done with you. Consider Her as your Inner Teacher, as your closest, dearest friend.

***Student:*** When you speak of the Goddess, there is true devotion and love in your voice. I don't feel that. I think of how my children love me so much; I was their universe for so long. And now the separation is beginning; they are moving away from me as they move more into the world. But there remains that spark of true connection and devotion that I think, I hope, I will always feel, and that I hope will remain with them.

Is this the process, to find that spark again as adults? Is it that I have been so far away from that pure love that I can't remember what it is, how it tastes, what it smells and feels like? Will the Goddess always love me, even if I do not love Her? I have heard the Goddess takes 1,000 steps toward you if you take one step toward Her. That has always sounded very nice. But in the midst of this practice, when I feel as if I am showing up to dinner with no flowers to offer mother and my dirty laundry for her to clean, I feel self-conscious, guilty, and not yet wanting to accept that and take in the love.

***Mukunda:*** Indeed, these concepts are there in the mind. The mind searches, and the Self reveals. The distance is nothing, but to the conditioned mind, it can seem insurmountable. By persistent seeking of love, it is felt and experienced with all its wonderful emotionality and passion. Cultivating passion and emotionality in all activities brings the Self closer to you. Patanjali says that, according to the passion you have for the divine, so is its closeness to you (*Yoga Sutras* I, 21–22). The more intense the urge, the greater Spirit's closeness. This is why the Tantrikas search themselves for ways to become increasingly passionate in all activities devoted to Her. It is that passion that pulls Her toward you. She is the prana at first, in lessons 1 through 4; later, She is the emotions; later still, She is the Shakti/Kundalini; then She is seen as the All.

It is a gradual process, until you fall into Her arms and She holds you fully there. Just search and you will find all that you are capable of holding at this moment. She is love; it is not a question of how much She loves you. Finding Her, you find that you are also love. The Tantrika uses all experiences as offerings, so give Her also your self-consciousness, guilt, and self-centeredness. These emotions—although negative to you—are received by Her as a gift of submission that allows Her to give you the only present She has, which is Grace. She accepts all that you don't accept. When you give to Her the undesirable as well as what you hold precious, you get the fullness of Her. She is all forms of maternity— disciplinarian, teacher, wise woman, sage, lust-filled whore, and scoundrel. As you are, so is She. Allow all these forms to manifest in your meditations. All is going quite well. Namaste.

**Student:** I know I had shared over the weekend about my image of the Goddess as Glinda, the good witch from the movie *The Wizard of Oz*. But I am having trouble in a conscious way bringing Goddess/Mother energy into my life. I have been chanting more to the feminine energy; I have been dreaming about women saints; I have been drawn to connecting to that energy. But, strangely enough, it all feels subconscious or unconscious. It is as if a part of my being *knows* and is just going there without the okay from my conscious rational mind. And that's good and nice. But I want to be able to act on this consciously and bring this feminine energy into myself with intention. Any thoughts on making conscious contact with the Feminine Goddess Mother energy?

**Mukunda:** Spending time with women spiritual teachers can definitely help. Ammachi, Anandi Ma, and Karunamayi do world tours regularly. Look to meet them when possible. Also, reading stories of women goddesses and learning their archetypal stories can promote that connection within you. See how they are, within you, also attempting to break free of your personality. Each goddess is within your first three chakras. Beyond that, they become without form. So it builds your devotion to feel them in any quality you perceive. See how your own first chakra manifests as creativity, your second chakra as nurturing, and your third chakra forms your mind's desire to become transformed or elevated as Goddess.

**Student:** As far as the energy you described in the chakras, can you describe more about the second chakra's nurturing capacities? I feel as if I am competent at being nurturing with others, but not with myself. How does that play out with second chakra?

**Mukunda:** As the water chakra, it is emotional in nature—crying, sadness, juicy feelings that also extend to saliva's enjoyment of taste (ojas) and the sexual moisture (amrita) of being aroused. As this region is ruled by Lakshmi, it is sensual and cultivates wealth and abundance. She has another dual form as Devis of Sri Dhari and Bhudevi; both are the nurturing consorts of Vishnu. They all take multitudes of forms. As Lakshmi, these are manifested as spiritual wealth, feelings of omnipresence of spirit, and being immersed in Her as a fish in the ocean. There is nothing but Her. Second is Mother Earth—voluptuous in another way, breasts fill and swell during your menstrual cycles, and also during arousal of the water element in a woman's body. Their consort is Vishnu, also called Krishna, Govinda, Mukunda, Gajendra, etc. This quality is one of nurturing the Shakti, taking care of His consort so She is encouraged to be fulfilled happily in all Her maternal and nurturing actions.

**Student:** I have been/am working on surrender. And then I realized that all that I am grateful for has been given to me by God/dess. How can I not surrender? She created me, and takes care of me; of course I belong to Her. Barrier discarded. And the other day, as I finished reflecting on *Yoga Sutras* III 1–3, I realized that it was your gentle, loving guidance that brought me to my morning practice and meditation—to this point where I understand why to practice dharana and where I can, at times, experience moments of stillness and emptiness. All this and what is to come is because of you. And then I thought, what if I surrendered to you in an hour-long hug at our next meeting? I am acutely aware that I pull away. Suddenly, a flow of energy entered me as I was doing the joint-freeing series. Grace was the only word that came to my mind. I stopped so I could be still with this flow and stayed with it until it passed. I don't know what it was, but it was beautiful. Thank you.

**Mukunda:** All is proceeding very nicely for you. I am delighted at your commitment to being immersed in such a profound Spirit-filled experience. Blessings.

***Student:*** I was rereading Tantra lesson 10 last night. It has been helping me to center once again. I've now been in Italy for four months, and I'm going through the monkey-mind process of Why did I quit my job? What will I do when I return in November? Did I make the wrong decision? Help.

I know the answers to some of the questions. For others, I know it is not the time yet to look for answers. I go in and out of trust, knowing I'm guided always, yet the new surroundings and being so far from home make it challenging at times. I make time for yoga each morning, as that helps me calm down and surrender to the beauty of life. I don't make enough time for meditation, which I want to do. I found such inspiration in Tantra lesson 10. I know a teacher will help to guide me along my path so that I will continue to progress. That was the guidance I found in you when I was in touch with you last year. I would like to continue this path with you. I recognized such peace and beauty in you. That happened from the first time I saw you in Phoenix. Also, your teachings resonate in me. I have a copy of *Vasistha's Yoga* with me—it is the only book I brought. I'm reading a bit each day. The area I want to work on most right now is acceptance; that is a challenge for me. I find that, once again, I am moving into an area of judgment.

***Mukunda:*** My main recommendation is to spend more time doing sadhana and reading *Vasistha's Yoga*. I especially recommend that you read chapter 1 two or three times before moving on with the rest of the book. I am giving annual ten-day retreats in India at my guru's ashram on this text. It is the most sublime text, as it contains all teachings in one. My guru called it a spiritual warehouse of his tradition.

Don't assign yourself to fate. The decisive factor is your self-effort to move ahead and connect more deeply to Spirit. Give yourself a stronger willpower by persisting in this sadhana. There is nothing that does transformation like these qualities. To be really ready for initiation, one must take all care and persist. Blessings.

***Student:*** I am writing you with great joy and warmth. As you are well aware of all of the signs I told you I was experiencing about fertility and the connection Tantra has given me to myself and my husband and daughter over the last months, I am pleased to give you the news that I am pregnant (less than a month)! I took an EPT test yesterday that confirmed what I was feeling. My husband and infant are in tune with the fertility as well. Imagine that! My husband saw a man stopping traffic for a mama duck and her ducklings a week ago and told me he thought I was pregnant for having seen the procession.

**Mukunda:** That is wonderful news! I am so delighted for you and your family. The Tantrik lessons are well-known for heightening fertility. My last spiritual teacher, Swami Prakashananda, taught me an energy transmission that a teacher can give a sincere student to promote fertility through the scope of Tantrik sadhana. He was renowned for having helped many couples conceive. He was a devotee of Divine Mother as Suptashring Devi. She has the form of a sacred mountain in Western India five hours from Mumbai, where an eighteen-armed image has manifested.

With reference to your husband's story, here is one from another student that connects Sight with Goddess:

> I recently had my first training show of selling jewelry in my house. It was a night of my family and friends enjoying adorning ourselves. I loved it! Well, that next morning at 4:30 a.m., Sierra woke up for milk and comfort. She lay beside me nursing, and I tried to rest back to sleep. I had a calling to lift my head up and look toward my altar, which is in our bedroom. I looked and I saw a shadow vision of a tree goddess. Her legs were roots in the Earth and her hips the trunk. It was a side view of a pregnant belly, with her left hand supporting her back. Her ample breasts were resting and her right hand rested on her head with the elbow lifted. The branches flowered from her head. I lowered my head and thought "Am I really seeing this?" So I looked up again and she was still there, so grounded, sensual, and statuesque. Then she disappeared.
>
> I put my baby back in her crib and wrote down what had happened. I drew the image too. I began telling the mothers in my life who I knew would understand, and kept it sacred within me. So wonderful and comforting to know that Goddess has given me a vision and now it is true. This is so amazing to me. I feel as if the mystical is here with me when I put all of these "peeks" of time into One. So many secrets that I have kept secret are starting to come into my consciousness and, instead of being afraid, as I once was of Sight, I now feel the music of my life's song. Thank you for opening the door to Goddess' gifts and the divine. Without you, I wouldn't be so grounded in this knowing, right now, of how connected we all are.

This is a wonderful story. God/dess indeed manifests—as *apsaras*, tree spirits, and many other forms. There are many stories of Devi manifesting, but the greatest is manifesting within you and evolving you into a unique expression of Devi, which means a "being of light."

The Goddess of fertility is primarily Lakshmi, who rules the second chakra, physically located at the cervix. Other aspects are Kamala—a Goddess who creates the beauty and love necessary for fertility—and Vajrayoni—a Goddess whose womb is filled with thunder. In each village, there are Devis unique to the needs of that environment; all are considered to possess the blessings of fertility. Normally, this cannot exist alone. A Devi temple that has a yoni as the *sanctum sanctorum* must be near to a Deva temple of some aspect of Shiva where the lingam is worshipped. The lingam is a naturally arising stone in the shape of a phallus from the Narmada River in North India and Nepal. Or to a Vishnu temple where the *shaligram* (a special spiral fossilized shell sacred to Vishnu) is honored. The lingam, the yoni, the shaligram, and the vajrayoni can all be empowered by sadhana and the blessings of spiritual teachers. A sign of a true spiritual teacher is that he or she is able to give tangible blessings to householders, whether they are seeking healthy children, health for family members, or abundance.

There are many books about Tantra as it relates to the Devi; you'll find a recommended reading list at the end of this book. Some specific ones I recommend are David Frawley's *Tantric Yoga and the Wisdom Goddesses*, which gives an overview of the ten major Devis, and *Devi: The Mother Goddess* by Devdutt Pattanaik, a lovely book on all the aspects of Devis.

**Student:** I was beautifully touched by all the students' questions and comments and how their inquiries are similar to mine. I feel connected to Bhadra Kali too, and I find the Bhadra Kali puja from your CD, *Mukunda Chants*, irresistible. I am chanting it with you all the time! I find that, when I am dancing or teaching dance, I feel the currents of energy, and I redirect them to specific parts of the body. They feel pretty big in mass and weight. However, when I am still, they become small, and I cannot totally tell where they are moving. They are hard to follow. Do you have any suggestions?

**Mukunda:** How sweet that you enjoy Bhadra Kali so much. It is most powerful and lovely to dance with Her also. That is a beautiful way to move, dancing to some favorite prana current in the Tantrik tandava dance. Tandava means "eternal dance." It is done from a standing or seated posture, as you allow stillness or motion to lead to a spontaneous shift in either direction. At this time, it has mass indeed. In seated meditation, the prana becomes subtler, as it is seeking to go to deeper koshas. When so doing, it is not operating from the chakras, which is their normal method of expansion for physical activities. So meditation is learning how to refine and yet sustain the energy connection. Thus, a way to enhance your sensitivity to deeper pranic currents is to alternate dance with seated subtle motions. By seeking, you can create a tandava dance that will also purify. A purification action (kriya) may create and release motions or emotions, which in turn will promote heightened consciousness of the eternal dance of life force. Just continue to train with lesson 7, and you will become more responsive to these forms of the Devi's language.

**Student:** There are still many memories coming back to me from the child abuse, but there is no emotion attached to them now. WOW! Blessings, hope all is well with you.

**Mukunda:** It is good to hear of your persistence, that is the key to success wit this sadhana. Namaste.

# PART IV

# Spiritual Awakening

# Initiation and Spiritual Awakening

With Great Respect and Love, I Honor
My Heart, My Inner Teacher.

Y ou cannot force or grasp a spiritual experience, because it is as delicate as the whisper of the wind. But you can purify your motivation, your body, and train yourself to cultivate it. Because we come from a culture that teaches us that there is always something external to be obtained that will lead us to fulfillment, we lose contact with our innate wisdom. As the Indian Tantric Buddhist saint Saraha says:

Though the house lamps have been lit,
The blind live on in the dark.
Though spontaneity is all-encompassing and close,
To the deluded it remains
Always far away.

Spiritual Awakening is enhanced by devotion to the Divine of your understanding. Let us review some aphorisms on Divine Love from Narada's *Bhakti Sutras*, presented in lesson 5. Notice how cultivating love and devotion, stillness and freedom from extraneous thinking creates the flowering of the heart of Bhakti. Encourage the blossoming of your spiritual devotion for the flowering of love. This quality is crucial. It needs to be protected from the twisted karma that may come up as you unwind and make your way through the unique mix of energetic openings and blocks. Safety is crucial as you tread the path, regardless of how far you rise. Here are some select sutras to reflect upon.

> Sutra 7. Spiritual devotion does not arise from desire. Its nature is a state of inner stillness.

> Sutra 8. The inner stillness consecrates the performance of worldly and traditional social duties.

> Sutra 9. Inner stillness, furthermore, requires a single hearted intention, and disinterest in what is antagonist to spiritual devotion.

> Sutra 10. When one is single-hearted, one relinquishes seeking security in anything other than God.[54]

The *Avadhuta Gita*, a text of non-dual Advaita Vedanta, begins with this sutra:

> It is only through the Grace of God that in people with knowledge, is born a desire to experience unity, a desire which also protects them from the great dangers of the illusions of worldliness.[55]

When awakening happens, a wide variety of signposts reveals the uniqueness of the path the seeker will take to cultivate the gift of Grace. One of these signs is that the awakened Shakti is contagious. This is why forming a meditation group or satsang is helpful, because as you experience the awakening of your neighbor, it is often accompanied by similar movement patterns in others. The experiences occur across all of the senses and will be detailed in the next lesson. There is an automatic protection for seekers, regardless of whether they are sincere or insincere. My favorite spiritual guidebook, the *Yoga Vasistha* says: "If the teaching falls on a qualified heart, it expands in that intelligence. It does not stay in the unqualified heart."[56]

Another major sign of transformation is the beginning of the loss of self-centeredness and the tendency to help others, regardless of their difficulties. Those

---

54. Prem Prakash, *The Yoga of Spiritual Devotion* (Rochester, VT: Inner Traditions, 1998), 19–25.
55. *Avadhuta Gita*. Ramakrishna Vedanta Society, Calcutta.
56. *Vasistha's Yoga* VI, 2:17, 16.

"spiritual" teachers without this sign are to be avoided. Being of service to others in suffering is a primal consideration for Yoginis and Tantrikas with integrity. This service arises from the innate love of the Self. Devotion is a naturally arising consequence of yoga sadhana. Spiritual practice redirects our thinking from seeking our own benefit into the question: How can I be of help? In chapter 31 of my book *Structural Yoga Therapy,* you will find a series of sutras that arise from a devotional approach to Classical Yoga meditation based on guidance from Patanjali's *Yoga Sutras.*

> To eliminate obstacles to concentration, practice of a single technique should be followed; the object can be any beloved object. (*Yoga Sutras* I, 32)

> Communion (Samadhi) is gained through devotion to your own chosen form of the inner Self. (*Yoga Sutras* I, 23)

> Consistent, earnest practice and dispassionate detachment can stop the persistent waves of a vacillating mind thus removing the clouds from obscuring the Self. (*Yoga Sutras* I, 12)

Awakening is rare, yet there is help available to those seeking it. Seekers need to distinguish between their search for a Yogi and a yoga teacher. According to Alice Christensen, "A Yoga teacher must be exceptionally conscientious and professional in their work of transmitting to others the exacting disciplines of Yoga."[57]

Most yoga teachers are not familiar with the signs of spiritual awakening. Most popular forms of yoga are Hatha Yoga given different names for marketing purposes. Classical Yoga incorporates Tantrik techniques dileneated in Patanjali's *Yoga Sutras.* Those who follow the teachers and texts of the tradition are more likely to experience a spiritual awakening.

A Yogi is altogether different from a yoga teacher. Yogis are individuals who clearly know and express that their path is a spiritual journey to God. While yoga teachers may know techniques for relieving pain and stress, creating health, increasing energy, or even providing therapy for psychophysiological issues, a Yogi is a yoga adept who lives a committed lifestyle of one-pointed yoga and spiritual practices. If this is what

---

57. Alice Christensen, *American Yoga Association Beginner's Manual* (New York: Simon & Schuster, 1987), 16.

you wish to develop in yourself, I highly recommend you spend time searching for these qualities in someone who has been a disciple of a spiritual teacher and has been given permission to assist others. I may not be right for you, but I am an example of someone to consider as a yogic spiritual mentor until you find the right one. If you truly wish help, just ask and it is freely given.

## Finding Your Inner Teacher

Contemplate the attributes, location, qualities, and presence of your Inner Teacher. Ask for guidance in some specific arena of your life that is challenging. Do this in the same manner as you sought prana in lesson 1. You know instinctively that your Inner Teacher is there; now seek the form that is most captivating. What you seek with sincerity, you will find. The spiritual community has a common saying: When the student is ready, the teacher appears. If that has not happened, consider the other possibility: When the teacher is ready, the student appears. Find your way to devotion and identify the qualities that generate love within you. Write down any insights or observations that occur during this contemplative meditation and continue to clarify them as you proceed through this lesson.

Put your hands on your heart and repeat the previous exercise, seeking the heart within your heart within that heart. Pray for your Inner Teacher to come to you. You may find that your outer teacher and your Inner Teacher are the same. If so, ask the outer teacher for confirmation. Consider the possibility that your Teacher may not be ready for you. But if She is, then you are doubly blessed. By regularly opening to your Inner Teacher, She (in the form of Shakti prana) will communicate to you on a consistent basis. Trust that process, yet do not hesitate to talk to your outer teacher or spiritual friends for confirmation. Always be alert to staying grounded; sometimes, what students consider to be the Inner Teacher is the ego sense masquerading. By persisting in reading and reflecting on the central text of Patanjali's *Yoga Sutras,* these reminders become ingrained, and your mind will be protected from excessive doubts and uncertainties.

"Success in yoga comes from consistent earnest practice of sadhana over a long period of time with dispassionate detachment from the results of that practice to have success."[58] From following the advice of Patanjali, Vasistha, and other sages, you can protect your attainment, thus increasing the nurturing quality of ojas. Continuing to develop your qualities as a yoga student will naturally bring you to your Inner and outer teachers.

Among the signs of being with your Inner Teacher is the natural progression of thinning the veils of the gross and subtle bodies (koshas). Insights come to the ripe student on a regular basis. Understanding the truth of your spiritual path is intuitive, a sign that the fourth (wisdom) kosha is being accessed regularly. The truth is that each kosha is a function of the Self. The experience of the fourth kosha gives wisdom as spiritual knowledge. The bound student knows this and seeks limited knowledge.

> Knowledge is inherent in consciousness, even as void is in space. However, consciousness now believes knowledge to be its own object. The diverse objects are limited by time and space. Such division does not exist in the Self, which transcends time and space.[59]

In a similar fashion, the experience of thought shows the function and limitations of kosha three (the mind—mano maya kosha). The experience of the senses and of the life force shows kosha two (prana maya kosha). Sensations of the body and health or lack of it reveal the functions of kosha one. Those ripe for higher knowledge, for the spiritual teachings of yoga, do not limit their search to the grosser sensations of koshas one and two. They focus their attention on seeking, not only higher teachings, but how to access the Source of those teachings. To know is good; to understand is better; to know how to find the Source of wisdom is sublime.

> Mind is a field. It is plowed by right action, it is watered day and night by right feeling, and it is nourished by the practice of pranayama. On this field known as the mind the seed known as samadhi, turning away from the world, falls of its own accord when one is alone in the forest known as wisdom. The wise person should endeavor constantly to keep this seed of meditation watered and nourished by intelligent means.

---

58. *Yoga Sutras of Patanjali*, 4.
59. *Vasistha's Yoga*, 396.

When this seed begins to sprout, it should be further protected by peace and contentment. At the same time, one should guard it against the birds of desire, attachment to family, pride, greed, etc. With the broom of right and loving action, the dirt of rajasic restlessness must be swept away, whereas the darkness of tamasic ignorance must be driven away by the light of right understanding. The sprout grows two leaves. One is known as study of scriptures and the other is satsang, company of sages of wisdom.[60]

## Two Forms of Initiation

There are two forms of initiation. In the first, your teacher decides you are ready for a spiritual practice and gives you a mantra, perhaps also a spiritual name, and their blessings to develop your sadhana into an effective path to your true Self.

> Know that all you experience in the name of mind, egosense, intellect, etc., is nothing but ignorance (avidya). This ignorance vanishes through self effort. Half of this ignorance is dispelled by the company of holy ones; one fourth is destroyed by the study of the scriptures and the other one fourth by self effort.[61]

When you find a spiritual mentor or teacher whose words and presence bring you peace, it is important to test them. From the moment that you meet, the event can be suspicious or auspicious. My spiritual teacher recommended testing such a person for a year by following the advice given, doing the practices recommended, and testing the validity of the teachings. Through this mixture of self-effort and devotion, you can discover the integrity of your experience.

How do you recognize your outer teacher? There are several characteristics: Teachers end your doubts; they are readily available to help you; you perceive them as good and wise; you feel safe with them; and you have a willingness to do whatever they recommend for your spiritual life.

---

60. Ibid., 529–30.
61. *Vasistha's Yoga*, 496.

Whoever wishes to enjoy unalloyed happiness, fame and long life, should by all means honor and worship good wo/men, by giving them all that they might wish to have. Wise wo/men, good wo/men, are indeed great benefactors of humanity. When encountering one it is best to utilize this opportunity to clear the doubts that are in the mind: for one is surely a fool who, having the company of a wise wo/man, neglects to clear his doubts.[62]

This is the proper attitude to have when you are testing someone to be your teacher. Baba Muktananda frequently used to say, "your spiritual teacher is the means to the attainment of whatever you seek." Though their actions sometimes seem bizarre, true teachers act only for the improvement of others.

The other form of initiation comes to those who have developed a devotional mind, described in the *Yoga Sutras* as being "consistently concerned with spirituality."[63] This can lead to immersion in God's Grace and the descent of the Holy Spirit. In this form, there is a transmission of the awakened spiritual energy into the student. This is the secret, yet true, form of all initiations. In the Tantrik language, the Holy Spirit is the Divine Mother. She manifests in the human body as an energetic force called *Kundalini*, which means "coiled serpent," an apt description of how its awakening may be felt—as the motion of a snake up or down the central energy channel near the spine. The upward-rising energy is called Shiva, hence the upward-pointing triangle or lingam is its symbol. The descending energy is Shakti, symbolized by the yoni-shaped triangle. Most students of willful Kundalini Yoga experience the ascending force of Shiva, while devotees of Shakti tend to have descending energies predominate.

For those who have had an awakening, what is often needed is a teacher who has undergone and sustained an awakening—one who can keep the lamp lit. The key elements for Tantrik transformation are a technique and a teacher who can impart awakened energy and guide your energy to its fullest expression. Only a Yogi or Tantrik master can give you the awakened prana Shakti that they have received from their teacher. In my own case, I received the awakened spiritual energy from my guru, Swami Muktananda Paramahansa. This occurred in 1974; it was followed by

---

62. *Vasistha's Yoga*, 99–100.
63. *Yoga Sutras of Patanjali*, I, 20, 6.

eight years of sadhana under my guru's guidance and continues to evolve thirty-five years later. Muktananda taught some advanced disciples, including myself, how to guide students through the process of Kundalini awakening and how to give *shakti-pat*, which means literally the "descent of Shakti."

Before my Baba passed, on October 10, 1982, he sent me to his chosen successor, Swami Prakashananda, who gave me teachings in devotional Tantrik practices to the Divine Mother in the form of Suptashring Devi. As a result of following their teachings for over thirty years, I now counsel students from diverse backgrounds to understand the mysterious process of their awakening. Since I am neutral, not promoting a specific lineage, students feel safer in having their own clarity in their personal sadhana. The task of the student and teacher is to transform both into a spirit-guided lifestyle.

Shaktipat initiation is a transmission that connects you to the siddhas, the masters of the Nath lineage. In my case, this has led to inner guidance that continues beyond the death of my guru in 1982. I have never felt myself without guidance since my initiation. Without such continuity, those who experience prana are merely given a taste, but do not drink from a deep well. In the secret Tantrik teachings, a student receives Shakti from his or her teacher; it then descends into the student taking the form called shaktipat. The prana moves downward and inward to these spiritually blessed students.

Spiritual awakening occurs in the spinal channel called sushumna. The sushumna nadi contains past-life memories, including the memory of previous awakening. Coming into consciousness with the unique form that this has taken in the past will enable you to merge in the sushumna to the place where spiritual continuity has left off. The force called prana has several forms and functions. As prana, it performs all the functions of health and consciousness. In the form called Shakti, its functions are concerned with Grace and the development of humility. In the form of Kundalini, the same prana awakens from its gross function to realize a spiritual direction. Kundalini prana moves upward, piercing the chakras through the seeker's effort, gradually opening the door to sushumna nadi. In contrast, shaktipat moves downward.

For some individuals, the prana Shakti has chosen them, rather than the reverse. Some feel that spiritual awakening without a teacher is dangerous due to the confusion and chaos that results from spontaneous energy moving in the body and mind. In my experience, fear of the unknown, without devotion to its source—the

Unknowable—is where the danger is most pronounced. When students can point to a physical source of the awakening (a teacher), they are relieved of their worries by the teacher's depth of experience. Those without a teacher need Grace and understanding in order to feel safe and nurtured by being in the hands of someone bigger than you.

There are other cultures in which spiritual awakening is described in a spiritual language that is similar to Indian teachings. In the teachings of Tibetan Tantrik Buddhism known as *Dzogchen*, this process is called a transmission:

> In the Sutras it is taught that enlightenment is only possible after many lifetimes dedicated to practice; in the Tantras on the other hand, it is said that one can reach enlightenment in one single lifetime, because the methods used are much more effective. The "Great Transference into the Body of Light" is spoken of. This particular realization was accomplished by masters such as Padmasambhava (the founder of Tibetan Tantra), involves the transference or reabsorption, with a physical death, of the material body into the luminous essence of the elements, in the course of which realization the physical body disappears from the sight of ordinary beings. . . . This realization depends not only on the specific methods found in Dzogchen, but primarily on the function of the transmission from the master.[64]

The second line here reminds me of the shifts into the subtler luminous koshas described in Patanjali's *Yoga Sutras* II, 52.

Initiation transforms the mind and our experience of the world. All the elements of the multi-dimensional body/mind/Spirit are restructured. The transformation is spoken of in the *Yoga Sutras* in several passages. In chapter III, sutras 9 through 13 describe the changes, not only in the stability of the mind, but also the constitutional elements that make up the physical body. This transformation also manifests within the three Ayurvedic doshas. Although the word *dosha* literally means "that which is unstable," following initiation, the mind becomes more sattvic, producing equanimity to the many changes that are occurring. An overview of the mind's new perspective

---

64. Chogyal Namkhai Norbu, *Dzogchen: The Self-Perfected State* (Ithaca, NY: Snow Lion Publications, 1996), 62–63.

when the doshas—kapha, pitta, or vata—transform into the higher dimensions is given in *The Yoga Vasistha*.[65]

The elements of the body are unstable; therefore, a return to the Source is an intriguing point of contemplation. Tantrik experience is a recreation of the primal sound resonating as your body. The yogic symbol for the primal sound, which is the source of all things, is *AUM*. The AUM phonetically begins with the sound "Aah" and moves to "Uuu," then the audible sound terminates with "Mmm." I call it the dial tone of the universe. When we hear this sound, we can dial the number (repeat our mantra) that will place the call straight to our chosen deity as the source of all sound. The sound continues beyond the audible into the state of transcendence, both symbolic and experiential. The practice of intoning AUM returns the elements to their source.

In striking a similar cord, the Christian Gospel of Saint John begins thus:

> In the beginning was the Word; and the Word was with God and the
> Word was God. She was with God in the beginning, and through Her all
> things came to be, not one thing had its being but through Her.[66]

The symbol for this unstruck sound is a dot. Around this dot is a downward-pointing equilateral triangle. This is called yoni, the Mother, whose subtle form is the feeling of "sacred space." A natural evolution from this sacred space is the manifestation of the male counterpart called the lingam, meaning first "form" or "wand of Light." His symbol is an upward-pointing equilateral triangle. When they are in harmony, the symbol of the Star of David is created. In yogic language, this is the symbol of the whirling vortex on the spiritual dimension called the heart chakra. When male and female are in harmony, the spinning chakra motion ceases and the unitive symbol is experienced as mind/bodies in communion.

## Balancing the Fulfillment of Worldliness and Spirituality

As I mentioned at the beginning of lesson 1, according to the first Classical Yoga text, Patanjali's *Yoga Sutras*, the purpose of life is the dual experience of enjoyment of

---

65. *Vasistha's Yoga*, 640–42.
66. Neil Douglas Klutz (trans.), *Prayers of the Cosmos* (New York: Harper Collins, 1994).

worldliness and spiritual liberation. This same message is delivered in three sutras; no other topic is addressed with such deliberate persistence.

> The seen world has the qualities of luminosity, activity, and
> stability.
> It is embodied through the elements and the sense organs.
> It exists for the dual purpose of sensory enjoyment and liberation
> of the Self. (II, 18)
> For the sake of the Self alone
> does the seen world exist. (II, 21)
> The mind accumulates countless desires,
> although it exists solely for the sake of being close
> to the True Self. (IV, 24)[67]

The *Yoga Sutras* is not unique among yogic texts in seeking the harmony of spiritual and worldly life. The same message is delivered repeatedly in the *Guru Gita*, the song of love from the guru Shiva to his wife and consort, Parvati. She reverently asked him: "May I know the truth of the Guru's role? Please initiate me as my guru. By which path can a human being become one with the Absolute? Have compassion on me!"[68]

Of its 182 aphorisms, many are dedicated to the fulfillment of all aspects of life, citing that worldliness and spiritual attainments are not contrary to each other. Here is a sampling of the aphorisms on how to attain the fulfillment of worldly virtuous goals and spiritual liberation.

> Preface. I sing this song to win the gift of love, as I fulfill the
> goals of life—righteousness (dharma), wealth (artha), pleasure
> (kama)—along with liberation (Moksha).
> Sutra 87. O great goddess, meditation on the Guru grants all joy,
> always brings happiness, and gives worldly fulfillment as well as
> liberation.
> Sutra 165. All life's pleasures will come to one who chants the
> Guru Gita,

---

67. *Yoga Sutras of Patanjali*, 21, 53.
68. Swadhyaya Sudha, *The Nectar of Chanting* (Ganeshpuri, India: Shree Gurudev Ashram, 1978), 7–8.

along with liberation, O Parvati.

Wealth and liberation belongs to that one

and on their lips dances the goddess of wisdom—Sarasvati.

Sutra 166. All the powers that can be gained,

All the pleasures that wealth can bring,

Along with liberation belongs to one

Who sings this sacred Guru hymn.

Sutra 177. Victory is assured to one devoted to their Guru

Who sings this song when they are facing death.

All their journeys are made with ease;

In all endeavors they will succeed.

Sutra 180. O Goddess reveal this mysterious text only unto that one

Whose mind is spiritually matured, filled with reverence and devotion

O dear beloved, you are my very Self forever.


This song from the Purana, Sri Skanda,

This song of Shiva to Parvati,

I offer Thee, O Gurudev —

A gift of the goddess Sarasvati.

Remember to persist in your practice, yet stay detached from expecting specific outcomes. Tantra is a personal spiritual practice. When you feel complete with this lesson, read the Dialogue section that follows prior to beginning lesson 12.

## With Great Respect and Love, I Honor My Heart, My Inner Teacher.

## Dialogue with Mukunda

**Student:** The idea and discussion of dispassion bother me when I think about it. Is passion by itself attached to an end result, or is it just a yearning that hopefully becomes experience? Is dispassion experiencing passion but not being attached to its outcome? In

Tantrik partner practice, it seems that passion is allowed to express itself, and be quieted to a sattvic place. Is sattva dispassion?

*Mukunda:* I appreciate your persistence at asking deep questions based on doing your sadhana with passion. Both passion and dispassion can be sattvic (harmonious), or rajasic (over expressed), or tamasic (suppressed). Passion that is rajasic is attached to an outcome. Tamasic passion is not really caring what happens, whereas sattvic passion is healthy non-attachment. In Tantrik practice, there is an intention to allow naturally arising passion to be expressed. In cases where it has been suppressed, or tamasic, it will naturally become balanced by moving through a rajasic expression, which is then to be gently guided into a sattvic meditation experience as an opening of the heart. It is this state of mind that is sattvic. Thus, when we experience a sattvic state and are free, there will be a natural expression of all the emotions—even passion—and the mind is empty of criticism yet fully self-accepting due to the presence of dispassion. *Vasistha's Yoga* comments on this subject (pp. 132–134):

> The seed of this world appearance is ignorance (avidya); without being seen as "this is it," this ignorance has the quality of truth! This mental conditioning dies when not fed by attachment to objects; but even in the absence of such attachment, it continues to remain as a potentiality. This ignorance or mental conditioning is acquired effortlessly and it seems to promote pleasure, but in truth it is the giver of grief. It creates a delusion of pleasure only by the total veiling of self knowledge; it perverts all relationships and experiences. It is desire that is ignorance of mental conditioning and the coming to an end of desire is liberation. This happens when there is no movement of thought in the mind.

What I hear from this is that dispassion is not a loss of passion, but a loss of the reactive mind that is attached to passions as a means to obtain pleasure. It is dispassion that reveals to the mind that seeking pleasure and believing that it comes from objects other than itself is ignorance. When this ignorance is seen, the mind naturally becomes dispassionate. The result is not non-action, but rather the freedom to act appropriately in all situations, caring to express the naturalness of your personality freed from the mind's self-centered agenda. That freedom is liberation from the reactive mind. Then the mind is self-loving, enjoying its own Self. Nothing is outside. All is One.

**Student:** I have just finished reading *Nothing Exists That is Not Siva* by Swami Muktananda, and I wept through it. I felt very connected to you and your India journey. Envisioning you and your heartfelt response to being once again in the presence of your beloved guru and his legacy and his offering to you! Something very big is happening to me, and I do think I understand it to a degree. My heart is opening; my pranas are reforming and stronger than ever; my tejas and ojas are cooking, to put it mildly. I need a photo of Nityananda (Muktananda's guru) and one of Muktananda. I feel their presence. I don't want to "do" anything but "sit." If this were another world, that would be great. However, it is not. The reading of the *Yoga Vasistha* will be very slow indeed. Anything I read, however small, seems to penetrate. Do you have any insights for me at this time on what I should or should not be doing to ground these energies for me?

**Mukunda:** Wonderful news. That is great. Mostly, just sit when you can and be with the Shakti that is awakening within you. Do not try to direct it; just let yourself be guided by it. For photos of my lineage, you can go to *www.shantimandir.com*. They will have options for you. That website is for Swami Nityananda, brother of Gurumayi. He is a Mahamandaleshwar, one who initiates swamis into the lineage of Hindu monastics. His ashram is in the Catskills of New York. Go there if and when you can. Yoni mudra can continue to deepen the energies that are opening in you, so do that too. Continue with the Tantra lessons and move to the next one. Blessings.

**Student:** It seems like a long time since my private session with you two weeks ago. When I got back home, I had a lot of work, but was able to stay pretty clear and enjoyed practicing your sadhana recommendations, enjoying the moments of devotion as they arose. Then last week, as with every month during the long workdays preceding a big monthly deadline, I lost touch with my Self. At times, I was overwhelmed with the contrast between my outdated, workaholic, entrepreneurial life and my evolving Yogini path. Once again, I am asking myself: What the hell am I doing working long hours at this desk using my mind for business? That's not who I am! Even though it is my business (and my husband's), it just feels like a job that I am trapped in—one around which I have a lot of emotional baggage and that splits my focus away from healing, learning, and teaching. Over those intense workdays, I could feel my body tightening and the prana being blocked from certain areas, no matter how much I tried to stay relaxed.

My thoughts kept turning to questions like: How can I have more freedom in my life? I reached a low on Sunday. With mind scrambling, I felt the old familiar tightness in my belly and pain in my right pectoral area, which I now realize is the long-held suppression of my heart of hearts. In the article on symptoms of spiritual awakening, I feel that I can identify most with #4—psychological upheavals, swinging from highs to lows. After hitting a low on Sunday, I woke feeling great on Monday and had a good practice, but it is still taking some time to find my way back to stability and devotion. Not sure if this emotional instability is my Inner Teacher starting to speak to me or an absence of a clear voice.

***Mukunda:*** Your letter is showing a great evolution. Learning about the process of how your vasanas, or latent impressions and unfulfilled desires, all lead you astray. But when you continue to focus on your pranic field, it inevitably leads to your heart of hearts. The Yogis say all the nadis end there. That is what is needed. The Tantrik practice that draws energy into the heart source will naturally create devotion. From this devotion, the emotional forms of prana—such as depression, exhilaration, arousal, disinterest, and emotional and mental states—will produce a state of indifference. The Tantrik lessons help you to follow these energies to their source or destination; either way works. The source is the spiritual heart, and the destination is your Inner Teacher.

As you acknowledge me as your outer teacher, my job is to help you navigate this pathway back to your heart of hearts, no matter what variation in prana is blocking you from getting there. As we do sadhana together, I sense where you are open and where you are sluggish. By gently encouraging your prana to move in the direction of its ultimate destination—your spiritual heart—you have emotional or mental translations to what is experienced as prana. The prana, when purified, is omnipresent consciousness—not spiritual, not physical. It just is. Thus detachment from momentary arousals or depressions is necessary for you to move on. You are doing well. I am pleased.

If the teaching falls on a qualified heart, it expands in that intelligence. It does not stay in the unqualified heart.[69]

***Student:*** I wanted to share with you my feelings over the last week or so, as they may have some bearing on which way to go for the next Tantrik practice I take on. I thought today that perhaps it is my feeling all the grief held in my body, being surprised at the amount and the intensity of it, that has made me all the more aware of the absence of joy and beauty in my life. Not that I have none; I am surrounded by it, with my two amazing children, the beautiful place we have chosen to live, the community I live in, and my

---

69. *Vasistha's Yoga*, 499.

yoga studio. But what I am lacking is a connection to it all. I am holding myself back and I don't know how to let that go. You said to me in one of my sessions with you that I am now learning not to suppress emotion. The grief part is coming easily now, but it's the opposite that I don't have a handle on. And, in recognizing that, I am filled with even more sorrow.

You said in one of our workshops that the presence of the divine makes up for the illusion of this life. I am missing this too, and have been frustrated by my lack of appreciation of how the divine manifests itself in my life. Rather then being in awe of the Grace that I experience, I am sulking about not having more. I feel as if I need to make a switch in my attitude—one similar to how Patanjali tells us to substitute negative thinking with positive thinking. What I am finding is that I just want to go do sadhana, because there, I have a better chance of recognition than in my day-to-day life. It's taking me out of my life rather than filling it, and making me resentful and cranky of what I have to do for my family and business. I have chosen to be a householder and know this is my path, but I am finding it's a difficult path to tread, especially coming back from a full weekend with you.

I have heard many stories from Ram Dass and Krishna Das of how, when they were with their guru, they only wanted to sit at his feet all the time and drink in that happiness, and were lost when they were sent away from him. Is this how you felt with your guru? I feel this way, although probably not to the same degree, when we have class with you, because you are the purest emanation of the Divine that I have ever been in contact with. This makes me want that more. So, in this emotional downswing, I wonder what I can do to make a shift in my perspective and touch upon the other end of the spectrum from the grief and the fear. I know it's in there. My kids and husband know it too, and they certainly try their darndest to drag it out of me. But I am not letting go.

**Mukunda:** More than any other quality, there is a need to persist at sadhana while in daily householder life. Sometimes, the need is to let yourself be vulnerable with the teacher or deity that you connect to the most. If that is me, then so be it. Use an image, photo, or statue that represents, or that is a doorway to, a direct relationship with the Spirit's presence. Being vulnerable will crack the shell of the emotional crust that has formed over your heart. Allow yourself to be truthful, revealing the truth of your fears, longings, and cravings.

Being with my teacher was wonderful, but I never stayed with him for very long—six months was my longest stay in eight years with him. I followed his pattern, for he also came and went from his guru. There was too much chaos around my teachers, which sometimes led to a loss of discernment with my own Spiritual path. Baba had too many devotees, and I longed for intimacy and personal connection. So that made me come and go; I did not want to get caught up in ashram politics or personality plays. I also had my own work to do—work he had given me. He made me a professional yoga teacher the second year I was with him, 1975. So my duty was to do my personal practice so that I could have some depth of personal experiences to share with those interested in a Spirit-filled life. The process of transformation happens mostly on your own. The teacher's job is only to open you and help you understand what goes on in the process of clearing your old conditioning (vasanas and samskaras).

Sometimes, the teacher must break your hard crust; that requires the teacher to push you in ways that are unfamiliar. Mostly practicing humility, asking for guidance, and following what is given is the best. In your situation, I recommend more time listening to Om Namah Shivaya tapes and having the intention to meditate deeply. When family-life duties are over, then you have time for more sadhana. Namaste.

**Student:** I have been reading the *Yoga Sutras* (your book) and *Where Are You Going?* by Swami Muktananda. I have a couple of questions. In regard to *Yoga Sutra* II, 12; II, 13; and II, 14: How do you stop the suffering if it has karmic roots into your future? How do you erase or change karma?

**Mukunda:** Karma is lessened every time we experience meditation. By experiencing even a small degree of samadhi, the karmic patterns lose their force and are impotent, creating detachment and the ability to make a different decision. This allows freedom from the impressions making waves of karma. That is the key to lessening the vasanas (subconscious programming that directs your predispositions). Karma is your previous self-effort. If difficulties arise, they can be overcome by making a resolution (sankalpa) for more self-effort (tapah). Tapah is the remover of all obstacles; nothing can stand in its way.

**Student:** In regard to shaktipat, on page 75 of *Where Are You Going?* Swami Muktananda says: "Only if you have become perfect can you give shakti to others." What does he mean by perfect?

**Mukunda:** By receiving blessings of a siddha (perfected master), one becomes elevated and can give Shakti only if the master siddha gives his or her blessing. It is a gift (siddhi) that they can give; they can take it away also. I have been blessed with this and taught how to be an instrument for my guru's Grace. I do not imply that I am perfect, but that Shakti is perfect and it chooses who receives blessing. Even a siddha cannot transmit Shakti, unless She chooses to give Herself. Shakti is the Divine Mother, and She is greater than a siddha.

**Student:** I understand that shaktipat is given to seekers at different times. Is it a matter of your journey and where you are on your path?

**Mukunda:** Yes. Mostly, it is a matter of connecting to a teacher or Spirit and being ready to receive what they have to give. When you are ready, then you have met all the prerequisites of the course to be given. In this case, the prerequisites are not rational, for all previous connections with the teacher and the siddha teachings are clear to the teacher, although not necessarily to the student.

**Student:** Tonight, while meditating in front of the pictures of the gurus after all students had left, I had the most extraordinary experience. I was sitting for a long time, doing my mantra, when a question came to me most vividly: Why do I know what I know? That question just hit me. It hovered there, hanging in midair. Yes, I have studied—observing you, observing physical therapists, dialoguing with psychotherapists and many other healers, etc. But, there are many times when I seem to "know" things that I have never seen, observed, experienced, studied, practiced, or even thought of. Tonight, I saw how often "something" happens. All I need to do is relax and be open, and these teachings, this guidance, just come. I feel as if I *know* what to do, what to say.

I felt, tonight, that I was blessed with a special gift. I felt very, very old, ancient, in a most wonderful way. I felt the wisdom of others before me coursing through me—their energies infusing mine. I can't explain it. It was as if there were others—invisible, but "there"—who were whispering to me, guiding my thoughts and my hands and my heart and my teachings and my speech. The less I thought, the better it was. It was a suspension outside of time, and it felt very "right." My energies felt at full throttle; there were no doubts in my mind. The guidance was there, almost like a physical force. I was very moved by this experience.

**Mukunda:** You have a nice way of putting it. When one is experiencing wisdom (the fourth kosha), it often feels as if a spiritual light or illumination (tejas) is present, that intuition is clear and given to uplift others. Or at least, I should say, this is my experience of guidance. It is clearly not my own thoughts, just that I am being told what to do or say. The ego is an illusion. This is a central teaching of *Vasistha's Yoga*. At times when this is clear, there is no thought. The inquiry that is given is blessed wisdom. It is a blessing to receive; and yet, who knows who is receiving and who is sending? When the fourth kosha appears, the next sadhana is inquiry. The path of Ramana Maharshi clarifies how to do this from his teachings *Who am I?* Namaste.

**Student:** The lesson I just received is so intense. I completely feel as if I am heading in that direction, of being committed and devoted to the path of the Yogi. I feel as though my seeking is genuine and disciplined. And I have a lot of faith right now, too. I was thinking about the part of asking the teacher to do the initiation. I feel so drawn to you and comfortable with you as my teacher and mentor, as you have been for the past couple of years. Can you be my mentor even if I do not know much about your lineage? Something that confuses me is that I also feel so drawn to the lineage of the teachers of Neem Karoli Baba. My point is that I do trust you as my teacher and, if you feel I am ready soon, I want to pursue the process of initiation. I just get confused about not having an actual guru with whom I have spent time. And that is something I want. I just don't know how or when it will come. Can I follow the teachings of this guru and pursue his teaching and devotees without having a "teacher" per se from that lineage? I am trying to just let go and let it all be taken care of by a higher source, and I know that it will.

**Mukunda:** Yes, I can be your mentor, even if I am not your spiritual teacher. Check out my lineage—the sage Vasistha, Bhagwan Nityananda, Swami Muktananda, and Swami Prakashananda—to perpetuate your self-observation and see if any of their teachings aligns with your needs. I have several of their books listed on my website's recommended reading list (*www.yogatherapycenter.org*). See what pulls you more consistently over a year. For some, feeling a connection to the lineage is more important than to others. Others find it is just the one person that they need to connect to as teacher. See who you are. Indeed, the true guru is your own inner Self. Having an outward teacher comes if and when it is necessary for the Inner Teacher to manifest. Wait and all will be made clear. When the teacher is ready, the student appears—and vice versa.

**Student:** My understanding of shaktipat is the descent of the Grace of the guru through touch, mantra, readings, and/or visuals. My awakening energy body is a result of this Grace, is this true? The tremors, the sweating, the crying, and then the subtle experiences of Shakti, the newfound ability to dance, write, and pray more effectively, my awareness of energy—are all signs of enhanced (awakened?) Shakti. One reason I decided to go see Gabriel Cousins in New York was to experience his shaktipat. There was very little in the experience for me that day. Two days later, however, watching your private sessions, I had an incredible tingling and some clarity for the morning. So my questioning mind wants to know, directly: Do you consider the work you and I have done in private over the last year or so to be a transmission of Shakti? And if yes, why the difference in my connection to your transmission as opposed to that from Gabriel, if it is, after all, the Shakti of Swami Muktananda, as you are both his students?

**Mukunda:** Shaktipat comes through all the sensory experiences from qualified gurus and/or their blessed disciples. Once it happens, kriyas are the natural result—shaking and spontaneous release of emotions, etc., that can happen at any dimension. These will tend to persist in the kosha that is currently experiencing opening. One can direct the sadhana to follow the kriya process and, in so doing, participate in it. It is similar in concept to what I gave as Tantra lesson 1. Learn to find the energy first, then follow the energy. Finally, learn to retain the energy so that it can be elevated to a higher kosha. With practice and surrender, the Shakti will completely guide and direct your spiritual life.

Shaktipat can come all of a sudden, in one strong burst of overwhelming experience, or gradually over time. You know it as the continuing source of Grace and connection to the Self. Its source is the Divine Presence. Its form came through Swami Muktananda to both Gabriel and myself. Being with a surrendered student of Muktananda is, for some, the same as being with Muktananda. However, depending on your experience, it may be strongly attractive or unattractive to the personality through whom Baba's Shakti is coming. If your experience is from a subtler kosha, then the gross or pranic form does not matter, because you experience wisdom or bliss of the fourth and fifth koshas in your Shakti.

The form to give your devotion is important, until you become so immersed in devotion that devotion is what you love rather than the form that gave it to you. So students of Shakti are encouraged to be devoted. Whatever form of teacher, God, or Goddess you connect to most easily is to receive that devotion. Over time, it deepens to pure devotion.

See my website for a recommended reading list on meditation, Tantra, and Kundalini shaktipat. I especially recommend *Science of Meditation* by Kripaluananda, *Play of Consciousness* by Muktananda, *Yoga Vani* by Swami Shankar Purushottam Tirtha, and *Devatma Shakti* by Swami Vishnu Tirtha. These all have the secret teachings of the siddhas. Reading such books can help answer the inevitable questions that will continue to arise.

**Student:** How does a student qualify to be initiated? Does the teacher decide when the student is ready for initiation, or does the student have to ask for it? Can one be initiated at a distance?

**Mukunda:** Initiation depends on being in a relationship with someone you take to be your spiritual teacher. Sometimes, the recognition is there immediately; for others, it takes a long-term commitment before the relationship is sufficiently deep to warrant a commitment to following the spiritual advice. My guru used to say that "you should not give in quickly if you feel a teacher's elevated state or power. One should test them by taking their advice for a year, and if by following their advice you feel transformed and doubts are removed, then they can be your spiritual teacher." So it is really a mutual decision. Initiation can happen in dreams, over the phone, or with a physical contact and the presence of Spirit.

**Student:** Regarding a spiritual name given by a teacher: I love the idea, but wonder what the meaning is behind receiving a spiritual name. From my previous readings, it was my understanding that a soul chooses his/her name prior to reincarnating into a physical body—a name that resonates with the soul itself and what it is coming to experience in this lifetime. What do you think, Mukunda?

**Mukunda:** Often, a spiritual name is given with energetic initiation; and yet, there are no standard rules. In my own case, I received shaktipat initiation at the initial meeting with my guru; a year later, I asked him for a spiritual name. The name transforms your self-perception. Its purpose is to help identify you in a new role, as a more expanded cosmic archetype. Indeed, it often feels that the spiritual teacher perceives the student's spiritual name and mantra. It is already there. They may hear it, see it, or read it in the pranic level of the radial pulse.

**Student:** When the teacher is ready, the student appears. I love it that way. I have always looked at it the other way around. Thanks for this, Mukunda. You say that you may find that your outer teacher and your Inner Teacher are the same. How is this possible? I thought that the Inner Teacher is the Higher Self—what we call our inspiration, our intuition, this little voice inside. What is your point of view on this, Mukunda? How can it be explained?

*Mukunda:* The Inner Teacher is the true teacher, and yet the outer teacher plays the role of the Inner Teacher for some time, to help establish the continuously inner relationship on solid ground. In my case, I heard my guru's voice inside for a full year. He guided me in the most basic ways—turn here, go there, don't do that. He revealed his omnipresence. Later on, the personality of my guru disappeared from inside me, and I experienced a much subtler voice calling and guiding me in questionable situations. Now it is always there when I need assistance—just not as persistent as it was in the beginning. I was dense and needed a lot of reassurance that he could really be with me and would not leave me, no matter what troubles I got into.

*Student:* You said that true Yogis never lose energy, but are always able to contain their energy. I am aware that I am learning how to do this more and more. I would like our work to go into this subject further. After our talk today, my whole body was vibrating with energy. I do understand energy, but feel I am being taught about it on a much more subtle level at this point.

I want very much to connect on a deeper level with you energetically as a teacher— even while we are not able to work in person—as you mentioned that it would deepen the level of the work. I grapple with wanting you to know that I simply want to deepen, and I want to connect as closely as I can with you for that purpose. I feel a connection with you in spirit that is quite profound and feels like a positive karma. I wish for you to know that. I have great respect for the level of work that we are doing. I know it is profound, as the energy is so strong, even if we are never together in person. I see the rapid rate that is unfolding unheard-of potentials in me and the work I am doing. I want to express this to you, because I am afraid that you will think I am just getting to be too much, too clingy, or not understanding our relationship. Please know that I do. I truly do understand the nature of our relationship and the work, and I just love you so much for what we have touched on so far. It is truly a gift for me. Do you understand what I am trying to express?

*Mukunda:* It is good to know that you are responding with energy to discussions about it. The energy will manifest in a fertile soil. The term for such a Yogi is *urdhvareta*—literally, "one whose prana only goes up." This is a sign of awakened Kundalini, from its physical prana function as udana prana that creates exhalation. Shiva is always seeking Shakti. The beloved prana wants the infinite romance, not merely the consummation of love.

I do not have any concern about you being inappropriate. Desire for healthy teachings and making them a practical part of life is the sign of a healthy spiritual heart. It is natural for devotees to feel love for their teachers, as the teacher is the embodiment of their teachings. The teachings last, yet the body doesn't. Nonetheless, a serious student has an innate desire to feel close to the teacher, regardless of physical proximity.

*Student:* How can I continue to work as deeply as possible with you, energetically and otherwise? I know I would like you to teach me about the Tantrik energy work when we come together to work in person.

*Mukunda:* Do all the Tantra lessons as if I were there with you. Inviting my energetic presence in your meditation and Tantrik practices will help you to connect more clearly and know the difference between me as your outer teacher and your heart as your Inner Teacher. You can also do this as you awake and as you go to sleep, using the yoni mudra as a magnet to keep us close. During these times, the subtle body is more readily able to travel through distances.

*Student:* You say to ask your outer teacher for confirmation. Do you mean that literally, in a verbal sense?

*Mukunda:* Yes. How else can I respond, but directly in person? Any other response you sense would be on the part of your Inner Teacher.

*Student:* Can you explain the difference between a spiritual teacher and a spiritual mentor? You offer yourself as one or the other to people. What is the difference in roles, or the relationship?

*Mukunda:* The mentor is one who helps you find a spiritual teacher or a tradition of depth. When that is found, you will build a sustainable relationship. The former is a more transient relationship—tilling the spiritual soil so the student is more prepared to follow the spiritual teacher and know what it is to test and be tested by the teacher. Together, a natural conclusion is met that is mutually beneficial—one that meets the needs and skills of both.

**Student:** I work with a woman spiritual teacher (a Tantrika) in my area. I have been with her for over seven years, and the relationship has always been mysterious to me. I do not feel the intense devotion to her that many in our circle do. But there is a definite connection between us. She sent me away for a year, and that is when I met you, which I wouldn't have done if she had not sent me away. Then she invited me back just after I began your training. The work I have done with you has been swiftly transformational and has been an asset to the work I do with her. You both complement each other all the time. As I read your using of the terms "spiritual teacher" and "mentor" more and more, I wonder if she is a mentor to me and you are a teacher to me. I don't know what the difference is or if it makes a difference. I wondered if you can work with two teachers at once.

**Mukunda:** One cannot work for long with two spiritual teachers. It is like a courtship; one or both must become either friend or mentor, and fade into the background. This is necessary for spiritual life, just as married life requires a commitment of monogamy. A common saying in India is: One guru, one wife, one mantra, one sadhana.

**Student:** I am aware that you are allowing so much with me. It is relaxing me on such a deep level. That is not even entirely what I mean. I feel you are so "there" for me that I am transformed by it. I have a sense that you are giving me everything that I desire on many different levels—from the energetic exchange to the teachings that I crave so much. And then, the greatly unexpected package that it comes in—Tantra. I do think I understand how that is so. I know you have done a tremendous amount of sadhana and inner work to be able to be there in this way. But it is so far beyond what I even expected. I feel you with me so strongly all the time. I don't know if you really are, or if I am just connecting myself so intensely to you. I would like to think that you are with me.

I don't expect anything from you outside of the professional teacher/student relationship, and yet I feel that you would give me anything that I needed or asked for if you felt I was in a place to receive it. Because of that, I am finding that I am strong and there is an increased potency present in my work because I feel you are behind me. I see the power in that. Please tell me if I am wrong about these things.

**Mukunda:** That is natural when you are connected, not merely to me, but to my guru, Baba Muktananda. His power flows through me and also that of his teachers. Relaxation comes from empowerment. This is especially true as we are getting closer to the anniversary of Baba's initiation day (Dhivya Diksha, which was August 15, 1947). This day sends more Shakti through all of Baba's students and into all those close to his students, as you are. Shakti is spiritual food. It nourishes in a way different from the way prana feeds the second kosha, or tejas feeds the third kosha, or ojas feeds the fourth. Shakti fulfills the desire for Spirit to be tangibly present in all life.

*Student:* I hope it is okay that I share this much with you. It is all these experiences that I have written about to you that are pulling me. The transmission is so strong during and after we work that I find I am thrown right into a Shiva state of profound stillness when I receive your teachings. I also find that, when I do any of the Tantrik practices, I am literally vibrating with ecstasy. It is the same when I sit with you. All I have to do is think about you, and I go right into that state. That is why I said to you that I feel, on a subtle level, that I have already been doing energy practices with you. Maybe that is just the subtle work that is going on while all these other workings and teachings are happening between us. I don't know.

*Mukunda:* For a receptive student, the subtle work of connecting to a teacher who is not present is as strong, and sometimes even stronger, than when the teacher is physically present. Shiva/Shakti as Isvara is the true teacher of all the other spiritual teachers, as it says in the *Yoga Sutras* I, 26. By having a deep relationship with your own Shakti, it can awaken you to experiences that do not need to come through the physical teacher's presence. Shakti's ecstasy and Shiva's profound eternity come together to show their desire for communion and a spirit-centered life. The hungriest students need profound experiences before they can commit to a spirit-centered life.

*Student:* Your advice to seek my Inner Teacher during one of our first sessions helped to identify and define the intuitive, guiding voice that I have been aware of for a while now. I just did not know what it was or how to connect to it. But now I know that She is my heart, my Inner Teacher, and I just need to ask Her for direction and guidance and it will be provided.

*Mukunda:* Good. That can deepen by just asking for Her advice and following what is given. It can be as simple as talking to your closest friend just to "run something by them."

**Student:** When you identified this *granthi* knot in my heart, I first felt "burdened" with this knot like a nut, so I asked Kali-Ma for Her help. It was then that my Inner Teacher reminded me that nuts are seeds; and seeds need love and care to sprout and release what is within. Furthermore, She pointed out that this was an orchid seed/nut, because She knew of how my orchid taught me a lesson in love by offering Her flowers of love regardless of what I did. From this orchid, I understood that, if She could offer such love and beauty, surely I could do so with my husband.

I bought another orchid to remind me daily to open my heart and to love him unconditionally. And my heart continues to open. So now, during my meditation, I imagine that the orchid nut is bathed in Lakshmi's ocean of compassion and love, and that Kali's fire burns off the softened barriers. One by one, the nut sprouts roots and leaves, until it is ready to flower. Today, She was not ready to flower, but I imagined Her flowering. As the first blossom opened, I felt a warm energy in my first chakra that quickly moved to the second chakra—even before the second flower opened—and then on to the third chakra. Only a small trickle made its way to my heart, but I imagined the flow and the opening of the flowers all the way to the top. Later, as I was praying to the Goddesses, I became aware that I was just warm flowing vyana prana within the skin outline of my body. I am no longer "burdened" with this nut because, in reality, She is a gift. I will care for the granthi orchid nut for as long as it takes for Her to flower. I am so profoundly grateful for your guidance, which has brought me much peace and love. And how do I possibly thank you? I can only send you my love and a very big hug!

**Mukunda:** You are doing so beautifully. I am pleased at your ability to shift your attitude about the granthi from a pranic knot, to a nut, to a seed seeking blossoming. Your mind is wonderfully positive. Persist at seeking Grace from the Goddess; surely that is all She has to give us. So why not yearn and be fulfilled? That is the best way to thank me—just as my teachers asked for thanks only by doing sadhana and reaching for the best. You're doing the same. Being loving to all in your life is repaying the debt that each of us has for our teachers. Blessings.

**Student:** I should be observing what is real beneath the thoughts, the initial spark of current to be unchanging, not what forms from that. After all, my experience of Bhairavi is changing daily. Does that mean it's not real? My experience of devotion is changing daily as well. Again, not real? Were I able to tap into the direct source of these experiences,

I might find an unchangeable element, but it is not clear yet to me what that source is, or what real is. I think when I find that, I will also find the Inner Teacher. I am questioning whether what I consider "positive" is real and what I consider "negative" is unreal. Or is this a big-time illusion? No, I am not questioning that. That is obvious. But can I consider these positive devotional experiences to be real (if they are not) and still get to the root of it? And how do I interpret a sensation?

*Mukunda:* This is good for you. Open to what comes naturally arising. That is key in opening to the many forms of Devi. She can assume many different forms until you fully accept Her for what She is—All. She wants nothing less than the fullness of your heart and all that you conceive yourself to be. Feelings are not permanent, any more than thoughts are. The common ignorance (avidya) they share is that you believe in them. You believe your interpretation of the sensations. The sensations are merely currents of sensation, or pranic vrittis; they are not the horrible significance your mind attributes to them. The secondary reaction to prana must be changed. The initial is merely prana, vrittis, thoughts. It is in the thoughts about those thoughts that the trouble resides. This is what you can change. The initial reactions are the waves of past actions. By not reacting, by waiting until you are clear, you change your karma's destiny. This is empowerment. Surrender that to Devi. As far as sensation goes, just call it an emotion, prana, or waves of sensation (vrittis).

*Student:* But these currents are to guide us toward truthful actions, are they not? In order to have an action come to fruition, there must be a thought to initiate it. Or is that where I am going awry—by looking toward the thought to guide me?

*Mukunda:* Yes. When you are connected to the prana, it is the energy that precedes the thought. The truth is not a thought. It is pure prana, without vrittis of considerations. By learning to be connected to that, guidance will be experienced as non-verbal, without thought. The inner Self is pure; that is what to listen to. Discernment is a muscle that gets exercised with sadhana.

*Student:* It has only been one week since we met in New York, yet it seems as if so much has changed. I can relate to the birthing of my new Self in the sense that I did give birth to three children. As at those times, one week is spent in a kind of euphoria of bringing a new spirit to life—and then comes the reality of caring for the new infant.

The only weakness in this analogy is that I myself feel completely different. I feel more as if I am moving and reacting as one unit, whereas before, I felt more separate. I am even getting comments that I am reacting to events in a very grounded way, without anyone knowing about my rebirth. All I can say is that, now, my mind would like to understand more of what transpired and what to expect. It is kind of like a new parent asking questions of the pediatrician. It is such a time of celebration, but is also a period of many adjustments. Last week, I was one way; this week, I am another. I would appreciate your comments. I was hoping you could both explain the changes in a general way—what happens when we change and grow—and explain what I may expect from my transformation. As always, I appreciate your comments and look forward to them. Namaste.

***Mukunda:*** Before illumination, feeding babies and enjoying your consort. After illumination, feeding babies and enjoying your consort.

What is there to say? Something has changed and that which has changed was inevitably to fall anyway. That which has come as a blessing was seeking you before you knew it. This play of the life force results in feeling the blessings of living a life in spirit. Persist with the Tantra lessons for more details and consider reading my Tantrik Yoga poetry book, *The Yoga Poet*. These can provide much nurturing food for your awakening and integration.

St. Francis said, "The One you are looking for is looking for you." My thought is to make yourself easy to find by the depth of your spiritual practice and longing, plus the intention to be free of your conditioning. Keep opening yourself and know that you are always safe, regardless of who or what is encountered along your path. Know that your spiritual teacher is close. The *Yoga Sutras* say "For those who have an intense urge for Spirit, it sits near them waiting" (I, 21). You are such a one. Know that One. Blessings.

***Student:*** I did want to share some of my experience so far, as you have asked. Immediately when I first started using the yoni mudra, my lower belly would gurgle. This is not usual for me. Also right away, I had pain stings/releases on my right side, where I've had ovarian cysts and scarring from a C-section. One morning, there was a surge of sensation in my hands. When it passed, my hands felt numb. On another morning, after moving my hands to the pelvis, my hands felt as if they were on fire. The yoni shape from my belly was burning into my hands. At the same time, my hands were burning the shape into my body. I've had increased energy, including sexual energy, and have needed less sleep when doing even a little.

Finally last month, for the first time in a couple of years, I got my period! I'm fifty-four, and my gynecologist just told me a couple of days prior to this that I was certainly over this stage in my life. I would also like you to know that I'm a dreamworker. I've had two dreams of you that I've recorded. In the first dream, I'm telling students—after first saying I didn't have a teacher—that I actually do. You. In the second dream, you are on a couch, kind of lounging. You are observing a situation I'm dealing with. You confirm that the inner and outer teacher are the same. So it appears you are teaching me on another level of consciousness. Thank you!

**Mukunda:** [This question arose in the mind of a student with many spiritual experiences in yogic sadhana after only the first lesson. I placed it here rather than in the Dialogue section for lesson 2 so students will realize that Spirit's path arises from Spirit as much as from self-effort. See *www.yogaforums.com* for a three-year-long series of dialogues that led to this book.]

You are a very open student to have such a profound shift from a short period of practice. Health and energy issues are normally the first to respond to Tantrik techniques, although in some cases, when students have been developing their spiritual natures, they receive a real boost in that aspect of life. When energy increases or balances, it tends to release suppressed functions—whether health-related or, as you described, sexual. This is indeed about connecting to your Inner Teacher. From that place, all aspects of your Self can become open to healing.

It is common for me to hear stories of students experiencing their teachers in their dreams or meditation practice. My spiritual teacher gave me many gifts that allow some students to experience me as I experienced him. I am willing to help on all dimensions. Whatever unfolds through the yoni mudra is bound to lead you to a higher perspective and deepen your spiritual practices as a dreamworker. All this leads to being more available to serve others selflessly.

**Student:** I have a very ardent desire to know/merge with God, which seems to be getting more and more urgent. In meditations at times, I feel very close to something, as if there is only the thinnest of veils separating me from this something. But then it disappears. Also at times, I feel as if a column of ice/heat were rising up my spine to my shoulder blades.

**Mukunda:** A wonderful sign of spiritual energies awakening in you. Persist in your desire and let it become burning or ice. Shiva's energy is seen in the cold Himalayas as Mount Kailas, shaped like a lingam, or in a cave as a column of ice that never melts. Shakti's energy, on the other hand, is warm to hot, manifesting as passion and illumination. As Victor Frankl noted in *Man's Search for Meaning*, "What is to give light must endure burning."

**Student:** I just want to thank you for sharing what you have with me for free. At this point in my life, my husband and I are living on his income while I take care of our beautiful daughter. So receiving this instruction is priceless at this time in my life. Our daughter is eighteen months old, and she is very spirited!

Recently, I saw my therapist, and she is helping me learn how to deal with my fears about death and about the deaths in my past lives consciously. I've always known that I'm sensitive, but now I know that I am much more connected with the Earth than I ever have been after giving birth to our daughter, Sierra.

So now that I'm doing the first lesson of the Tantric lessons, I'm beginning to face some of my fears of feeling by taking the time to connect with my sexuality. In fact, in the past life that came to me after doing the eagle pose, I saw that I was stabbed in the chest and back and belly after being completely used and abused. Just writing this brings the sorrow to the surface. And I'm so tired of being numb to this deeper side of my soul. I'm starting to feel the whole. The feeling of losing the sacred is what I feel I'm grieving in my writings.

When I did the first lesson for the first time, I felt a rush of energy through my chest and back once I put my hands there after starting with the yoni mudra. I felt heat that could penetrate almost through the bed. (I was lying down because I do the lessons before I go to sleep.) Then, I felt a swirl of energy in my lower abdomen. It was a counterclockwise swirl and I saw the inside of a calla lily flower. The funny thing is that I get dizzy spells sometimes. But during this lesson, I stayed very grounded during the spiraling down.

In fact, the other night a friend of mine put me under hypnosis, and I started swirling above and I really didn't like it. So I was about to take myself out of hypnosis, but then I just surrendered to the feeling of confusion, of being lost, and started to find my center in the middle of the confusion. Luckily, he touched my head and brought me back down. Then, he took me into the beginnings of the past life I just described in which I was stabbed. But I didn't feel completely comfortable going there. I felt chills in my legs, but I felt such a draw toward the river where I was getting water. The earth was red, and I saw small pyramids far away in the distance.

***Mukunda:*** [This very moving email came in response to doing only the first lesson. I did not wish to share it at the beginning of the lessons. Instead, I decided to share it here, where a linear mind can conceive of stronger response to the spiritual quest. Of course, we cannot attribute such a response to a novice, but rather a long term of preparation seeking a life of Spirit. Those with prior spiritual training often have profound reactions to the first few Tantrik Yoga lessons. I felt many would need to see progression before they could understand how a life could be as transformed as this woman has shared. When you are open to Spirit, there is nothing but Grace. All difficulties bring Grace; all blessings bring the humility of Grace. There is nothing but Grace.]

How very amazing that you had such a profound release of past-life experiences from the first lesson. I wonder what will happen by the time that you get to lesson 18! Continue, by all means, and don't concern yourself with the pacing. Just do as Spirit is obviously doing. Blessings.

# Signs of Kundalini

With Great Respect and Love, I Honor
My Heart, My Inner Teacher.

Kundalini is best understood as the purifying force of prana whose job is to remove the ego sense and restore one's consciousness to its original nature. Just as when we cook food it becomes transformed, sometimes making it more delectable and sometimes not. In the same way, when we are cooked by spiritual awakening, others experience us as being more serene while we may be boiling over inwardly, stressed by the loss of a familiar perspective of ourself. Once prana becomes spiritually awakened, the same energy no longer is experienced as personal or biological prana, but rather as Divine Grace in the form of Kundalini Shakti. These terms are also associated with forms of the Divine Mother. She takes many forms, acting subtly within us hidden behind the mask of the ego sense. The purifying effect will resemble kriyas that are taught by a teacher, yet acting more effectively and spontaneously. In such cases, an experienced mentor or teacher can be of great help in clarifying what is happening. The major work of Kundalini is to remove the distractions from your mind so that you can see your True Self clearly—distinct, yet transcendent from your body and mind. It is Kundalini's task to remove, not merely the outer signs of distraction, but also the inner source of them.

The *Yoga Vasistha* describes Kundalini as a force that generates health, illness, and death, as well as being the spiritual force of life.

Kundalini functions in the body composed of the fivefold elements, in the form of the life force. It is this same Kundalini which is known variously as conditioning or limitation, as the mind, personality, movement of thought, intellect and egosense, for it is the supreme life force in the body. As the Apana it constantly flows downward, as Samana it dwells in the solar plexus and as Udana the same life force rises up. On account of these forces, there is balance in the system. If, however, the downward pull is excessive and the downward force is not arrested by appropriate effort, death ensues. Similarly if the upward pull is excessive and it is not arrested by appropriate effort, death ensues. If the movement of the life force is governed in such a way that it neither goes up nor down, there is an unceasing state of equilibrium and diseases are overcome.[70]

## Eight Categories of Awakening

In some cases, the awakening of spirituality comes unexpectedly, spontaneously arising without the student doing a spiritual practice. There are therapeutic organizations formed to assist those who may be confused or bewildered by the unusual events accompanying this phenomenon.[71] The awakening of Kundalini can be a dramatic experience, and the resultant shift in consciousness may be accompanied by periods of physical and psychological upheaval. The process of Kundalini awakening varies greatly from person to person. Some have intense physical symptoms while others experience mainly emotional or psychological symptoms. It is as if the new energy invites a spring cleaning throughout the entire system, with unresolved physical or emotional conditions coming up for resolution and release. The life-transforming changes that accompany a Kundalini awakening can cover the entire physiological, emotional, mental, psychic, and spiritual spectrum—collectively known as the koshas.

An article covering the signs of spiritual awakening along with an extensive bibliography is summarized below.[72] You will note that many of the signs lead students

---

70. *Vasistha's Yoga*, 429.
71. Spiritual emergence network at *www.spiritualemergence.info.*
72. For those confused by the process of awakening in contrast with therapeutic issues, see *The Stormy Search for the Self* by Christina and Stanislav Grof.

to seek medical, psychotherapeutic, or psychiatric help to alleviate the symptoms. Unfortunately, some seekers only tend to look for spiritual guidance when medical intervention has proved ineffective. In such cases, only a Yogi will know the difference between spiritual awakening and medical dysfunction, as they can read the signs of the Kundalini Shakti. A yoga therapist with a spiritual background can cover territory unknown to these other professionals. Dr. Greenwell (1990) has noted the following categories of symptoms that have been observed during spontaneous Kundalini awakening. The last category, one that I added, is also very common.

> **Pranic movements or kriyas:** An intense energy moves through the body and clears physiological blocks; a person may experience intense involuntary, jerking movements of the body. As deeply held armoring and blockages to the smooth flow of energy are released, the person may re-access memories and emotions associated with past trauma and injury. When the kriyas have purified the subtle body, the movements become graceful, and beautiful spontaneous asanas may arise in sensual Vinyasa flows.

> **Yogic phenomena:** Some people find themselves performing yogic postures or hand mudra gestures that they have never learned or could not do in a normal state of consciousness. Similarly, they may produce Sanskrit words or sounds, or have an awareness of inner music or sound, mantras or tones. Unusual breathing patterns may appear, with either very rapid or slow shallow breathing. Some people may not breathe for extended periods.

> **Physiological symptoms:** A Kundalini awakening often generates unusual physiological activity as intense movement of energy releases toxins in the body. Symptoms include apparent heart problems, pains in the head and spine, gastrointestinal disturbances, and nervous problems. Sensations of burning, oversensitivity to sensory input, hyperactivity, or lethargy, are also commonly reported. Symptoms can be erratic, coming and going without provocation, and are generally unresponsive to medical treatment.

**Psychological upheavals:** Awakening offers a direct challenge to the primacy of ego consciousness and the myth of separation. It brings with it a challenge to move beyond the unconscious responses ruled by drives and instincts, to remove ego consciousness from the center stage of the psyche. It comes as no surprise that such a challenge produces a period of confusion and unbalance. People find themselves beset by inexplicable emotional states as they move to clear out unresolved issues. The emotional roller-coaster may swing from feelings of anxiety, guilt, and depression to compassion, love, and joy, with accompanying bouts of uncontrollable weeping.

**Extrasensory experiences:** As perception expands outside of consensus reality, people experience atypical visual phenomena, including visions of lights, symbols, or entities, or of past-life experiences. Auditory input may include hearing voices, music, inner sounds, or mantras. Even the olfactory system may be stimulated, with perceptions of scents of sandalwood, rose, or incense. There may also be disruption of the proprioceptive system—losing a sense of self as a body, or feeling bigger than the body, or out of the body—with resulting confusion and disorientation.

**Psychic phenomena:** With the awakening of psychic abilities, a person may experience precognition, telepathy, psychokinesis, awareness of auras and healing abilities.

**Mystical states of consciousness:** A person may shift into altered states of consciousness where they directly perceive the unity underlying the world of separation and experience a deep peace and serenity accompanied by a profound knowing. Many clinicians still regard phenomena associated with spiritual emergence as indicative of pathology because the signs are so easily confused with the indicators of psychosis, mania, depression, schizophrenia or borderline personality disorder. Some people undergoing spiritual emergency are misdiagnosed and treated with suppressive medication that further complicates their process.

**Heightened sexuality:** Great variations in sexual desire, as well as latent or repressed sexual desires may surface, bringing about arousal, sexual fantasies, lust-filled dreams and increased orgasms. Women may begin to ejaculate with a force greater than their partners, and there may be spontaneous orgasm for either sex. Often, the increase is not due to any obvious stimulus. The prana seems to settle in the genital region, regardless of the student's mental state. In contrast, some students have a diminished sex drive due to awakening. There are no rules just variations seeking a sattvic harmony.

Swami Muktananda experienced a tremendous psychological and psychic upheaval when he was sexually aroused for months on end as prana persisted at moving upward in his erect lingam.

> I was afraid of the force of sexual passion. It is difficult to describe the agony of my organ. I tried to reason it out but could not succeed. A ravishing naked maiden filled me with fear and remorse. I thought I had made my organ lifeless and inert through mastery of Siddhasana. But it had sprung to life again. I was utterly astounded.[73]

The reason for his disturbing vision became clear once spiritual knowledge arose and he saw Her as Goddess Kundalini. This feeling of devotion and love for the Divine God/dess is the crucial factor in creating safety in spiritual awakening. In this case, seeing the Divine Mother and thus becoming devoted to Her freed Muktananda of the burden of failing to control his sexual energy. Indeed, control is impossible, for it is not a personal power, but the power of the Supreme Being's Grace.

Swami Vishnu Tirtha Maharaj, in *Devatma Shakti (Kundalini) Divine Power*, notes that the astral fluid is an involute form of prana; from brahmacharya (normalization of sexual desire, not necessarily through celibacy), one gains the ability for

---

73. Swami Muktananda, *Play of Consciousness* (S. Fallsburg, NY: SYDA Foundation, 2002), 104.

astral travel and for knowing the blessings of beings of other realms.[74] This is one of the most authoritative books describing spontaneous Kundalini experiences that arise from the preliminary development of your heart. Another book I recommend is *Kundalini: The Secret of Life* by Muktananda. Books alone are generally not helpful, however, because they make Kundalini into a mental rather than a devotional practice.

The eight signs previously cited are naturally arising in the case of spiritual awakening from an initiation. In either event, whether or not you have had an awakening, practice of the Tantrik tools can enable the hidden doorways to higher consciousness to be opened. Spiritual experiences can bring disruption or harmony to your lifestyle, fulfilling what was previously lacking and removing what is no longer beneficial.

In true spiritual awakening, the resulting experiences produce peace, inspiration, and love. Difficulties in life simply fall away with a minimum of self-effort. The spiritual force itself guides you from within and will lead you to an outer teacher if necessary. The counsel of an experienced spiritual teacher who was a disciple of a spiritual teacher is most beneficial for one to understand the inner workings of Shakti and how to safely enter a spiritual relationship with a teacher. In this manner, you can be assured that the quality of the advice is connected to a lineage of tested spiritual practices that lead to peace. Without such fundamental positive signs, consider that what is occurring is simply the removal of energy blocks, leading to a more natural self-expression.

## Awakening Your Heart

Among the most obvious signs of Kundalini Shakti is that the prana Shakti energy moves undirected by your mind. It has a mind of its own and reveals where you need to be purified for your evolution. In the teachings of Classical Yoga from the *Yoga Sutras* (I, 2–4), we are taught to direct the mind. And yet there is the paradox that, while it is good to direct the mind, without direction it is experienced as omnipresent.

---

74. Details of yogic subtle anatomy and its evolution can be found in Swami Vishnu Tirtha Maharaj, *Devatma Shakti (Kundalini) Divine Power* (Rishikesh: Yoga Shri Peeth Trust, 1980). A companion text is Swami Purushattam Tirtha's *Yoga Vani* (Bayville, NY: Ayurvedic Holistic Center, 1992). This is the book Muktananda found helpful to him when he was confused by these sexually arousing experiences.

It is through pranayama that we uncover the source of our thoughts, whose roots are called *adhya prana*. It is this primal form of prana that creates the experience of omnipresence. When this awakening arose in me, I experienced my guru's presence within me—speaking to me in a unique voice, guiding and directing me in all aspects of life—for a year. I literally had conversations with him, until, eventually, the guidance and my mind began to come into harmony. It continues to this day as a source of assistance when I feel unable to connect on my own. Faith and persistence are crucial, but more important is to develop the power of love and devotion.

> If the teachings fall on a qualified heart,
> it expands in that intelligence.
> It does not stay in the unqualified heart.[75]

Unlike willful masculine Shiva energy, which moves upward piercing the chakras, Shakti Kundalini tends to descend. Begin to feel your energy sometimes piercing you and sometimes flowing within, connecting disparate parts into an awareness of unity. Within the context of your daily meditation practice, seek your spiritual heart as you meditate. Practice following your pranic energy to its source in your heart. Begin to look through the multi-dimensional heart to its three levels: physical organ to the left, heart chakra in the center, and spiritual heart to the right of center. Let the meditation proceed at its own rate and move with awareness to each of your hearts. Find your way to devotion and identify the qualities that generate love within you. Write down your experiences from this contemplative meditation and continue to clarify them over the succeeding period.

## Congratulations!

You have just completed two-thirds of the Tantra lessons. May you persist to the end of these eighteen lessons.

Remember to persist in your practice, yet stay detached from expecting specific outcomes. Tantra is a personal spiritual practice. When you feel complete with this lesson, read the Dialogue section that follows prior to moving to lesson 13.

---

75. *Vasistha's Yoga*, 499.

## With Great Respect and Love, I Honor My Heart, My Inner Teacher.

# Dialogue with Mukunda

*Student:* I continue to have extreme pranic movement in the practice. It was warmth through the diaphragm that shot up to my heart center. There was a lot of fear mixed with joy during these upward-moving waves. There was a good deal of resistance to the movement from my mind. It reminded me of the first time I had an orgasm, accompanied by lots of fear of not knowing what was happening, but thinking that, if I relaxed, it would be okay. But still, there is much resistance, still jerking in my shoulder, although not as much. I was able to detect a "shifting" last night during my meditation japa practice and, as you suggested, I questioned whether it was a movement from one kosha to another. I don't have a question here, just logging in, but if you have any comments, I, as always, welcome them.

*Mukunda:* All is going well. I take these as signs of pranic awakening. As prana moves from being physical energy for health to Shakti energy for spiritual awakening, these sorts of deep-seated fears will arise to be removed. Interesting that you mention a resemblance to the fear you experienced with your first orgasm. It is like that for others as well. One needs education or sharing stories with others who have had these experiences to feel comforted enough to know that they are naturally arising. I recommend you read Swami Muktananda's book *Meditate* to be educated about how meditation spontaneously arises, and, with it, these sort of spontaneous kriyas to purify mind and emotions.

*Student:* I have studied, practiced, and reviewed the exercises and techniques of lesson 4 and found them very useful in channeling vital energy in removing/reducing some tamasic thoughts limiting progress in sadhana (e.g., getting out of bed early). Now, my tongue is stuck deep in my throat (kechari mudra) for prolonged periods during the scanning of pranic energy between my throat (vishuddhi) chakra and my heart (anahata) chakra. My difficulty is that, after getting out of sadhana, this mudra also takes place involuntarily—while walking or at any time during work. Should I allow it to happen as it is, or otherwise? Please guide me in this regard.

*Mukunda:* [Although this student is only at lesson 4 it is possible that awakening has happened from her previous spiritual practices. Therefore I will address this question here rather than at the lesson where the awakening occurred.]

When mudras occur spontaneously, it is a sign of Kundalini awakening, as described in lesson 12. One should submit to what is naturally arising and, if any effort is there, it is to be sattvic in harmony with the awakened prana. This particular kriya kechari mudra is seldom mastered by the physical practice to suspend breath alone. In fact, it is rarely known, as yoga teachers are trained to keep the students doing an audible, deliberate breath pattern throughout their sadhana. Instead, when this arises, the breath becomes so subtle that it is misperceived as having stopped. Definitely allow it to continue, unless it is interfering with daily tasks. Spontaneous mudra, bandhas, and kriyas often have a life of their own. Nonetheless, they are submissive to your discerning mind.

*Student:* I have been able to focus on the physical heart and the spiritual heart, but not as clearly on the heart chakra—or at least on sensations localized in the center of the chest. There is a feeling of overall expansiveness when I focus on the chakra. I have been experiencing sensual pleasures on an energetic level at times over the last couple of days during asana class and during sexual intercourse with my husband—not on the physical level, but as if the energetic is overriding the physical sensation. Is this a response purely on the subtle-body level of prana maya kosha, having left the physical body (anna maya kosha)?

*Mukunda:* Indeed, as the sensual becomes less distinct, it is elevated to experiences of prana. It is not always easy to distinguish, but if the enjoyment has increased and the energy of desire is gone, then prana is being elevated through the koshas as you suspect. There is a feeling of wanting the subtleties of expression rather than the gross hunger of sensual or sexual pleasures. Cravings gradually drop and natural expression of your self becomes more available. There is less stress, less striving, less seeking something that isn't present. Desire is said to be the root of duality in *Vasistha's Yoga*. Namaste.

*Student:* Everything is going well with the lessons. I just wanted to clarify a few points: Shiva energy runs up and Shakti flows downward. So would Shiva tend to feel like a light and airy sensation, while Shakti is heavier and more grounding?

**Mukunda:** Yes. In general, that is true, especially when these qualities are sattvic, harmonious, though the descent of Shakti energy called shaktipat can be intense, strong, and accompanied by a sensation of being filled with light. It is often so tactile that it feels as if you are physically being entered by the light. Not a subtle light.

**Student:** Is Kundalini the same thing as Shakti? That was a little confusing to me, because I had heard about Kundalini described in other contexts as an upward-moving energy, as in the phrase "rising Kundalini." I feel as if, intellectually, I am not getting a piece of this.

**Mukunda:** The Kundalini energy can move both up and down. Most authors on the subject are male and their tradition of sadhana is focused on controlling the Kundalini, sometimes even speaking of arousing it with self-effort. They often do not use the devotional Tantrik language of devotion and surrender. Thus, they are working with the male, or Shiva, aspect of Kundalini. In this form, it feels grosser than prana; it gives a sense of elevating yourself from lower chakras to higher. With the awakening of the heart of devotion, the movement, accompanied by feelings of Grace, arises as Shakti descending. Effort becomes effortless. Blocked energies begin to relax and may disappear, without effort.

**Student:** Overall, I have been working on the lesson and, energetically, everything feels as if it's moving in the right direction. Thanks so much for your guidance. And I just bought a book today by one of the disciples of Swami Muktananda, my first read of this lineage!

**Mukunda:** I highly recommend *Meditate* or *Play of Consciousness* by Swami Muktananda. They are more central texts of this lineage. The former is a wonderful short exposé on why and how to meditate; the latter is his spiritual autobiography, containing many experiences of Kundalini and spiritual awakening, with explanations of the states of consciousness leading to the fullness of Shakti Kundalini.

**Student:** Greetings, Mukunda. Lesson 12 gave me so much to process. When sitting for meditation, shortly after receiving the lesson, I saw the body of an Indian Yogi sitting on a raised platform the way gurus do. Just a torso, no face. It was startling. After rising from meditation, I had a heightened sense of physical sexual awareness. I admit to being disturbed and uncomfortable about it. In the midst of feeling quite vulnerable after that meditation, I've been able to resolve some old family issues with my stepmom and my dad. I never thought I'd have the strength to see them again, but it went very well and lots of healing took place. It was the easier issue, it turns out, because dealing with sex again has made me look at all sorts of entrenched hang-ups, body-image issues, and attachments. Talk about clearing out the cobwebs!

Now (a few months later), I feel brave enough to persevere, continue the lessons, and focus on your helpful reminders to seek answers from my Heart. While practicing awareness of the multi-dimensional heart, I had a sense of the physical heart as more dense and the heart chakra and spiritual heart feeling more light and expansive as I moved my awareness toward the right. But that's all I was able to feel or sense. Thank you for the gift of your teaching.

***Mukunda:*** Wonderful for you to have so much to open to. The process of spiritual awakening is indeed about clearing out all the cobwebs. Baba used to say that Kundalini Shakti primarily functions as the supreme housecleaner. Divine Mother's energy, unlike Shiva's, descends and clears—especially suffering and pain mostly due to misunderstanding. From this comes a deeper clearing than from Shiva's energy. His moves up and tends to be aroused quickly for spiritual, physical, and sexual pleasures. The benefits from the last six lessons arise primarily as a result of this house- or karma-cleansing. Encourage yourself to be courageous and move through this, knowing that any challenging situations you encounter are really formed from misconceptions. Persevere to the end. Blessings.

***Student:*** I was meditating on my karmic knot (granthi) orchid that resides on my chest. I had my hands over it and asked for your hands to be under mine. During this meditation, I visualize the hard layers of the nut softening and falling off, which allows roots, leaves, and one flowering stalk to sprout. The flower stalk has seven buds and each bud opens; I visualize it opening over a chakra. In doing this, I am beginning to feel energy in my first chakra, which sometimes moves up and fills all of me and sometimes not. Yesterday, I felt it move into the second and maybe the third chakra, but I continued with the visualization of the entire flower opening. After the seventh flower opens, I lie down and continue with the Tantrik practice of opening suppressed energy.

Then I did the three variations of the yoni mudra but, without thinking, in reverse. There was quietness with the yoni mudra over the first chakra. With the yoni mudra over my bladder, I was filled with love and gratitude for you and your guidance, which has taken me to this point. And then I realized my hands were over Lakshmi's domain, so of course I would feel love emanating from there. But then the energy changed, and I experienced anger spirits rushing away. At first, I was taken aback, but I was reassured that Lakshmi and you were taking care of me so I stayed with the experience.

When all of the angry spirits/energy had gone, I proceeded to my navel and gave thanks to Kali-Ma for Her guidance. At this point, I felt a huge block emerge and I became concerned again, but reassured myself that Kali and you were present and that I could stay in this moment and let it flow. And it flowed. At first, I could not name this torrential outflow of negative energy, but then I recognized it as fear. And I let it flow out. My abdomen was jerking and a deep sadness exploded and I cried from the very bottom of my heart. Then I was exhausted and empty. Absolutely empty. I crawled into bed and wanted to be loved. And then I remembered what you had said about being love and learning to hug my own Spirit.

Would you please explain to me what I experienced? To be honest, I am intimidated by the intensity of the experience. Did I do something wrong when I inverted the order of the yoni mudra variations? Is this experience related to the chest granthi or do I have another in my abdomen? When I do the Tantrik energy practice, I don't ever really feel any "flow"; I just experience regions that radiate or glow and those that are quiet. And at times, I feel overall or region-specific vibrations, as if I were cold. Is that because the energy is all suppressed? Thank you for being there with me. I was scared at times— sometimes, I'm just like a little girl.

**Mukunda:** You are doing beautifully. It is natural as you evolve from being a Yogini to a Tantrika that changes occur. Yoginis focus on discipline and control over the body and mind. They are taught to follow exactly the teachings of yoga and their teachers. Tantrikas focus on opening to the Divine Feminine as the Shakti and Her many forms, as your teacher, Kali Ma, and even your own body can be the source of guidance. Hence the Tantrika path is much more unpredictable than the path of the Yogini.

So that means you did nothing wrong when reversing the order of yoni mudra. Spontaneously, She will guide you. It is the heart granthi knot opening. This is the knot on the third heart, in a dimension beyond the heart chakra.

The feeling of being overwhelmed is actually not true. As you explain, you gave thanks to Kali Ma for Her guidance and also feelings of love and gratitude for me. These acts of surrender allow you to take the pressure off the granthi. It is that opening that releases the suppressed love, fear, and other emotions. Some people flow with prana; others radiate it. Different pranas arise; with the inhalation comes adhya prana (primary), then the pranas of exhalation that govern elimination arise—udana (upward moving) and apana (releasing waste from the pelvis). Other prana currents are there also, glowing, as in samana (circulating and digesting) and vyana prana (aura, glowing). Your sadhana is going very well. Your attitudes and connecting to your helpers are appropriate for deeper, more profound changes in the psyche and subtler koshas. It is very nurturing and healing to allow yourself to be so vulnerable—to be like a little girl. And yet clearly, you know you are in a loving embrace by the Divine Mother. Blessings are with you.

**Student:** I have a question regarding a non-spiritual friend. Gloria is the same age I am—thirty-four—and full of "tiger-like" energy. She has been through emotional turmoil and we often have conversations about the deeper aspects of life, to which she appears to relate. She is quite wild; she works daily with young people with behavioral problems, encouraging them into becoming mechanics. She is self-determined and recently competed in an eight-day rally across the Moroccan desert on a motorbike.

Last year, she decided to do Reiki, without any prompting from me, as I had no idea this would be something she would be open to. This was her first introduction to any energy work, although she practices asana and has done a meditation course. I've given her a number of Reiki treatments to try and help her through this unsettling period. I gave one to her before the rally to help her feel connected and safe for this dangerous endurance event. She later told me that her experience of the session was seeing a horrible snake that had been asleep for a long time at the base of her spine awaken. The snake woke up and twined round her body before shooting up her spine and out of her head.

She didn't like the experience and, since then, she has been crying a lot, feeling very unsettled, confused, and unbalanced. She feels totally full of energy and doesn't know what to do with it. She feels as if her body has had a spring cleaning. She had a one-day menstrual period (having not had any for months), suffered from a cold, and is now starting to have insights about herself. The addiction to obsession came to her during relaxation pose (savasana after asana) on Monday. She said she hadn't known who to talk to or what to do about it and thought she was going mad. We talked for several hours after yoga and I talked her through the signs of Kundalini from lesson 12. She definitely connected with some of the explanation and felt better afterward.

I explained that I wasn't sure if this was what was happening to her, but recommended that she do the wave breath and yoni mudra, and recite the Ganesh mantra to which she also feels drawn. She had never heard of Kundalini or the serpent image, etc., before. Do you have any advice on this?

**Mukunda:** You have done very well with her. She needs a spiritual practice and more understanding of Kundalini experiences that come with spiritual awakening. In spite of her awakening from a Reiki session, her experience is classical Tantrik Kundalini, with the snake "shooting up her spine." Shiva is accompanied by cobras that move up from the chakras at the base of the spine. This is often confused with sexual arousal. That is quite good of you to share lesson 12 to help comfort her and let her know that she is not alone. Ideally, the next step would be spiritual counseling with one with whom she feels safe and connected. This could be over the phone or in person, depending on availability.

If you send her to my website (*www.yogatherapycenter.org*), there are several reputable contacts for her to consider. I am willing to assist and can counsel her, if she wants to contact me by phone. There are also plenty of excellent resource books on my recommended reading list. I suggest she look at meditation, Kundalini, and spiritual life titles. Swami Muktananda's *Play of Consciousness* or Swami Kripaluan's *Science of Meditation* and *Dhyanyogi Madhusudantas* would be a good starting point for showing the variety of experiences. Definitely not Gopi Krishna's writings, as they are confusing, even frightening, due to lack of humility or devotion. With these qualities, spiritual awakening is Grace-filled.

**Student:** Please help me clarify my experiences of this lesson. I have three issues:

You say: "Begin to feel your energy sometimes piercing you and sometimes flowing from you." My flowing energy is okay, but there is no piercing.

You describe moving energy from the "physical organ to the left of the chest, heart chakra in the center, and the spiritual heart to the right of the center." It is not natural for me to move left to right across the chest. It is more natural in a circular motion. Is that too literal?

You say: "Identify the qualities that generate love within you." Yuck. I find myself identifying qualities that relate to the perception of others toward me! Please expound.

*Mukunda:* First, piercing is there if there feels to be a block for it to pierce. If so, this would be classified as an energy block. If there is no block, then only flowing is felt. Next, the circular motion I describe is the natural motion of the gross chakra in kosha two. This is the grossest form of the subtle body. What I am describing is a much subtler level of this subtle body at kosha four. This is not felt physically, rather more sensed or seen. It is the home of your intuition, the voice of your Inner Teacher. Finally, identifying the qualities that generate love within you helps you to find the experience of love as it is emanating from yourself to yourself—not to others or from them. Seek what you can deliberately do, imagining or remembering experiences that generate love to and from yourself only.

*Student:* I now understand what you meant when you said I was a Tantrika and not a Yogini. I had to read this lesson three times before I saw what I needed to read. That is, I am experiencing what you have described. Is this so?

You are a disciple of Baba Prakashananda and Swami Muktananda; are you also a swami or guru? Are you an adept? At some level, I have such questions. On another level, I understand that you are my guide and that I have a lot to learn from you. And then such questions are not so important to me. But they came up, so I ask.

Also, I have been reciting Baba Prakashananda's beautiful prayer at the end of the book that you gave me—*Storytellers, Saints and Scoundrels* by Kirin Narayan. Do you know what it is called so that I may find the Sanskrit version? I have also begun to read *In Praise of the Goddess: The Devimahatmya and Its Meaning*. I just finished the introduction. This book and *Kali's Odiyya* found their way into my hands a few months ago at the bookstore. Am I ready to study this book, or is there other material that I should read before starting?

*Mukunda:* Yoginis are committed to physical sadhana. But when the Shakti (spiritual) energy draws you more than yoga discipline—that is the main feature distinguishing a Tantrika—this sadhana can go much deeper. It is good to do all the eighteen lessons to see which ones suit you for that depth of practice. Then, with discussion, I can provide guidance more specifically for you.

For your other questions: Yes, to the first part. A swami is a celibate person who has taken vows for life. I am committed, but not celibate. There are different terms to explain. My main role is as a spiritual *mentor*, counseling and explaining the experiences that arise from awakening. A spiritual *teacher*, or guru, is one you feel you have been with before and have a spontaneous deep truth in their capacity to direct your awakening through spiritual sadhana. A true guru, more properly called a *satguru*, is one's inner spiritual teacher. It will feel as if they are inside you or with you in all situations. In contrast, a mentor provides outer guidance and answers questions. My role varies between these first two roles. Yes, I am adept at what I share; if not, then my sharing would be unethical and would not prove to be of spiritual benefit.

Your questions should be asked until your mind is satisfied with the answers. Only then can you see how committed this relationship is and where it may evolve if there is a feeling of wanting more.

The prayer you mention is a different translation of the Universal Prayer that I sing at the beginning of each day's classes and seminars. The books you mention are good choices for you. It is especially great to read what you find in being open to Shakti's guidance. Both these books can help promote your consistent inner guidance. For clarification of the Tantrik student-teacher relationship, I recommend reading *Tantric Quest* by Daniel Odier and *Tantra* by André van Lysebeth, in addition to *Kali's Odiyya*.

# PART V

# Deepening Your
# Tantrik Practice

# From Pranayama to Bandha to Mudra

With Great Respect and Love, I Honor
My Heart, My Inner Teacher.

*ranayama* means to "regulate the flow of life force" and *ujjaye* means "to be victorious." With persistent practice and reflection on the effects of that practice, the all-pervasive nature of the Divine prana can be uncovered. Then you can regulate the flow of your internal life force as it moves through your subtle, non-physical body.

## Advanced Pranic Breathing

To develop the energy body, it is necessary to train your breath. Begin by breathing down through your torso and exhaling to create an upward motion. This is the natural wave of the diaphragm. For some people, this may not feel natural, but with practice it will enable you to coordinate the pelvic and thoracic diaphragms. Feel the motions of your breath like a wave flowing down from the nostrils as you inhale, and up from your lower abdomen as you exhale from bottom to top. Consciously tone the abdominal muscles by contracting them during the exhale and relaxing them in reverse sequence during inhales. By allowing your belly to become soft during inhales, the breath can gradually descend its full range—and eventually, to your yoni. This will take time, so please be patient. This breathing exercise is called *ujjaye pranayama*.

Begin to connect the rate and rhythm of pranic breathing exercises with your pubococcygeal (PC) muscle contractions at your pelvic floor. As you inhale, consciously relax the PC region. Begin the exhaling motions with a mild contraction of the PC muscles; gradually increase the contractions so that the end of each exhale features a full-force contraction that pulls upward from the pelvic cavity into the abdominal cavity. In this manner, the pelvic floor contractions will meet the wave of the abdominal contractions during the exhale motions. With practice, the wave of the breath joins the wave of pelvic and uterine contractions in a harmonious flow, increasing pleasure as it removes any subconscious barriers to heightened pleasure and ecstasy. This practice enables the root of your energetic subtle body to hold and lock; these two concepts of holding and locking correlate to the experience of mudra and bandha. As the prana becomes more dense from holding and locking it is experienced as both personal and impersonal—yours and not yours. This is one of the secret Tantra exercises that will help your spiritual experiences to stay with you. By cultivating a memory of the difference between worldly and spiritual states, both are fulfilled more readily. Consciousness must be trained on both the physical and subtle levels through cultivation of a proper attitude of openness to your Spirit.

For men, a similar ability to isolate the urethral muscles from the anal sphincters can be gained. Men can do this by repeatedly stopping the flow of urine. This practice is not recommended for women, due to their tendency for urinary tract infections. Men who can isolate their urethral muscle sphincters develop this from a gross to a subtle level. The subtle body retains prana through the practice of *vajroli mudra*. The same practice for a woman is called *sahajoli mudra*. These two mudras begin to open a subtle channel of prana that leads inside the *sushumna* (the central nadi channel). Analogous to a tube within a tube, the sushumna is the grosser dimension of pranic flow corresponding to the first level of the chakras, the pranic energy body, the prana maya kosha. Inside it is the vajra nadi, which leads to the second level of the chakras, correlating to the mind as the mano maya kosha.

By refining these pelvic floor practices (mula, vajroli, sahajoli), sexual energy is transformed from its grosser level into ojas (the essence of Spirit as matter).[76] As you heighten your sensitivity, you may also uncover a third tube of consciousness called

---

76. The details of these practices are described in the third chapter of the *Hatha Yoga Pradipika,* translated by Swami Muktibodhananda of the Bihar School of Yoga.

the *chitrini nadi* (literally meaning a "thread of light") inside the vajra nadi. Those who control the urethral muscles with detachment begin to have access to subtler channels within the pelvis and, specifically, the first two chakras. Over time, persistent practice facilitates access to the subtler koshas.

## Advanced Root Lock—Mula Bandha to Mula Mudra

Through the deepening of mudra and bandha, the feeling of holding and locking is enhanced. In much the same way as when we embrace a dear friend, we hold them until the point of locking on to their vital force. Thus we feel that we are carrying them with us. In contrast, brief hugs are natural for relations that are superficial yet fond. The sites of the chakras can, in much the same way, be deepened by holding and locking. The first practice we will deepen is the subtle shift from mula bandha to mula mudra.

The muscles of your yoni will now be sufficiently developed to move to the next level of training. At this point, you will be training yourself to find the androgynous energy within your pranic body. The lingam spoken of earlier as a "wand of light" is already available within you. It is easier to develop it with a loving man as your spiritual partner, but it is, nonetheless, crucial that you know yourself as both masculine and feminine energies. By pulling upward from the yoni, you will notice that your body responds above the physical place of your exertions. Relax and open yourself to experience the energetic or emotional aspects of these sensations.

This is a doorway to the second body—the body of prana, an energetic life force composed of love and light. At first, the sensations may be a wide range of emotions, from sexual arousal to pleasure to frustration, or even anger or fear. With persistent practice, the energies and emotions become purified into their subtler spiritual components. Know that these lessons are for the purpose of moving through yourself to find your deeper energy that leads you to Source. With this comes a transformation of your mind and a heightened ability to enjoy the sensory world.

Remember, by developing pranayama through these various techniques, problems with the lower back, pelvic organ functions, and sexuality will arise. Hence, your problems come to the surface to be alleviated and resolved. These muscles, like all others, can suffer due to these underlying problems: loss of tone (hypotonus) where mula bandha is needed, or excessive tension (hypertonus), in which case the lingam stone will release that tension from within or in painful spasm. In the latter case, pelvic-floor pain may prevent comfort during intimate relations. Some physical therapists are trained to free this web of internal and external muscles called the pelvic floor manually.[77] Personalized therapeutic guidance may be necessary before proceeding with these practices.

One of the most experienced yoga therapists I have trained is Uma Dinsmore-Tuli, who has some remarkable considerations for pelvic-floor training based on her experience and those of her students, who have assisted at 5,000 births.

> Reflecting on the different tone of the muscles of the thousands of women she has examined, and upon their birth experiences, [Uma's mentor, Gowri Motha, MD.] considers that the thickened pelvic floor that results from sustained practice of Mula Bandha can lead to difficult birth experiences—specifically to a lengthened second stage, where the thick muscles take so long to "give" that even once the baby's head has crowned, the rest of the head finds it hard to be born, and keeps disappearing back up the birth canal. I am utterly convinced by Gowri's arguments on this one.
>
> I believe it is really best for pregnant yoga students to cease all practice of classical mulabandha (i.e. using the exhale to draw up /in) until after they have birthed their babies. From Gowri's evidence, I am convinced that strong practice of that 'uplifting' kind can overdevelop the muscles of the pelvic floor to the extent that they become an obstacle to the baby's exit.[78]

Before we develop your mula bandha to a more advanced level, let us look at gross and subtle anatomy more closely. In yogic anatomy, the ten gates or openings are the beginnings of gross pathways that lead to the subtle body's nadis, on the prana maya kosha level. By the practices of pratyahara, sense withdrawal cited in lesson 4, energies that normally are lost through speech and lack of grounding are recycled inwardly for spiritual elevation. For all yoga practitioners who are not celibate, emotional, psychic,

---

77. See *www.pelvicpain.com* for descriptions of the procedure and certified therapists.
78. Uma Dinsmore-Tuli, *Mother's Breath: A Definitive Guide to Yoga Breathing, Sound and Awareness Practices for Pregnancy, Birth, Post-natal Recovery and Mothering* (London: Sitaram and Sons Limited, 2006), 127. For more from Uma Dinsmore-Tuli, go to: *www.sitaram.org*.

sensual, and sexual energies are encouraged to have natural expression. This is both for health and vitality, and for the enjoyment of love.

For the Yogi, the evolution of the chest pranas—udana prana flowing upward and adhya prana flowing downward—becomes the Shakti and Shiva forces. Thus, by opening to the subtler dimensions, this practice can lead to thinning of the veils of the five bodies, experienced as detachment and a profound yet naturally arising spiritual awakening to the Source as the union of Shakti and Shiva. While teaching at Integral Yoga Institute's Yogaville ashram[79] in central Virginia, I saw a beautiful quote in the majestic Lotus temple to the unity of all religions. It is from the Sikh faith, popularly known by its practice of Kundalini Yoga. Its initiates wear white clothing and head coverings (men wear turbans).

> If you close your nine doors, lo, the Tenth Gate opens to you.
> Know this, for this is the Essence of Wisdom.[80]

Closing the nine doors implies keeping the senses inwardly directed. The tenth gate is the crown chakra leading to a sacred door and the Divine Presence.

Any lying or sitting posture can be used for developing your mula bandha. But for a stronger pranic response, sit in one of two tantrasanas. Equal pose (samasana) is done by placing your right heel if you are a man (left for women) against the perineal root of the pelvis (between the genitals and anus) and the opposite foot in front of it so your heels are aligned with both ankles on the floor. This posture can be quite stimulating to the first and second chakras, as its pressure can be regulated for increasing your root lock's power. An even stronger position is siddhasana (perfect pose), which for men begins as in equal (samasana) pose, with the right heel pressing the perineum, and the left foot placed above the lingam so that pressure is applied to both the base and the root of the lingam (i.e., at the top and bottom of the pubic bone). Then pull the right toes upward between the calf and thigh, and the left toes downward to lock the posture. For women, the feet are reversed.[81]

---

79.  Learn more about Integral Yoga at *www.yogaville.org*.

80.  *Guru Granth Sahib*, the holy book of the Sikh religion, Gauri M 145, p. 151.

81.  For details, see Swami Satyananda (Bihar School), *Asana Pranayama Mudra Bandha*, 64, siddha yoni asana. Regardless of the posture chosen, practice isolating the various muscles of the pelvic and abdominal region until they can be isolated. See *Hatha Yoga Pradipika* I, 37–43 for more details.

Look in a detailed anatomy atlas, like *Human Anatomy* by Camine Clemente, to see how your muscles lie; the end points are called their origin and insertion. The end points move toward each other to tone a muscle. The gluteus maximus, the posterior buttock muscle, is attached from the sides of the sacrum at the sacroiliac joint to the lateral sides of the upper thighs. It is usually the first muscle felt when you make a pelvic contraction. The anal muscles are two sphincters—round muscles similar to those that form the mouth into a pucker—composed of an outer ring and an internal ring. Contract this region in and up, then relax; repeat the sequence. Locate the distinct feelings of controlling and separating these two sets of muscles. The ability to do this is called *aswini mudra*, "horse seal," for it heightens virility.

Then locate your vaginal sphincter muscles. With practice, you can isolate these from your rectal muscles. Gradually, this differentiation of the pelvic-floor muscles will lead to a heightened awareness of pelvic and lower-abdomen organs, including your cervix. This, in turn, will lead to the discovery of your vaginal coils, a series of rings that contract like a wave ascending toward the cervix and subsiding again, guided by the rhythm of your consistent practice of yogic breathing. This practice is called *sahajoli mudra*, seal of spontaneous psychic awareness.

The same practice for men that isolates the urethral muscles, is called vajroli mudra, the thunderbolt seal. A simple way to develop this and lessen your tendency to leave dribbles after urinating is to start and stop the flow of urine several times. For men, the psychic point to tone is just internal to the perineum. For the Tantrik male, ecstasy becomes a naturally arising state. In order to become whole, a man must surrender to a woman, for she will naturally be drawn toward the expression of a continuum of waves of Shakti. The evolved man will surrender fully to the primal Shakti as it manifests in his beloved.

In a similar manner, women will direct their contractions from the external muscles to the internal muscles. With consistency, the entire length of the vaginal canal can be toned. While the base of the penis (upper border joining the top of the pubic bone) is the second chakra for men, the cervix is the physical location of the second chakra for women. Thus, a gentle and loving physical or energetic penetration by a man to this point, accompanied by relaxation for the woman, establishes the inner yoni mudra for both. It is that internal point that is the psychic location for mula bandha. Practice tightening this canal to narrow its circumference, as in closing a fist one finger at a time.

## Yoni and Lingam Puja

The honoring of the primal female and male is called yoni puja and lingam puja. There are several varieties of this practice of devotion to honor the primal couple. In the outer form, the use of an image will help ground an unstable mind so that attention can be held on both the spiritual heart of yourself and the essence, spiritual heart of your partner. This practice consists of elements from several of the previous lessons. From lesson 2, you have the offering of the five elements, both within and outside. Here, one can use a sculpture and offer five liquids, representing five elements, that are poured over the Shakti yoni of Devi or the Shiva lingam of Deva and collected in a container below.

The element earth is represented by yoghurt, water by blessed water, fire by honey, air by milk, and ether by a form of edible oil like sesame oil. By cultivating feelings of love, opening your heart, and encouraging the entire chakra field to expand, the offerings become sanctified. The final mixture of liquids can be given to devotees as blessed food (*prasad*) that promotes the transformation of matter into Spirit. Variations of this outer ritual are common in Indian temples throughout the world. It is wonderful to be able to go on pilgrimage to India and experience the cultivation of love and humility that this ancient tradition evokes in us. It is also quite possible to experience a taste of India outside the subcontinent, as there are many Hindu temples worldwide. These temples are open to all spiritual seekers, regardless of their cultural background.

The main practices are puja, which can be performed to serve three different purposes: rituals of adoration, rituals of magic, and meditation rituals. In the first, devotees chant mantras and prayers, showering their love of this form and quality of the Divine Presence. In the second, they ask the deity to grant them what is missing in life (children, health, money, husband), thereby placing their burdens at the feet of the divine form. Such practices are common in most religious traditions.

*The secret form is where these practices are done for the purpose of becoming One, establishing the feelings of communion with yoni or lingam.*[82] The outer practices of lesson 10, as the Divine Couple born of the Mother, become the inner lesson in lesson 15, with Devi/Deva communion. All are encouraged to find the Tantrik sadhana that is naturally attractive for them.

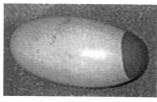

Shiva Lingam Stone

Tantriks encourage expression of suppressed feelings until they become natural. In Tantra, the orgasm is neither encouraged nor rejected. Reporting what you feel, whether the feelings are repeated or irregular, will help clarify to yourself and your partner what connects you to your highest feminine expression as God/dess, the Divine.

To develop the ability to create, contain, and sustain the experience of "sacred space" (yoni) is the object of a woman's Tantrik spiritual practice (sadhana). The word *sadhana* means the method of "Truth realization." For a woman, the Truth is that She is the microcosm of the macrocosm, as the Divine Mother. She can reach out and become transformed into what She already is.

## Enhancing Fertility for Conception

In India, sages are renowned for their ability to help promote a deeply satisfying life for both renunciants and householders. If they are unable to do so, they are of little regard. Among the ways I was shown by these sages to aid fertility are by giving a blessed banana *prasad* (offering) and personally modified sexually enhancing bandhas and mudras. These practices can heighten one's ability to fulfill any aspect of life's four dimensions. For those seeking children and the ability to allow a soul to incarnate as their child, fertility and passion are necessary to prepare the soil of their loving bodies and hearts.

*Sahajoli* is a perfect practice to increase a woman's fertility, as it increases ojas from the elevation of kapha. It is among the practices recommended for creating a fertile sacred space within you that will be inviting to an elevated soul consenting

---

82. Rufus Camphausen, *The Yoni* (Rochester, VT: Inner Traditions, 1996). Yoni puja is described in chapter 4. See also Alan Danielou, *The Phallus* (Rochester, VT: Inner Traditions), 1995.

to be born as your child. The sequence for its development is to do yoni mudra first, then sahajoli mudra. For men, the sequential practice is: *agnisar dhouti, uddiyana bandha*, and *nauli*. This is the optimal practice for enhancing male libido, as it increases tejas and ojas once they have learned to create a harmonious mental state of sattva. Nauli can help a man learn to direct his energy through his lingam, so that energetic intercourse can be felt by his partner. This practice is especially beneficial for infertile couples, as the energetic arousal touches both beloved partners in an unpredictable manner.[83]

Remember to persist in your practice, yet stay detached from expecting specific outcomes. Tantra is a personal spiritual practice. When you feel complete with this lesson, read the Dialogue section that follows prior to moving to lesson 14.

### With Great Respect and Love, I Honor
### My Heart, My Inner Teacher.

## Dialogue with Mukunda

**Student:** We had a Homa/Fire ceremony on Saturday for healing. At the ceremony— can you imagine—there was a basket *full* of Shiva lingam stones of all shapes and sizes! Boy, I tell you, the universe was promoting this practice! I chose one, as you said, that was as close in size to my partner and put it on the altar to be blessed during the ceremony. Talk about Shakti! The stone called to me and I went. Wow! How do I relate this without it sounding racey? Wow is all I can say. I felt lots of tremors and releases of my emotions during the experience. I had no trouble retaining the stone or expelling it. I was left feeling so sensual and so like a woman that I can't even explain. I did it again the next day. The second time, I experienced a large release of suppressed emotion. I can see how this is truly healing for stress issues for me. A great deal of sexual trauma was released during my second session with the stone. All I can say is that I truly was left with an experience of the Divine and feeling really at one with my beloved Shiva. What an experience!

The only questions I have are: How often should you do this and how long is it recommended to "hold" the stone? I could get hooked on being intimate with Shiva.

---

83. Mukunda Stiles, *Ayurvedic Yoga Therapy* (Twin Lakes, WI: Lotus Press, 2009), 72–76, describes these techniques.

**Mukunda:** Treat it with respect and love, as all sacred practice is intimate, personal, and sacred, then the amount of use will be clear to you. It is a very personal practice, so not for all. Those with naturally more sexual energy or those with suppressed emotions will need more time with the practice to find their own harmonious sattvic place.

**Student:** I had a dream in which I was told by a friend that I was confusing the energy of the yoni with the energy of the heart. Since then, I have been having this very specific sensation in my heart. It's in the center of my chest. It is small and shaped somewhat like a leaf or a diamond with smooth edges. It is all pink—darker and lighter shades. Inside it, I picture what looks like a clitoris. The visual image is quite similar to that of a beautiful yoni. And when I feel it in my heart, it is very deep, soft, and sensitive. Very tangible. I experience it for brief moments, from ten seconds up to one or two minutes. I am learning to contact it, and it keeps coming more and more consistently. The sensation is not at all sexual, but the feeling of it is so similar to the pleasure that I experience deep within my yoni. Is it perhaps similar to what we might call the G-spot of the heart? I hope you don't mind my graphic details. Do you know what this is?

**Mukunda:** Graphic details are helpful in clarifying your experience to me, as it is non-physical. And yet, your use of physical analogies does help me clarify your experience. The variety of experiences is huge from faithful Tantrik practice. It is beautiful that your heart is opening in this way—so unique and yet so sensual that pleasure arises. Kama, that is sexual and sensual pleasure, is one of the four natural arenas to be fulfilled according to the ancient Vedic teachings. Without fulfillment of physical pleasure, one cannot open spiritually to find liberation (*moksha*), as the passion of one is not different from the passions of the other. When it is naturally arising, I encourage you to open your prana and do whatever motion your prana Shakti wishes.

The process of helping you see the G-spot that is both in your yoni and in your heart can raise you to a fulfilling whole-body level of pleasure. According to Ramana Maharshi's *Ramana Gita*, chapter 5, there are three hearts. The physical heart is to left, the chakra heart is in the center of the chest, and the spiritual heart is two finger widths to the right of the breastbone. It may be that you are confused, but I encourage a different perspective—that what is coming to you is lovely and both places are seeking fulfillment. So open both seats of pleasure and fulfillment. See if you can encourage your awareness to go back and forth and to blossom. The sense I have is one of a unique yoni flower that is the essence of your womanhood blossoming to your Beloved. This is a great blessing.

**Student:** In the root lock with pranayama, I am having some questions. When we inhale, we release all of the pelvic and abdominal muscles. Then we exhale, contracting the pelvic floor and abdomen, trying to do outer ring to inner ring. What I am finding is that, when I contract the pelvic and abdominal muscles, I feel that I am contracting my neck and shoulders, which is causing tension. Simply stated, when I contract those muscles, I feel tension. I feel contraction everywhere, not just in the lower part of my body. Something about this practice feels blocked for me. Any thoughts? I also think I am overdue for some of your energetic yoga bodywork around my heart.

**Mukunda:** Do your best to stay relaxed throughout your body. This is normal for pranayama, that the upper body contracts when sending breath lower. It is a sign that you need to go more slowly into opening the lower abdomen where it becomes the pelvis. The distinction between the two is not clear, but the abdomen is pitta- and the pelvis vata-predominant. The meaning is that pelvic sensations are subtler and thus more challenging to feel and to discern their true significance. When Tantrik energy bodywork is received from me, it tends to go where needed. In some ways, it is the same when you do energy work on yourself. It is just that I can help you with your discernment about opening where you are suppressed and hungry for sensation and aliveness.

**Student:** You instruct us to sit by placing the heel just below the pubic bone. Due to limited range of motion of my knees and hips, I cannot sit in any of these poses that put pressure around this region. Do you have any modifications for applying pressure there without the use of the heels?

In terms of the siddhayoniasana seated position, placing the heel inside the labia and the modification of hero pose, I am uncomfortable at this point even doing a modified hero pose with a cushion. I am hesitant to put that much pressure on my knee just three months after surgery. Any further modifications available?

**Mukunda:** If neither knee bends to that point, then you can do the hero pose while elevated on a cushion or wooden meditation bench to protect your knees from bending beyond their capacity. To do what is asked, heel to pelvis, is beyond normal knee flexibility. Sitting on a wooden meditation bench is done with the heels toward the sitz bones.

Basically, connecting bone to bone tends to increase energy flow, so the heels are brought to the pubic bone in cross-legged poses or to the sitz bones for the hero pose (virasana). This is similar to the yoni mudra option of wrists on the iliac bones and fingertips on the pubic bone. Bones can retain prana more than soft tissue, so regular practice can sustain raised energy levels. If physical contact is not possible, extend prana beyond physical contact into your bones.

As for a sitting position, try sitting in a chair with your injured leg down and your other knee folded so your heel comes close to your yoni. If your chair is comfy enough, it can work. If it does, then you can tense the vaginal muscles around the heel and notice the sensations distinctly. With practice, this can create an inward-drawing sensation, one that, ideally, is more inward then upward. Doing this rhythmically—that is, with coordination of breath to tone your muscles—can help differentiate the pubococcygeal web of muscles from the vaginal and rectal sphincters. Attempt to do them separately after you can locate the vaginal muscles. You do not need to sit on the floor to do this practice.

*Student:* The instruction about yoni mudra hand placement reminds me of a challenge I am having. I have mostly practiced yoni mudra on my back until recently, and have been doing more seated in siddhasana or samasana. When in siddhasana, I have to bring my hand placement higher than where I feel I would like it because of the placement of my upper heel. Should I just go higher, or is there another option for what to do with my fingertips?

*Mukunda:* In siddhasana, because the upper heel is on or above the pubic bone, your hands will have to be higher than normal. The option is to elevate your pelvis with a pad so that both heel and fingertips can be on the bone. The ideal is to use *siddhayoniasana*, the variation given in the *Hatha Pradipika* (I, 32–45) for women. [84] In it, the lower heel goes to the perineum, the upper one adjacent to your yoni or underneath, but touching, the lower border of the pubic bone. With increasing comfort, the fingers can be on top of the pubic bone for yoni mudra. For this to work, both feet need to be angled so they are relatively parallel to the floor, not heel going upward. Because the pubic bone varies in height and width, there may be adjustments needed to your legs. A helpful adjustment from Iyengar is to roll your calf and thigh muscles away from each other upwardly, which should both make your knees more comfortable and allow your hips to relax.

---

84. *Ayurvedic Yoga Therapy*, 72–76.

This tantrasana practice is to help you connect with the vajra nadi (of the subtle body within the urethra/urinary canal). For that to happen, you must have first connected with your deeper Shakti in sushumna (central nadi). The process is one of connecting your physical body to Devi's outer form as a physical body; then you seek to connect your subtle body of Shakti prana to her subtle body. Thus, unveiling yourself leads to Her unveiling Herself—very much like the Middle Eastern dancer of seven veils lifting one veil off at a time, until she reveals her natural form. Eventually, primal Shakti Devi (yoni) is dancing only with Shiva Deva (lingam) in the Shiva/Shakti pose of consort yoga, an "eternal dance" called Shakti/Shiva tandava.

I am delighted how you are actively pulling energy in a way that generates insights. That shows you are doing well with sadhana. The more hungry you are, the more juicy ojas can get. That will pull what is needed to you, whether it appears to come from an outer or Inner Teacher. Always encourage yourself to pull, pranically or mentally, to give you more. The hungrier you get, the more will be given to you. Blessings.

**Student:** You said "mostly this practice is to help you connect with the vajra nadi. Though of course for that to happen, you must have first connected with your deeper Shakti in sushumna." Where exactly is the vajra nadi? I found a really stable siddhasana with firm heel pressure, practiced some wave breath with subtle spinal and sacral undulations, then, with hands in yoni mudra, I concentrated intently on drawing energy from my extremities and beyond to this place. My yoni mudra practice has been in a plateau for a while, but no longer! I experienced a clear intense throbbing sensation radiating behind the pubis that lasted ten minutes or so—very powerful! Is this the vajra nadi? I believe it allowed me to feel sushumna up to my solar plexus area, but not as strong above that. And I experience it now as I recall it. I just found connection between my pelvis and heart—between the second and fourth chakras! Namaste.

**Mukunda:** Your experience of "a clear intense throbbing sensation radiating behind the pubis" is the movement of vajra toward the second chakra. Later on, you say you found connection of that to the fourth chakra. Wonderful. Persist with this sadhana. Don't pay too much attention to my descriptions, as the uniqueness of your unfolding is due to devotion, not intellectual understanding. Nonetheless, read the lesson thoroughly, as it may trigger more openings.

The anatomy is peculiar, as we are talking of the subtle body, which extends to koshas 2, 3, and 4. It is intense and hot when it is in vajra. Vajra means "thunderbolt" or "diamond." When it awakens, it will tend either to move up (Shiva lingam energy being increased) or down (Shakti yoni energy predominant), piercing the chakras. Eventually, it moves to subtler dimensions that transform pitta into qualities of luminosity, light, piercing, or flashes like lightning. If the nadi is opened outward, it becomes a sexual arousal with plenty of ojas juice. In men, if it hasn't yet turned inward to subtler koshas, it makes the lingam as hard as a diamond. This is the experience that Swami Muktananda described in *Play of Consciousness* that was confusing to him. By maintaining the yoni mudra practice, experiences are short-lived, as the prana is pulled by the mudra to the inner chakras and, ultimately, to their source at the inner heart.

Vajra is inside sushumna nadi, yet in the second dimension of the subtle body (kosha 3). They both begin at the base of the physical pelvis. But sushumna begins at the perineum in kosha 2 with a kunda, or coiled energy, above it. Imagine a snake coiled between the second and third chakras in the region of the small of the back. It is wrapped three times around a column of light (lingam). The lower tail of that Kundalini (coiled serpent) is in the mouth of the sushumna at the pelvic floor. Inside sushumna's mouth, there are four tubes, or nadis, that are the openings to the final four koshas. The first is vajra nadi; located in kosha 3. Vajra begins at the urethra, but from there enters the subtle body into a channel deep in the pelvis located at the cervix (lower edge of the pubic bone, root of the lingam, for men).

**Student:** It came from your instruction to "persist in the Tantrik sadhana and learn to hug more deeply your own Spirit." I have a newly uncovered block with that instruction. It seems that I can freely and openly hug others, but not myself. Does this diminish the love that I give to others? Or will sharing my love and energy with others help me to love myself?

This block is a small hard kernel nut that resides in the center of my chest. I feel discomfort where it is right now, and sometimes it catches my breath and I cannot breathe deeply. At one level, the outside layers of this nut, is my little-girl spirit that feels rejected, dejected, unloved, and unworthy. I would like to say it is the result of the poor relationship that I had with my father. But now he lives in my heart, and I have forgiven him and love him. Nevertheless, this feeling still persists, and it colors my responses to any perceived rejection by a man. I identified that I was holding on so tenaciously to this discomfort, to a perceived rejection by a possible male employer. Of course, I just released a deep sigh and the discomfort is reduced. At least, now identified, I can let it go.

*Mukunda:* By sharing hugs, one can experience three possibilities: giving, receiving, and/or being love. A Tantrika has all three options. But they usually choose the third. The first two are foundations for Tantra, teaching others how to give or receive. The third is rarely available with another person, so it must be shared with a partner or consort as a sadhana, until it becomes naturally arising from the Devi's Presence living fully as you. This is learning to experience only love; then it can be available to others, who are hungry for love.

The source of this constriction does not matter. What matters is that you remember the process of energy-block removal as taught in early Tantra lessons and apply the same basic procedure. Sometimes, the blocks are not merely knots in the pranic flow; they can encounter what is known as a granthi. This is a much deeper knot of karma that can be located in heart, gut, or pelvis. They are on the level of the fourth kosha, at the level of the root of physical karma. They are removed by persistence just to be love. By making amends to some imagined harm in this life or recent past lives, it fades away. Seeking the source of love as your innermost heart will resolve all limitations, even those considered as destiny or fate. This level of Tantra clears even the blocks in the astrology chart.

*Student:* Last night during mula bandha practice, I had the sensation that the bandha was engaging on its own, subtly, and wanting to stay—this morning as well, although a little less intense. I assume, in this case, I should do as you always suggest—follow what is happening. So I just let it stay as it wants and, when it releases, continue the pulsing of the bandha with the breath.

*Mukunda:* Mula bandha has many variations that arise spontaneously. For me, I use the term mula mudra when the root lock stays engaged without self-effort. Details were given in lesson 13. This is a sign that the Shakti is supporting your awakening and She will naturally take bandhas from a physical expression to their energetic form as mudra. Mudra creates a sealing of prana into the cavity or chakra, enabling you to retain a much higher level of prana in both physical and subtle bodies. Remember, the subtle body is the second through fourth koshas, so many variations of experiences are likely to arise as you persist into transforming the pranic koshas.

**Student:** I have had a few students come to me after final relaxation and ask what it was that I was doing to them energetically. Today, one student said she felt as if I were pulling a string out of her throat. I know she has been having thyroid problems, and my hands were guided there. But I am not sure what I was feeling. It was something, but I don't know what, while I had one hand on the back of her neck and the other hovering over the pit of her throat. I don't often get feedback from students like that, so I don't know what else, if anything, is going on. Sometimes I feel a strong reaction from someone that I can't sort out. I don't really have a question here; I trust it will come together someday. I sometimes wonder if I am being appropriate working this way without knowing what I am doing, and I have asked you about this before. I guess what I really need to develop more than anything else is trust in my Self.

**Mukunda:** What you are describing is what I called Tantra Prana Bodywork in Tantrik lesson 6. I can teach variations of body postures and hand gestures (mudras) through a seminar; but most effective is the naturally arising Shakti. This is healing and promotes the end of suffering, even forms that you don't perceive while seemingly "working" on someone else. Now that you are at lesson 14, an advanced variation of lesson 6 is arising spontaneously. This occurs when one does the lessons with devotion and surrenders to a higher power. Doing higher lessons brings about new realizations and experiences of the gross methods of previous lessons. It is definitely good to trust in your own guidance, as only beneficial results can come of this. But learning to understand what is happening can be helpful and, most especially, will allow students to relax if they feel your self-confidence in Shakti.

**Student:** I am finding that, as I move from practicing ujjaye breath to the breath with mula bandha, the breath moves from being very fine without contraction to being more defined as breath and less so as just prana. As the effort increases, so does the need for grosser breathing. There are times when the breath remains fine and the contraction seems more on an energetic than a physical level. Should I practice this, moving from the gross to the fine, or the fine to the gross? Does it matter? While I like the refinement, I don't want to ignore the very physical part of this practice. I know my pelvic-floor PC muscles have not regained their strength since my last child four years ago.

**Mukunda:** For sadhana purposes, one should always be taking progression from gross to subtle. Allowing for the fact that having children has diminished the muscle tone of your PC group and pelvic diaphragm, you should balance practice with gross toning of your muscles. If physical tone is more desired than energetic, then practice longer or more often throughout the day. Doing practice at intervals, such as prior to meals, can give you more time without longer single periods of practice. The longer periods of practice are for the energetic benefits of mula bandha.

**Student:** I need your help. I have a conflict between promoting non-violence and a need for fulfillment in love-making and wanting to be as pure as possible so I cause no harm (*ahimsa*). I met a very loving man. Our connection is without effort and deep on all levels. He has great nurturing kapha qualities that I realize I have longed for for a very long time. I have not been intimate for a long time. I just had not met a man I wanted to share that with. Now I meet this wonderful, loving, humorous man with whom I connect deeply. The sex is "love-making," even though I don't want him to penetrate me because it feels sacred. Without movement intercourse, there is a subtle vibration I cannot explain, only that it feels like Tantra, which I have never experienced. He is the most honest man I have met in my life. It sometimes hurts to the bone, but he is crystal clear.

He wants to have children; I don't. So we already decided we cannot step into a relationship, but both feel the need to connect. He is seeing other women to find the partner with whom he can have children and marry. We both have to cry, as our connection feels so intense and he is scared of "throwing away" something precious. His love is nurturing and healing for me; I feel it inside, but also I am in conflict, because I don't want him to have sex with another woman. It feels to me that this love-making could not hurt anybody. It is not wrong because it is so honest; that's where he triggers me. I don't know what to do.

**Mukunda:** It is a Tantrik relationship you are blessed with. So you must treat it as different from ordinary sexual relations. This is healthy, as there is honesty and truthfulness. I am sending you more advanced Tantra lessons related to this topic. It is okay to skip ahead, as you need advice now. Read through all this and see what feels naturally arising and appropriate for you and him. Find a way to be intimate with your energies. In Tantra, energetic sexual intimacy is there. Sexual penetration is another topic. The former is always safe; the latter is often questionable. So question what is needed and fulfill each other with what is needed and not what is inappropriate. If he is having sex with other ladies, then you need to protect yourself from that and know that this is different. He needs to find the sacred in this intimacy with you, and you both need to find a boundary that makes this healthy for you both. Talk a lot before intimacy. Use the Tantrik agreement form to find out what you can offer each other.

**Student:** Lesson 13 is where I have a block. I noticed it at lesson 9, but I was not really aware of it until I reread lesson 13 (rereading is something that I have been doing a lot of lately—apparently I don't always read what I need to). Over last weekend, I had begun to feel lower-back pain and pain in my right hip. After practicing the exercise in lesson 9—mula bandha, with the four variations of the yoni mudra—this pain was much reduced. In fact, when I was moving away from our loving hugasana, my pelvis and lower back felt very heavy compared to everything above it, but I did not know what it meant at the time. Now I realize that that is where I am blocked.

After our session, I was able to feel more energy in the first chakra than ever before, so I became more confident in facing this block. So then, is physical pain the result of an energy block? As always, I am deeply grateful for your presence, guidance, and love.

**Mukunda:** Yes, it is often a sign of grosser energy blocks. Sometimes, the range of blocks is wide, reaching throughout the spectrum from insensitivity to over-expression. Doing mula bandha with yoni mudra is always beneficial. It can greatly help to invite feelings into consciousness. Often, internal practices of mula with the Shiva lingam stone can produce a much more complete release of your energy block there. The first and second chakras are so close to each other that one cannot really distinguish them, so the best procedure is to do something that deliberately goes to both regions. I am happy to serve you and deepen your ability to connect with your own spirit and higher powers. Namaste.

**Student:** Last night, I practiced the sadhanas in Tantra lessons 1 through 3. After nyasa, I did seated yoni mudra at first position, low belly—I usually place my hands a little lower on my pelvic bones. My neck was really uncomfortable. I tried to soften the rigidity in my neck, shoulders, and arms; when I did, my head started bobbling. I realized that this neck tension is me trying to be in control and not flowing with life. I wanted to just let the kriyas come out freely, but fear came up that, if I let go and just flowed with it, I might hurt my neck. It is hard to soften at times when my spine feels more crooked and restricted. With my scoliosis, softening can feel like collapsing. Much energy has been used just trying to carry my structure around, so staying upright took great effort that is hard to let go of now. When the fear came up, some tears followed, as I remembered other times when I let go and got hurt. I realized I may have some unresolved feelings about being out of control, unprotected, and misunderstood. I moved my thoughts to the present and recalled from reading the *Vijnana Bhairava Tantra* (VBT) that all is possible in the space between the in breath and out breath (*kumbhaka*). So I tried to allow kumbhaka and realized that I can stay safe and protect myself if I just allow more consciousness in my life in general.

***Mukunda:*** Some practices for you to do based on the VBT:

> Sutra 43. At the beginning of sexual passion, be in the fire, absorbed into her by the flames of passion. Allow the burning, persisting with the nectar of intimacy, then merge into Spirit.

> Sutra 44. When, in such an embrace, your senses are shaken as leaves in the wind, enter this shaking as you merge with the celestial bliss of ecstatic love.

> Sutra 45. O Goddess! Even from remembering the intimate bliss of sexual communion, without Shakti's embrace, the radiant pleasures of kissing, hugging, and embracing again swell into a flood of delight.[85]

I find that Sutra 44 is especially good to work with the naturally arising kriyas as you unwind your scoliosis and its multi-dimensional layering of stress. Trust is important, and yet you are not likely to know that it is safe unless you have the feeling that you are fully embraced preceding the trust. So look for that sense of being embraced by Shakti or hugged; it really doesn't matter, just see what gives you the feeling of really being held lovingly. If that is sufficiently enhanced, then trust will naturally arise and, with it, the safety to be vulnerable. Be gentle, as this is a most delicate edge to play with the dance of Shiva/Shakti tandava. Definitely keep deepening the kumbhaka, as that will naturally arise in this blossoming process you are engaged in. I am delighted to have you stay in touch so deeply. Blessings.

***Student:*** My experience so far with the Shiva lingam stone has been amazing. When I was holding it to wash it for the first time, I felt twinges in my right hip. I began with the energy-balancing and, when I laid the stone on my belly, I felt a warm gush/flow of energy from my feet to my forehead. Over time, it dissipated into little eddies of energy that I felt all over, but most intensely at my forehead. When I held the stone at my belly with my left hand

---

85. *Vijnana Bhairava Tantra*; sutras, adapted from the appendix in *Zen Flesh, Zen Bones*, by Paul Reps and Nyogen Senzaki.

and placed my right hand on my left, I felt energy surging on the left side. When I reversed the position of my hands, I felt energy only on my right leg and my upper body. All was quiet with stone and yoni mudra at the third chakra, but at the second chakra, there were palpable "pulsations" and then there was an adjustment of my lower spine. Much quieter at the first chakra, but with the yoni mudra over the sacrum and the stone on the second chakra, there was a flow of energy from sacrum to chest. Yoni responded to the external massage, but was not ready to accept the stone. So I left it there for a while and then placed it in its bag, but kept it close by so that yoni would become more familiar with the lingam stone. I will continue to do this practice with the lingam stone. Do you suggest that I do anything differently?

*Mukunda:* You are doing quite well. Just persist with your loving intentions and let the lingam and yoni become familiar with each other. In time, they will be more receptive to each other, and will know the unknown that is currently their yoga. Love is expressed in the feelings of being captivated and fully embraced as if the Beloved is all around you. A unique reaction like the one you are having is the Beloved's form. All is going well.

*Student:* Are there lingam stones sold specifically for the purpose of both external worship and internal vaginal toning? The stone resembles my husband's shape, so I wonder about size. Is it something that fits into the canal completely, or is it longer than the canal? Do you know of a good website from which to purchase one?

*Mukunda:* The Shiva lingam puja practice is a secret technique revealed to me by my inner connection with Devi, so you will not likely find others informed of this method. There are no stones sold for this purpose, though I recommend a stone that is three inches in length and circumference.

The stone is to be treated as your own Shiva's lingam, revered and gently massaged with hands and placed against the chakras or any energetic reaction that you experience. Some ladies' physical yoni may wish to receive it. Once inside, by relaxing the muscles, the lingam stone will descend. It should feel comfortable and fully inside your canal and sink with gravity to release the pelvic floor. In contrast, it can be used by repeatedly pulling upward and relaxing to tone the pelvic floor. Optimal practice will draw both physical and energetic sensations from your first to your second chakra, thus increasing udana prana (the source for Kundalini Devi's Shakti). Doing this regularly can greatly enhance your response to your husband's loving.

The stones can be used for this purpose, as well as for worshipping the first form (the literal meaning of lingam) of Shiva. They can be found at many Indian import shops. Some websites that provide education about lingam or Shiva stones include *www.bojis-tones.com, www.sanatansociety.org*, and *www.dragonsreverie.com*.

You can find yoni wooden or stone bases to hold your lingam vertically at *www.pilgrimshandicrafts.com*. While this may be the only option for those students in remote areas, I do not recommend purchasing that way. The ideal test is to hold the stone to get a feel for its size and weight, and also for the prana of the lingam. In India, the larger the lingam, the more revered the temple. (The greatest of these temples are called Jyoti Lingam. There are naturally occurring sites. I take students to Trumbakeshwar, located midway between my two teachers' ashrams, each January.)

Shiva lingam stones are naturally formed in the Narmada Rivers then polished to the form that is sold. They can contain and increase prana when they are of the highest quality. In this way, they are more suitable for your altar's worship (puja). The outward puja is to Shiva with a yoni-shaped circular base, shaped like labia with a trough from which offering fluids can flow. The word *yoni* means source, as well as sacred space. In this case, the sacred space of yoni allows the lingam to take shape. This means the Goddess is the Source of Creation. She provides the space and the energy required for Shiva (Her husband) to come into Her yoni as the microcosm of the macrocosm.

**Student:** I have found various problems cropping up as I do the readjustment work on my pelvic floor. My pelvic floor muscles had tightened up almost to the point where they had been when I went for my physical therapy appointment to release them two weeks ago. I had noted some tightness and used a small black egg-shaped rock in the way you suggested. Playing the scientist, I will bring my body back to a better muscle balance, then will try using the weight again to see whether it helps or aggravates.

**Mukunda:** I suggest using the Shiva lingam stone more and perhaps getting one weighty enough to drop your pelvic floor when it is inside. The key is to relax the pelvic diaphragm and, once you are as relaxed as possible, gently pull the stone upward and fully release it. Practice pulling mildly and releasing more. The key is to encourage the relaxation reflex so that the internal musculature spreads and releases. With full relaxation, it can reach as far as the pubic bone. If this doesn't provide relief of pain and openness, look for a pelvic-floor physical therapy specialist. (Try *www.pelvicpain.com*.)

# The Colorful Paths of Tantrik Yoga

With Great Respect and Love, I Honor
My Heart, My Inner Teacher.

A way of sharing yoga practice is partner yogasana practice. This practice is especially beneficial for same-sex friends who share a common physical practice. This is a lovely way to share stimulating and enthusiastic emotional expressions. The range of techniques goes from partner practice of popular asanas that deepen the physical benefits, to opening your heart in hugasana. This is described in several books: *Double Yoga* by Ganga White and Anna Forrest; *Doubles Yoga* by Shar Lee and Dawn Mahowald; and *Dwiasana Yoga* by Professor Fernando Estevez Griego and Iris Stein from Buenos Aires (published in Argentina in Spanish). All these manuals share delightful partner poses that are a lovely way to share asana reactions, whether or not they move you into a deeper physical tone or stretch. This can be a jumping-off place for sharing prana as a Tantrik partner practice.

## Yoga and Tantrik Partner Practices

Tantrasana partner practices generate emotionally "colored" Tantrik practices that run the gamut from White to Pink to Red. While White Tantra is the most commonly practiced form, Red Tantra and its less passionate variations may be approached using partner yogasanas that lend themselves to moving into meditative stillness. Red Tantra, also called the left-hand path, is for those who seek to merge into a spiritual life, even if it moves in a direction contrary to public opinion. According to *Vasistha's Yoga,* "the left handed ritual reveals the supreme truth."[86] This method seeks to free the practitioner of all self-restraints and limitations and fully enter the innermost Self and its field of Divine Love. This path seeks to break through all blocked energy patterns, whether they are emotional, sensual, conceptual, or karmic.

Seekers who follow this path have the experience that all energy is sexual, in the sense that it is creative and naturally attracts its polar opposite. It is the path of passion and self-acceptance, encouraging all of one's energies to be directed toward spiritual awakening. The extremists on this path do rituals with substances forbidden in Classical Yoga practices. Through their rajasic practice, they seek to remove the negative charge to these substances. Aghora Tantriks engage in transforming all aspects of life that are disgusting to orthodox Yogis and Tantriks. They vehemently pursue the five prohibited substances and acts (makaras, described in lesson 7)—alcohol, sexual intercourse, meat, fish, and parched grains—and may meditate in graveyards to be free of their lust, the duality of addiction, and/or aversion to the body.

The awakening can create a colored Tantrik expression. When seekers have spiritual partners or spouses, they naturally shift into Pink or Red forms, as it is natural to express your spiritual awakening in all avenues of life, including sexuality. One of the signs of a Yogi is that his energy only moves upward. This state, known as an *urdhvareta,* will not permit prana or sex fluids to drain. Yogis gain this state from discipline and renunciation, while Tantriks gain it by surrendering to the Mother or Her representative as their consort. Without a consort or a firm conviction of the Mother's presence, Tantra partner practices are on unstable ground. They can be stabilized by going slowly, increasing the level of communication, and establishing clear boundaries on what acts are questionable or forbidden for each partner. The fundamental difference is that White Tantriks do not share their energetic practices; they will more than likely be celibate or monogamous in a committed relationship.

> If you wish to be sexually active and do not yet have someone to teach
> you Tantra, the best path to follow is to the path of the happy home.

---

86. *Vasistha's Yoga,* 348.

Select a partner and commit yourself to a relationship, and when you have experienced full enjoyment, begin to experiment with periods of sexual continence to deepen the relationship and enhance your spiritual development. At all times, in all interactions with your partner, offer all your pleasure to the Divine and let That One guide and direct you. It may not be the highest possible expression of sex, but spiritualized sexuality can become the beginning of a sexual sadhana.[87]

"Pink Tantra" is a term that I coined. It is a compromise form of Tantra communion midway between White and Red Tantra. Like other valid paths, its fullness is not attained without consistent sadhana over a long period, and its stability requires the guidance and blessings of a teacher. It often takes the form of a lingering hug, in which there is an exchange of elevated prana. It differs from Red Tantra in that its practitioners do express all their energies, including sexual, but do not act upon an emotional or energetic rush to sexual intercourse. They may agree to a variety of expressions, such as caressing the Beloved or "energetic intercourse."

In directing yourself toward the Deva/Devi spiritual communion, I recommend the use of the Tantrik partnership agreement that follows. This will prevent stress by helping you make clear agreements on what boundaries you need to feel safe. This will deepen your ability to communicate clearly to your partner, even a spouse with whom you have a healthy rapport. It is important to express your concerns about difficulties with previous traumas, whether they are physical, emotional, sexual, birth traumas (your own or a child), or spiritual in nature. In addition, have a face-to-face discussion about sexually transmitted diseases (STDs), including revealing your history. If you feel like proceeding, have an STD test to assure yourself and your partner of your health before any romantic, ritualistic, or sexual arousal that involves removing your clothing.

Read the Tantrik partnership agreement carefully so you can establish safety. Spend plenty of time formulating this agreement. Make sure you both feel in complete agreement so that when revisiting it, you continue to agree with it. A primary reason why Tantrik partnering is unsuccessful is a lack of communication. Both before and

---

87. Robert Svoboda, "Sex, Self-Identification and the Aghora Tradition," in *Enlightened Sexuality*, ed. Georg Feuerstein, 197.

after each session, take all the time you need to share your feelings and thoughts, and talk about anything that may be confusing. Repeat this at the beginning of each future session to clear the naturally arising after-effects of a Tantrik Yoga partner practice. If you wish, you can change the agreement anytime, following insights you gain as to your needs. One cannot spend too much time on this, as it promotes depth in your shared sadhana.

## Tantrik Partner Agreement

The purpose of this agreement is to manifest our intentions and define the boundaries of appropriate and inappropriate conduct during Tantrik Yoga prana sharing. Clarify what you agree to and remove what feels improper for now. These practices are for our spiritual and energetic elevation, so that we may be of greater service to our spiritual selves and others.

We agree to share our knowledge, pranic/Kundalini energy, and healing gifts fully and freely to assist each other in the removal of blocked and restricted patterns, whether they are physical, energetic, mental, emotional, or sexual in nature. In essence, we agree to be of selfless service to the Spirit of guidance through our intimate connection with each other. We further agree to maintain a balance of detachment from personal self-serving agendas, yet cultivate openness to naturally arising creative self-expression. It is understood that this Tantrik partnership will increase our energies and will likely take the form of arousal on the different dimensions (koshas) through these elevated states of consciousness. As such, it is crucial that we have discussions to assure all levels of safety—emotional, physical, and sexual. This will include the release of fear, anger, attachments that no longer serve us, and traumas from prior relations. We agree to take the time necessary to communicate our feelings and desires prior to and following each exchange. These sessions may run beyond the scheduled time.

Tantrik energy sharing works with clothing on or off. Vyana prana flows through the skin; thus stillness or skin-to-skin contact can facilitate that subtlest of pranas to open their sensitive channels. We can choose what supports our comfort and safety. We agree to abstain from sexual intercourse, yet will encourage all energetic and physical openings to run their course via energetic "inner course" and sexual "outer course." Thus, there will certainly be a free sexual and spiritual energy exchange, but not physical penetration. We will support each other and create a space of safety to allow the complete expression of these memories and/or expansive energies and emotional states. We understand that all such expressions are temporary in nature and will encourage the development of a stable mental and spiritual state in each other.

## Clarifying Your Personal Path

If you wish to proceed on this path, I encourage you to clarify your marriage or partnership vows with your significant other, so that you can maintain your integrity. For the yogi and yogini, being aligned with the Divine as the source of all teaching creates the greatest relationship. When writing the partnership agreement, bear in mind that you can extend this to the vow of *brahmacharya*. Brahmacharya means behavior that respects the Divine as omnipresent. When we act as if God/dess is always watching us, our response is a passionate life.

You will have difficulty if you do not feel your husband/wife is your spiritual partner and does not share your interest in spiritual practices. If this is your situation, I advise you to honor your marriage vows and commit to White Tantra. Do not seek another partner.

Tantrik partner practices enhance both your ability to be intimate and your desire to live an empowered spiritual life. By connecting energy centers through meditative "hugs to the melting point" and pranayama techniques, fears and limitations can dissolve. Women learn to become receptive vessels of their own and their partners' transformed Shakti energies. Men become solid, grounded in their Shiva nature as a commitment to stability. In the *Amritanubhav: The Nectar of Self Awareness* by Jnaneshwar, a 14th-century spiritual master and poet, adepts learn to merge, as well as to "separate just for the pleasure of being two."

The process of communion leads to a balance of the subtlest forms of the dimensions (koshas) of our bodies and the Ayurvedic instabilities expressed as doshas. In yogic language, we call this *sat/chit/ananda,* or serenity-vitality-ecstasy.

"Ecstasy, from the Greek root ekstasis, means to stand outside of oneself," Geralyn Gendreau tells us. "The term comes to us, quite literally, by way of the Dionysian tradition, in which ritual ecstatic sex was practiced as a means of communing with God."[88] The persistence of this experience over various cultures and centuries shows the potential for the inseparability of Divine Love and human love.

Partner Tantra is best learned, like all spiritual practices, with a teacher's guidance. Partner practices enhance the spiritual life of couples currently enjoying a fulfilling intimate relationship. It is known in the formerly secret teachings of both Tantrik Yoga and Buddhism that the proper use of sexual energy can penetrate the multi-dimensional layers of the chakras, aiding in the pursuit of liberation (*moksha*). Among the earliest texts of Tantrik Hatha Yoga is the 14th-century text the *Hatha Yoga Pradipika*, translated by Swami Muktibodhananda of the Bihar School of Yoga, Practices of vajroli and sahajoli mudra that permit a profound energetic exchange are described in III, 83–103. Note that, of the six other editions available, only the one published by Kaivalyadhama Yoga Institute in Lonavla, Poona, India has the fifth chapter, which describes Ayurvedic recommendations for treating the root cause of injurious yoga practices.

Some detailed stories of this sadhana include a contemporary story of a male Hatha Yoga teacher with a female student told by André van Lysebeth in his book *Tantra Yoga: The Cult of the Feminine*. The story of a Tantrika teacher with a male student is shared in *Tantrik Quest* by Daniel Odier. Miranda Shaw, with the Dalai Lama's blessings, gained access to Tibetan Buddhist lineages that share sexual spiritual practices for their mutual evolution. She shares these in *Passionate Enlightenment: Women in Tantric Buddhism* (see chapters 6 and 7).

Men need to learn how important it is to make sure a partner is safe first (grounding the first chakra) and focus on pleasing the Beloved second (opening the second chakra), as only she can create the sacred space necessary to bestow blessings. They will learn karezza (prolonged intercourse with restraint of male ejaculation), enabling them to detach from the heat of prolonged passion to give selfless service to their partner.

Women learn to become receptive vessels, retaining their own and their partners' transformed higher energies. They can then exchange energies that make available experiences that neither can attain on his or her own. This occurs by connecting

---

88. Gendreau, ed., *The Marriage of Sex and Spirit*, 7.

marma points on the skin with pranic energy centers and learning how to give and receive "hugs to the melting point." From this, fears and limitations of natural self-expression can dissolve. It doesn't matter what your level of experience or attainment is; just being in the field of influence of another spiritual seeker will elevate both of you. By sharing your love of the mystery of life, you open new fields of exploration within yourself and your spiritual partner.

## Choosing an Appropriate Partner

Give your teacher plenty of feedback if you need help for these more vulnerable practices. Communicating to your journal or teacher is especially important as you move to more intimacy with your True Self. Remember this practice is for Communion with that One.

This lesson will focus on the development of your natural sensuality into a spiritual expression. The practices herein can be taken as Pink (clothes on) or Red (nude) Tantra, in that they seek to help you transcend sexual emotions and expression. Hopefully, you have decided which practice is for you and your partner. The most important prerequisite is to be assured you have found an appropriate partner and have clear agreements that you both respect and follow. The ideal partner is someone with whom you share a loving relationship and whom you mutually wish to take to a higher level.

What are unhealthy choices for Red Tantra? A novice, a new romantic partner, or your teacher. What are unwise choices for Pink Tantra? Those people for whom you have a romantic attraction but who are in a committed relationship, and those in dissolving relationships who have not achieved a complete clear resolution with their previous partners. Among the many challenging situations is when you do not perceive your relationship partner or spouse as your spiritual partner. This is due to incorrect perception, for clearly you are having spiritual lessons in addition to intimacy lessons.

If your romantic partner or spouse does not share in your spiritual practice, this will make for an emotional and energetic distance. If this is your situation, I recommend that you only do White Tantra group practices. It is imperative in spiritual practice to keep your integrity and truthfulness intact. Students who hold that a spiritual relationship is more important than a marriage tend to suffer greatly, and that suffering then extends to others. I encourage you to keep your marriage vow as a tangible form of brahmacharya, and not engage in Red Tantrik practice with anyone other than your spouse.

When sex without love happens, it opens the door to unhealthy energies and entities; the diseases that result can be difficult to treat as they exist on multi-dimensional levels. Your partner, like yourself, should already have a consistent spiritual practice, so that the increased energy from partner practice will deepen your sadhana. The ideal is for your partner to be your romantic partner as well. That way, what you will share is unbounded great respect and love of Spirit. Other healthy choices include someone on your spiritual path, or someone in your yogic or meditation community whom you know well. The same ethical standards that you hold for healthy personal relationships apply in finding a Tantrik partner. If you have a romantic sexual partner, do not seek someone else as your Red Tantrik partner, but consider if you would be respectful White Tantrik partners. If you cannot imagine yourself keeping your clothes on with this partner, then do not propose a Pink Tantrik practice. Instead, consider the person as a member of your White Tantrik community and maintain healthy relationships.

Major considerations are to find a partner who can hold the energy openings and create a feeling of safety. This is especially true in a male partner. He should hold Shiva state, minimizing his physical motions, and encourage his Shakti partner's responses without trying to create physical or sexual arousal. The partners, while not necessarily fully illumined, must possess a strong motivation for this sadhana to transform them, and must seek to serve you. Most important, they should have an openness to communicate about anything that is a concern. From that respectful foundation, you can both move to become neutral with regard to four categories of challenge:

> Energetic and emotional blocks
> Sexual history
> Concerns, criticisms, and doubts
> Strong motivation to help you hold an increased prana Shakti

Sharing Love is the key. By Love, I do not mean romantic love of your partner's personality, but a mutual spiritual Love of the Divine Presence. If this quality is being shared, you have a good foundation for healthy practice. In this way, you must be assured that you are safe—a condition that the first two chakras require before opening their tremendous storehouse of latent energy. This safety comes through making a clear partnership agreement (see the example above). Your mutual connection to a higher Presence must be cultivated; it does not come naturally. We are self-centered beings and will continue to remain so until final Self Realization.

One way to test a potential partner is simply to ask for a prolonged hug. "Hugasana" is a beautiful way to see how energetically compatible you are before opening yourself to challenging energies and emotions. This person can be of either sex. The ideal candidate for regular energy practice will have an immediate and natural opening to you, and your energies will spontaneously produce one of the techniques you learned in the first three lessons. Your hug takes both of you to a deep relaxation or "melting point," yet you remain grounded in spiritual energy. The optimal partner may not know the Tantrik lessons, but will be able to follow the patterns of training when you describe them. This includes the polarity balancing of two-hand placements, breathing rhythmically together, opening energy blocks so you physically relax, connecting heart to heart (both lean your head to the right), and grounding each of the five elements. If both of you can relax and open to the pranic currents, this is a strong indicator that you can share more deeply.

Keep in mind that the Devi (Goddess) is more important to please than the Deva. The Cakrasamvara Tibetan Tantrik system "emphasizes that a female practitioner of the yoga of union should be one who keeps the Tantrik vows or 'commitments' (samaya). Thus, an appropriate female partner is often specified as a 'possessor of vows,' or a 'non-breaker' of vows."[89]

Simply put, women are more likely to maintain an ethical relationship and will be upset easily when boundaries are disregarded. Her comfort is to be maintained regardless of the practice.

## Preliminary Guidance

Before proceeding, be sure that you both fully agree to encourage all energetic responses for as long as possible, so that you experience your practice not only as sexual, but as a

---

89. Miranda Shaw, *Passionate Enlightenment: Women in Tantric Buddhism* (Princeton: Princeton University Press, 1994), 171.

sacred energetic ritual that connects you to the Divine in a personal way. As the energy increases, it will normally generate kriyas, spontaneous movements, and energy rushes. When your partner is having these, do not stimulate them, but rather keep your hands and body motionless to allow them to process their release into openness. In this way, both of you will be more likely to retain the elevated levels of Shakti. On a practical note, that means Devi women are encouraged to slow down and focus on being the object of pleasure, so as not to overstimulate their Deva partner to the "point of no return."

Once a man is aroused to a point of heat, his energy will drop unless his prana is trained to be sustained as a continuum regardless of his lingam's state of arousal. Without training, this can spell the end of communion. Men need to assist their partners by letting them know if they are feeling overly stimulated. This is true for both Pink and Red tantra. Through Devi/Deva communion, we are seeking continuous connection with our partners to manifest the eternal pulsation (*spanda*), also called the primal prana (*adhya prana Shakti*). With practice, Deva men can keep their attention on what brings pleasure and ecstasy to their Devi female partner. That will always increase the capacity for both to retain their elevated Shakti prana.

## Tantrik Practice for a Couple

In Tantrik relationships, what's important is clarity of agreement about where you're going before you go there. Tantra is not better sex. Tantra is sadhana to be free of karma. That's the skipped-over piece. Teachings that increase our sexual energy regardless of our emotions and thoughts are popular. The question is: Are we really honest in maintaining integrity with all of our energies?

Pretend you're starting all over again, with the question of how can we open to infinite love. It's healthy to start over, to be a consummate beginner. It's a process, with plenty of courtship of your True Self. In the yoga ethics of Patanjali's *Yoga Sutras*, the first imperative is to do no harm (*ahimsa*). The second is truthfulness. So, let us begin again with clear karma. Begin your dance of intimacy on the energy level, ethically courting each other's prana. Know that you are participating in the dance of eternity—Shiva and Shakti tandava—with your partner. This is, all at once, a spiritual dance, an energy healing, and an exchange of the essential energy that arises regardless of form. Play with this for a few days. Then slowly come together, standing close, then sitting together. Now closer. Slowly, deliberately. The whole intention is to have a relationship with Spirit. By immersing in the True Self, literally see the Self. That is the essence of Tantra-darshan, the vision of the Beloved's form.

Sit and face each other—close, but not touching. Close your eyes. Come deeply into your selves. Pull your selves away from each other and into your own selves. Move to your core. Breathe into your core and acknowledge your core. You can use your hands or not. The core is not a static place; it is dynamic.

> She: hands to heart
> He: hands to belly and sacrum

Now, come to a pathway, or door, or light. What's in there? Someone? Something? Be there. Now bring your hands to that place. Look more deeply into that *sanctum sanctorum,* that holy place. Affirm to your self that you are holy and sacred; know that your inner place has everything. Listen inwardly and feel into what is there.

Slowly open energies with each other. Keep your hands in place. Two energies becoming one; two rivers into one. Relax whenever you feel tension, and breathe into it. Vocalize your breath, with a sigh. See where you can get more physically comfortable.

Now, open your eyes. Don't move your hands. Bow, Namaste to each other. Keep your hands in place. Do what you want to do with great respect and love.

Bring your right hand into place on each other's heart. Put your left hand on your partner's right hand. Close your eyes. Go back to your core. Find the core. Part of you will be with your partner. Most of you will be in your own core. Your partner's intention is to be rooted in your core. Each helps the other deepen connection to the other's core.

Breathe, move, and let out emotions and feelings, but no words. If the posture needs to shift, that's okay. Most of your self—80 percent—is a watery core. Begin to replenish yoni mudra without using your hands. Begin to rejuvenate your pranic mind fields. Go to the core as a place of renewal. Let more of your body energy go to your core. Sigh, moan, and yawn. The body may have little jerks and responses. Kriyas may come up and dissolve. Encourage what is actually arising.

Slowly, bring your hands away, to your own lap. Sit and breathe. Encourage a lingering connection. Feel safe; know that feeling is the truth. Let the breath go through the chakra fields, becoming a column of light (lingam) opening into the third eye for some time.

Now sit back to back. Connect chakras to chakras with breath and body. Feel free to move and play, or to be still; let naturalness happen. Occasionally, sigh, moan, and yawn. Play. Discover how to be comfortable being with each other. Spontaneously dance, back to back.

Don't do anything else. Just be.

After a while: "Hugasana!" Lingering into what naturally arises.

Partner Tantrik practice is beneficial for committed spiritual couples, and even more for those seeking to conceive. It heightens fertility in both partners. For all others, it is best to proceed slowly into partner Tantrik practice. I recommend you do the energy-work practices from the last lesson as you visualize yourself sharing your energetic evolution in a group hug. Begin to open your energy fields more, so that there is a feeling of deeply receiving and sending your pranic currents. As you evolve this practice to the next koshic dimension, it can become *prana prathista*, in which the prana is deliberately installed and retained in the gross body tissues or in a statue. Constantly cultivate an attitude of openness and receptivity, and seek to discover which practice offers you the most opportunity for growth. At the conclusion, spend time discussing your experiences with your spiritual partner and teacher to uncover which aspect of the Tantrik Yoga path is best at this time. And if needed, seek clarification on how to adapt these general teachings for your unique situation.

If you are not comfortable or don't have a potential partner, then you have the choice of visualizing the partner practices or simply skipping over lessons 14 and 15 and moving to lesson 16 as you continue to become openly exposed to the range of Tantrik practices.

## Preparation for Lesson 15

The next lesson is about opening yourself to love and sharing it with your partner. I recommend that you share a loving and erotic videotape called *The Secrets of Sacred Sex* (produced by Living Arts, available at *www.gaiam.com*), as it reveals the use of Tantrik arts in the loving presence of real-life couples who share, not only awakened sexuality, but also guidance and dialogues for increased intimacy. Consider also *Freeing the*

*Female Orgasm—Awakening the Goddess* by Charles and Caroline Muir, available on audio or videotape from *www.sourcetantra.com*, which explains a loving method for freeing repression or traumas via a loving massage of the sacred G-spot. When this is shared lovingly, the yoni responds by spiritually awakening and producing the elixir called *amrita*. This powerful sexual nectar flows freely once the Yogini experiences herself as a Goddess.

Remember to persist in your practice, yet stay detached from expecting specific outcomes. Tantra is a personal spiritual practice. When you feel complete with this lesson, read the Dialogue section that follows prior to beginning lesson 15.

**With Great Respect and Love, I Honor
My Heart, My Inner Teacher.**

# Dialogue with Mukunda

**Student:** I spent a good part of the weekend with Ammachi's (the hugging-Indian-woman guru) crowd in New York. I received darshan on Sunday evening and attended the all-night Devi Bhava program. After both experiences, I felt very much in my heart, with huge expansive heart sensations. The other thing that was coming up for me all weekend was second/third chakra weakness/depletion. It was my first time really out of the house since surgery; I was around lots of energy—especially attractive, openhearted single men.

When I noticed myself make eye contact with someone or found someone attractive, I came immediately out of this heart state and felt energy going into my lower, mostly second, chakra. This was accompanied by a feeling of desire and anxiety. I was aware that, instead of seeing all individuals as my brothers and sisters, I was seeing many of these men as potential lovers. When I noticed this happening, which was practically all the time, I became aware of my breath and tried to breathe the energy in, back up to my heart, and exhale, directing the breath through my third eye and then all the way down to my root, along the front of my body. It did help somewhat, but it did not feel like the most effective "technique." I felt as if I were just trying to do anything to change the pattern or flow of the energy.

This type of occurrence happens frequently for me: instead of staying heart-centered on men, I go to the lower chakras. My second gets thrown off; then my third tries to compensate and they both get all messed up. Is there any specific technique for this type of "dysfunction"? Is this something that many people experience? I think that mistaking heart energy for sex energy (or the other way around) must be quite common.

***Mukunda:*** Indeed, it is a common issue. With Tantra, the intention is to follow the energy, not to try to change it. So that means when you feel the second chakra, just feel it. To do that is not to act inappropriately. Changing the energy into something more acceptable for your mind will always displace the energy of prana Shakti—if not deplete it as if it were a "leaky bucket." Emotions of anxiety are often a projection of the "what if ..." thought. What if they don't like me? What if they are not single? What if they are not the One I am looking for? You are, most likely, jumping ahead of feelings of attraction and desire into some other space.

Shakti energy is always seeking an expression. In this case, the expression is flirtation. Enjoy the attraction to those men who are potential partners for you. There is nothing wrong with that. Remember lesson 1, on the yoni mudra, is simply to find your energy and allow it to direct your attention to where it is most plentiful. So if it is sexual attraction, enjoy it. That is certainly not a dysfunction. Take your time to feel the sexual energy of yourself and others. You are clearly a thoughtful woman and your thoughts will serve to protect you from partners who are inappropriate due to uncomfortably long periods of celibacy. Move slowly into the expression of your sexual energy. Feel it; enjoy it, by all means. But that doesn't mean you must act on it simply because it is present. You are single, available, looking for a partner. How you find one will require you to move through a mixture of all sorts of emotions. All the chakras will be open when there is optimal opportunity for partnering. It will be mutual. Until it is, enjoy yourself coming back to life after some time of not dating. All is going well. Be gentle and stay with your energy rather than trying to change it. Bless it and you.

***Student:*** Is it advisable to share this lesson with my husband and see what his thoughts are on proceeding with Pink/Red Tantrik practices? The focus of my doing this practice has been to try to extend whatever I have been feeling in the spiritual heart outward during meditation. Although I haven't gotten a sense of which practice is more suited for me, I would like to proceed to the next lessons if my husband is interested as well. I can't say with certainty if he is my spiritual partner. Is there a difference between having "a" spiritual partner (as in many) and having "the" spiritual partner (as in one)? Do we have many or is there just one true partner?

*Mukunda:* These practices are best shared only with your husband, who is to be seen and known as your spiritual partner. Do not go looking for a spiritual partner if you are married. In the case of those who are not in a committed relationship, one who is your spiritual partner is unlikely to become your significant other. This partnership can evolve them to a more complete level of personal and spiritual intimacy. Best is to have only one spiritual partner whose commitment is to spiritual practice shared only with you. Having more than one partner is confusing to both mind and prana, and takes you from your spiritual path, not to it.

*Student:* I wanted to share with you that I dreamed about you for the first time three nights ago. I dreamed that I was asking you for initiation and that, when I met you for the forthcoming yoga therapy course, you gave me an enormous hug. There was not a huge energetic exchange, which I must have expected. It was as if, in some way, I were holding back, which surprised and disappointed me.

*Mukunda:* So let it be a message for you not to hold back when the opportunity for energy exchange arises. Make yourself into how you wish to be; dreams are both foretellers of past karma and guides for how to be in future. I am scheduling private sessions on the day prior to and the day after my workshops.

*Student:* I found this lesson quite extraordinary. I read, some years ago, the *Gospel of Ramakrishna*, and he describes this same partner practice meditation, shown to him by a Tantrik Yogini. I always wanted to learn this same meditation after reading that book and voila! Here it is. I was so moved by Ramakrishna and his teachings, and by the fact that he seemed to practice something very hidden and not so obvious to others (even his students). At the same time, he taught the Vedanta, chanted, immersed himself into other traditions, prayed, and did pujas.

*Mukunda:* Ramakrishna was a remarkable Spirit with a unique destiny that led him to experience the validity of the popular phrase "all paths are one." His woman teacher successfully led him through all the sixty-four Classical Tantrik sadhanas in only two years. Subsequently, he did the spiritual practices of all the major religious spiritual traditions. At the culmination of each, he experienced the living presence of the major teachers—Jesus, Mohammed, and the Buddha—who all merged into him. What you seek with a pure heart is always given.

276

***Student:*** [This sharing came in response to doing the third lesson, though it brought the student to a much deeper level than those teachings.]

I got a rose and placed it on my altar, but visualized it in my heart chakra for offering to God. Then I sang the Guru mantra for my Inner Teacher. I felt God in everything around me and in me. And more often, I realize there is nothing else. I felt so complete and connected with everything and everyone. So whole. I was always desperately looking to find God; and all the time, it was here. All I had to do was put my trust in your teachings and in God. Thank you for sharing. I love you so much for that. And yes, I am a bit euphoric at this point. Hope it will not become an obstacle. Please tell me if it is and what to do. I feel so hungry. I study Patanjali's *Yoga Sutras* and borrowed *Vasistha's Yoga* from the library. All I want to do is read teachings and meditate and worship.

***Mukunda:*** You are doing great. Please deepen and stabilize this lovely state by doing all of the lessons. Blessings.

# Devi/Deva Communion

With Great Respect and Love, I Honor
My Heart, My Inner Teacher.

n his article "Sex, Self-Identification and the Aghora Tradition," Robert Svoboda tells us:

> A Tantrik's view is simple: God has created all of us and all of us are part of the Ultimate Reality. If every act we perform is first offered as worship to God, the karmas involved in self-identification with our actions are minimized: not eliminated, but rendered less harmful. Sex, the expression on the human level of the union of the universal male and female principles, is a fit offering to the Divine.[90]

Evelyn M. Brown concurs:

> To become holy, you must first of all desire to be holy. You are born for that alone.[91]

---

90.  Robert Svoboda, "Sex, Self-Identification and the Aghora Tradition" in *Enlightened Sexuality*, ed. Georg Feuerstein, p. 197.

91.  Evelyn M. Brown, *He and I* (Paris: Editions Paulines, 1969), 34.

## Sharing Your Love

An important reminder is for your male partner to focus on retaining his role of nurturing and keeping his consort safe from any challenging emotions and difficult kriyas, providing for her comfort so that pleasure will arise naturally and effortlessly. A Tantrik will do anything that increases his partner's passion, so that she knows she is desired, above all else. "The purpose of desire is to increase your ability to receive."[92]

Devi is the source of pleasure. The Tantrik role for a woman is to increase her goddess energy, then she will naturally increase and express her nurturing, compassionate nature. Tantriks heighten the best of both sexual archetypes by encouraging spiritual elevation to hold them in subtler dimensions (koshas). In Tantrik Yoga, we say that the highest place in the body is not the head or the crown chakra, but the third dimension of the heart—not the physical heart nor the heart chakra, but what is called the spiritual heart, hidden within us all. The route is to seek the Shiva/Shakti mudra that holds us in "the cave of the heart."

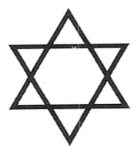

Shiva/Shakti mudra
(Devi/Deva mudra)

The male energy of Shiva is an upward-pointing triangle, while the symbol of the female's Shakti energy is a downward-pointing triangle. The symbol of harmony in Christian and yogic teachings is the intertwining triangles forming the Star of David, or the heart chakra symbol (shown here). In both, the Buddhist and yogic tradition is the communion of male and female bodies in seated meditation. Buddhists call this the *yab/yum* position, meaning union of cosmic father-mother. In this pose, you begin to move into the archetypal quality of the primal masculine and feminine. From a Tantrika's perspective, it is Deva below Devi. The masculine assertive force is dominant in man, while the receptive force is dominant in woman. The former creates a penetrating force within the lingam, while the latter manifests as a receptive force within the yoni. Partner yogasana practices can be mutually beneficial through sharing of their uplifting udana Kundalini pranic force.

---

92. Evelyn M. Brown, *He and I*, 3.

By reversing the socially acceptable roles and encouraging the woman to be assertive and the man passive, the shift in polarities moves both to a sattvic harmony.

> Devi is to Deva what movement is to air.
> Just as in empty space, air moves as if it has form,
> She moves in the infinite consciousness executing the will or the wish
> of Deva.
> When there is no such movement of energy,
> then Deva alone exists.
>
> While she continues to dance in this fashion in space,
> then by accidental coincidence She comes into contact with Deva.
> The moment this contact is made, She is weakened, made thin and
> transparent.
> She abandons her cosmic form and becomes a mountain,
> then she becomes a small town and then a beautiful tree.
> Then She becomes like space and lastly
> She becomes the form of the Lord, like the river entering the ocean.
> Then the Lord shines as one without a second.[93]

# The Requisite Mind for Devi/Deva Partner Practice

For this and future lessons to be sustained, one needs to condition the mind to reflect on the essence of Tantrik Yoga training. *Vasistha's Yoga* once again clarifies the mindfulness necessary for communion.

> When the mind does not crave for pleasure it is absorbed into the Self,
> along with the life force of prana. If the mind remains absorbed even
> for a quarter of an hour it undergoes a complete change, for it tastes
> the supreme state of self knowledge and will not abandon it. Even if the
> mind tasted it for a second, it does not return to this worldly state. The
> very seeds of the illusion of the world and the cycle of birth and death
> (samsara) are fried. With them, ignorance is dispelled and the unstable

---

93. *Vasistha's Yoga*, 575.

mind (vasanas) is utterly pacified; one who has reached this is rooted
in truth. He beholds the inner life and rests in supreme peace.[94]

Contrast this with the transformation of the mind described in *Yoga Sutras* II, 51 and
III, 13.

In the same way, the mind embraces ideas and is constantly active, searching for
satiation. It will never be content without finding the inner Self. Similarly, a lover seeks
this state of absorption in the embrace of the Beloved, knowing and trusting that,
when the Beloved is found, the embrace will reveal the goal of luminosity and wisdom.
The yab/yum and Devi/Deva are symbols of this "knowing luminosity." Mystic art
conveys mystic experience. The inner Oneness subsides and arises simultaneously,
like the peaks and valleys of the ocean's waves. They will continue to embrace others
until that One is found. The true consort is the one with whom this quest for the True
Self can be shared. Each supports the other in their quest, selflessly seeking what is as
naturally arising as the prolonged love hug of the consort.

Remember a central teaching in the lessons is that, when sexual or emotional
energy is allowed to build, it will naturally become neutral energy, pure prana, Shakti.
When passion is increased, spiritual energy will naturally arise. Know that these lessons are for the purpose of finding, remembering, and rejoicing in that essence and
knowing it as the Divine Presence.

What I have shared with you in the early lessons is no different from what I share
now. The process of seeking your energy and letting it guide you to the place of communion is now to be shared in the most intimate fashion with your partner. When
you or your partner are processing negative emotions like guilt, fear, anxiety, or self-
doubt, it is crucial for your mental and emotional well-being that you hold them in a
very sattvic place—loving them unconditionally, suspending your own reactions. It is
that dispassionate mind that will generate a truly compassionate love that is healing,
nurturing, and transforming to both of you. Being in that energy of transformation
is what Tantra is all about. Being unconditional is the essence of this communion,
partnering practice.

What you are to do from this loving sadhana is to run prana that is mixed with
guilt, fear, or other feelings through you both, until it passes and returns to its primal
nature as unconditional love. All fear (and other vata imbalances), when surrendered,

---

94. *Vasistha's Yoga*, 418.

becomes peace. If you persist, whatever starts as a negative thought or emotion will become supreme peace (suppressed or overly expressed vata becoming sattvic prana), or high vitality (rajasic or tamasic pitta becoming sattvic tejas), or unconditional love (imbalanced kapha becoming sattvic ojas). Given a deep commitment (sankalpa) and a willing, motivated partner, you can run the energy through all the Ayurvedic doshas and yogic koshas. I wish for you to become adept at Tantrik transformation. This Devi/Deva practice is essential to cultivate in the most natural form. When your partner is not with you, or you are not in an intimate Tantrik partnership, remember that the universal consort is always with you. Practice with that One.

When you initiate Devi/Deva practice, it is so nurturing for your partner. You will quickly see how you both long for communion—if you have the correct partner for you, that is. A gentle reminder is that your romantic partner is not always capable of being or motivated to be your yab/yum partner.

When you are with the optimal partner, you will be healing each other of the deepest wounds. When we do a simple hugasana practice, the mind goes to noticing blocked energies seeking resolution. The energy of self-criticism or negative emotions that comes up in you or your partner is the fuel for this sadhana. Regardless of the emotion or thought, see it all as prana seeking to return to your personal yoni space and be held there with the loving mudra of self-acceptance. If there is sexual energy between you and your partner, then that is what you must move through to get to the place of Devi/Deva communion.

It may look as if one or both of you is being sexually aroused and seeking only sexual expression. The skill comes in learning to seek what is a healthy natural expression of all your emotions and energies. No matter what they are, if you remain neutral and allow the expression to be received fully, it will pass to a higher pranic level. And then the deeper drive of the spiritual level of pranic energies will be revealed as they seek resolution in the higher koshas. It becomes fuel for the refinement of vata/pitta/kapha to evolve into prana—tejas and ojas, as described in the Ayurvedic model of yoga therapy.[95]

This is a spiritual practice. You must practice it in this context for it to achieve the high intentions that it is capable of fulfilling. Each partner needs to be in the role of serving the other as their own Self. Encourage sharing from the deepest place possible, by your mutual willingness to transcend any fear of rejection, self-doubt, suppressed

---

95. *Ayurvedic Yoga Therapy*, 250.

sexuality, or whatever unknown may become present. Any thought or feeling that is expressed while in communion with your dear beloved is meant to be given to the divine Devi/Deva through your communion. Grasp the significance of this instruction. I want you truly to deepen your spiritual practice. If you commit without any hesitation, you can deepen the mutual benefit that arises to heal your wounds and those of all beings you encounter. I pray for you to manifest the divine Devi and Deva. I want for you to become living examples of the loving kindness, compassion, and spiritual wisdom that are Deva and Devi.

## Indian and Tibetan Tantra

This communion is both symbolized and realized in the lovely depictions of yab/yum in Tibetan Tantrik art introduced in lesson 7. The Tantrik teachings are juicy with double meanings and twilight language to veil secret attainments from the uninitiated. This is especially true in the Buddhist branches of Tantra, Vajrayana. In his comprehensive overview, *Lust for Enlightenment: Buddhism and Sex*, author John Stevens reveals many insider insights.

> The female is an embodiment of prajna, transcendental wisdom; the woman's yoni is the abode of pure bliss. The male is upaya, the skillful means to compassionate enlightenment; the man's lingam is the diamond hardness of Buddhist emptiness.[96]

There are major differences between Indian Hindu Tantra and Tibetan Buddhist Tantra. The practices mean something different to each, and it is important to make some distinctions as we proceed in clarifying our spiritual path. The path leads to different goals for Hindus and Buddhists. The Tibetan Tantra specialist, Herbert Guenther, puts it this way:

> This difference is borne out by the underlying metaphysics and similarities are purely accidental, not at all essential. Hinduist Tantrism, due to its association with the Samkhya Yoga system, reflects a psychology of subjectivist dominance, but tempers it by infusing the human with the

---

96. John Stevens, *Lust for Enlightenment: Buddhism and Sex* (Boston: Shambhala Publications, 1990).

divine and vice versa, Buddhist Tantrism aims at developing man's cognitive capacities so that he may be, here and now, and may enact the harmony of sensuousness and spirituality. Dominance or power has a strong appeal to the ego, as it enables the ego to think that it is the master of its world. But unaware of the fact that the acceptance of power as the supreme value is the surrender of one's true individuality, a person who feels insecure and is afraid of becoming himself may turn to anything that seems to promise him the attainment of power. Because of this slanted view and because the word Shakti "creative power," is frequently used in Hindu Tantra, but never in Buddhist Tantra, the Buddhist Tantrism concepts are misunderstood. In contrast, it stresses individual growth and the struggle to realize the uniqueness of being human.[97]

Tantrik Buddhism expresses the divine feminine in many forms, perhaps the most predominant of which are Tara and the Dakini. Tara is of various colors (passions) and is the archetypal ruler of the heart, the fourth chakra, whose element is air. For the Yogi, Tara is the energy of protecting the integrity of the Classical Yoga and Tantrik sadhanas from corruption by short-term gain seekers. Dakini means "she who enjoys and flies through the sky," or "sky dancer." Her masculine counterpart is called a *daka* or *vira* (fearless warrior). When the male heroes have full realization, they are called *herukas*. The heruka is a complete perfected form because "he" is the inseparable pair of "she and he."

> In the Dakinis highest aspect she is called the formless wisdom nature of the mind. On an inner, ritual level, she is a meditational deity, visualized as the personification of the qualities of Buddhahood. On an outer, subtle body level, she is the energetic network of the embodied mind in the subtle channels and vital breath of Tantrik Yoga. She is also a living woman: she may be a guru on a brocaded throne or a yogini meditating in a remote cave, a powerful teacher of meditation or a guru's consort teaching directly through her life example. All women are seen as some kind of dakini manifestation.[98]

---

97. Herbert V. Guenther, *The Tantric View of Life* (Berkeley: Shambhala, 1972), 2.
98. Judith Simmer-Brown, *Dakini's Warm Breath* (Boston: Shambhala, 2002), 9.

The core element of Indian Tantra is its devotion to the divine feminine as Devi, the "shining one." In Tantrik practices, one honors the Goddess in all Her forms—as every woman, as Mother Earth, as food, as Divine Light, and most importantly as our spiritual energy of Shakti Kundalini or the Holy Spirit. Tantrik tools described in lesson 7 include spiritual geometry (yantra) to build grounded energy fields, Shakti yoga postures (tantrasana), words of power (mantra), and vital points (marmas) that open blocks to fluid energy. Together, these tools lift the veil from personality to reveal the luminous nature of the True Self. With a spiritual affirmation, Tantra renames us as hermaphrodites— the male organ is a lingam, which literally means a "wand of light," while feminine sexuality is blessed with a yoni or "sacred space." The Tantrik path seeks to unify these primal male and female aspects. That harmony creates, within one's own sacred space, an illumined spiritual light, empowered by the source of guidance.

> The Tibetan mantra *om mani padme hum* is a condensed form of the same teaching: om is the origin of life; mani is the jewel of the male organ; padme is the lotus of the female; hum is the union of the two in undifferentiated consciousness, and the reintegration of emptiness with form, wisdom with skillful means, nirvana with samsara.[99]

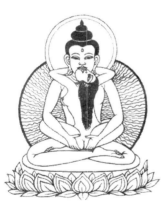

Yab/Yum (Tibet)—Devi/Deva (India)

The Tibetan Tantrik tradition is ripe with the stories of masters who had consorts to "assist them in the final production of co-emergent bliss and wisdom in enlightenment. Wherever the Master finds his consorts, his great bliss awakens the Dakini's natural insight. Saraha, after a long tenure at Nalanda University, took an arrow-smith's daughter (a Dakini) as his consort, and said 'Only now am I a truly pure being.'"[100]

Although a madman in the public eye, Drukpa Kunley, was a secret Buddha who fought the demons of Bhutan and—like his predecessor, Padmasambhava—freed the country of their

99. Ibid, 64.
100. Keith Dowman, trans., *The Divine Madman: The Sublime Life and Songs of Drukpa Kunley* (Kathmandu: Pilgrims Book House, 2000), 22.

influence. One Demoness had the capacity to change forms and became a beautiful and seductive woman seeking his assistance. She said:

> I beg you to lead me to a blissful release. Am I not a celestial ornament? Above my waist my form is entrancing while below my waist in my Mandala of Bliss my muscles are strong, and my up thrust is skillful—I offer you my art in milking! For you who delights in love making, and I a serpent with fervent lust, this meeting today offers great joy. Please stay with me and I'll offer you my body in devotion, I beg you to grant me your godly favor! Then she promised to serve the Tradition thereafter and vowed never to harm living beings. Finally to prepare her as a suitable candidate for instruction on higher spiritual union, he purified her through divine sexual play.[101]

Tsultrim Allione, author of *Women of Wisdom*, tells us:

> The Tibetans recognize the importance of sexual yoga in opening up further fields of awareness and insight, and in bestowing the blessing of long life on the Tantrika. Besides the sexual contact, living with a wisdom Dakini brings intuitive insights in daily life situations. . . . It should be noted that this contact with a consort does not come at the beginning of the training when the passions are still out of control and distraction is rampant. Rather, the taking of a consort is suggested as one of the final measures for complete enlightenment. Emotions are very powerful, and unless we can truly use them for further depth of awareness, intimate relationships can become a big obstacle instead of a boon to the practitioner. . . . All Tantrikas must be tuned into the energy of their own bodies and that of the world around them. This means they must have a positive relationship to the Dakini, who is energy in all of its forms. She acts as a spiritual midwife helping the Tantrika to give birth to the wisdom which she embodies by cutting through conceptualization and working directly with the energy promoting illumination.[102]

---

101. Ibid, 134.
102. Tsultrim Allione, *Women of Wisdom* (London: Arkana, 1984), 39–42.

Other masters include Guru Rinpoche Padmasambhava, whose mission was aided by his two consorts, Princess Mandarava of Zahor, India, and Karchen Yeshe Tsogyal of Tibet, and Milarepa, who was aided by Tseringma.[103] Historical and contemporary examples are cited by Miranda Shaw in her book *Passionate Enlightenment: Women in Tantric Buddhism.* Padmasambhava, considered the second Buddha, passed on his teaching through his consort, Yeshe Tsogyal. His teachings were left in hidden forms to be found by future wisdom treasure seekers.

## Summary of the Devi/Deva Partner Practice

Now you are ready for Tantrik energetic partnering. This is a long meditation, so you may choose to break it up into more than one practice session. I have written this so that each paragraph can serve as a separate practice session.

1. Before the practice, repeat the Ganesh and Karuna kriyas described in lesson 8. Let Deva give Karuna kriya to Devi, and She will reciprocate with Ganesh kriya to her Deva. Practice being in an elevated state as you give and receive. Perceive that both of you are perfect beings—loving, kind, and compassionate with your partner, who is the embodiment of the Devi (feminine) and Deva (masculine), which literally means "beings of light."

2. This lesson can be done as a visualization if you lack an appropriately trained and willing partner, or if your partner is the divine Being. As the location of the external sex organs is different—the male organ being at the top of the pubic bone and the female below this two-inch vertical bone (described in detail in lesson 5—men and women should use different postures. This will facilitate fully opening sexual energy, thus clarifying its uniqueness from spiritual energy. Both are forms of prana, but there is a difference. I suggest that you sit opposite your Deva when he is doing his most perfected form of tantrasana, ideally siddhasana. Devi should be resting in her most regal seat of tantrikasana siddhayoniasana (described in lesson 9).[104] Deva places his right heel against his perineum and the left heel above his lingam, so that a steady even pressure is exerted on both his first and second chakras. Devi places her left heel against

103. Shaw, *Passionate Enlightenment: Women in Tantric Buddhism.*
104. *Hatha Yoga Pradipika*, chapter I, 35–43; 102–16.

her yoni, with her right heel directly above it, applying a mild yet tangible contact against the lower pubic bones. Any close approximation that is comfortable will suffice.

3. Begin with the wave breath for some time until you both feel relaxed. Send the waves from your nostrils to the region of your navel. Gradually slow down to deepen and prolong your breath, so that it reaches to both your higher and lower chakras. Encourage relaxation as you open yourself. Create a state of openness and gratitude. Ask your higher power or the Divine Presence to come into the sacred space within you. Take your time with each step. When you feel emotional or energized, take some time to breathe into the experience and allow yourself to remain sattvic-centered, regardless of what it may bring to the surface. Remember that Tantrik practice is healing on a multi-dimensional level, so persist as you invite healing and sacred presence. Once you feel relaxed and centered within yourselves, begin to connect your breaths so they flow at the same pace, inhaling downward and exhaling the breath from the lower abdomen upward. Continue this until you feel a connection to each other. After some time, open your eyes and gaze into your partner's eyes. In Tantrik vajrayana practice, "The male should visualize himself as Buddha, and the female should imagine herself as the Lady of Transcendental Wisdom. They should first sit facing each other and gaze upon their partner with intense desire."[105]

4. Just be present with your partner/consort. If there is tension arising, gently close your eyes and do the wave breath through it until it dissipates. When you are ready, open your eyes and gaze again. Repeat this as many times as you wish until you are fully comfortable in your openness to both yourself and each other. Look softly at the energy field of your self and your partner until you perceive the separate fields of Devi and Deva. Stay connected to yourself; avoid the tendency to merge or surrender your field of energy to each other. Just practice being together.

5. Next, practice the elevating of the primal elements (nyasa) given in lesson 2, while facing your partner. Touch your own chakras from the top down to invite Shakti's life force to descend into you. Take your time with this; move on only when both feel ready to proceed. Upon reaching the root region, repeat

---

105. John Stevens, *Lust for Enlightenment: Buddhism and Sex* (Boston: Shambhala, 1990), 65.

the procedure, moving upward and encouraging the Shiva's stillness quality to ascend within. Then sit in the field of each other's charged energies and allow a sharing of your energies of Spirit and Love. Feel free to follow whatever is a naturally arising impulse. Through this process of nyasa, your bodies are consecrated—no longer personalities, you become the cosmic couple of Shiva and Shakti, Deva and Devi.

6. Repeat the process with your right hand on top of your partner's left hand, which is placed on his or her chakra regions. Again, focus only on your own energy, not on sharing yourself. Simply use your right hand to encourage your partner to feel all of his or her feelings, regardless of whether they are gross or subtle, physical or energetic, mundane or spiritual. Give your partner permission to be with you fully and with all the potential present.

7. When you feel ready for communion, let Devi, the Goddess, sit in her Deva's lap with her legs around his waist. Embrace each other lovingly. Gently hold each other, with your right hand on your partner's sacrum and your left hand at the back door of the heart. Begin to connect your second and fourth chakra energies. This is an optimal beginning and concluding practice when doing Tantrik partnering. Continue this hug, surrendering to the warmth of your hearts. Sometimes, this will lead you toward a "melting point" in which "you" may disappear. If this happens, allow the hug to open itself to your spiritual connection to reveal a third presence, that of Spirit, who will continue to guide you both. Just immerse yourselves in this field and allow Shakti to direct Shiva where She will.

8. Now Devi gently positions Deva's lingam against her yoni so that the lingam is external and vertical to it. The state of passion or dispassion does not matter. The practice is to linger here while connecting hearts and placing the yoni mudra on the lower back of your consort over the sacrum, as in the Devi/Deva illustration.

> At the place where the tips of their sexual organs touch, or "kiss" in Tantric metaphor, the drops of sexual fluid that have gathered there mix and intermingle, creating the ultimate libation. Details sufficient to perform the practice cannot be found in any text, but in its general outline the drops of sexual fluid (called "red" in the case of woman and "white"

in the case of the man, referring not to their color but to their respective concentration of female and male endocrinal elements) intermingle and melt, inaugurating each partner's successful gathering location of the inner winds into the central psychic channel. The exact location of the inner hearth may differ in different yoga systems, although a consensus places it at the navel, where it is imagined as a short "A" that is ablaze. Regardless of where the inner hearth is visualized, the real fire is understood to be the higher form of consciousness that devours any lesser forms that are fed into it or sacrificed for its sake.[106]

9. This quote is from a remarkable book on sexual practices to elevate both partners. The author was given permission from the Dalai Lama to interview monks and nuns sharing these spiritual practices.

10. The secret men need to learn is to continue to develop karezza, prolonged intercourse. This is so that Devi should be completely satiated and filled with her own Shakti. From this, Deva learns to manifest more of his Shiva nature. Through patience and persistence, they will become transformed into a living presence of Shakti. Just learn to be with the primal energy of Shakti as yourself. It is enough to stay steady in your own Self. This session needs to be free of time constraints. The more adept you are at being with the prana Shakti, the more it will guide you to unique, indescribable experiences that reveal the omnipresent form of the formless. Surrender to that One.

11. When Devi is comfortable and wishes the next step, it is up to her to initiate it. She can then lovingly bring her Deva's lingam into her yoni. She will maintain a firm mula bandha mudra to hold the lingam inside while both seek an ever-deepening stillness. Remain in that stillness regardless of the lingam's arousal or lack of passion. Encourage a communion of energies and the contentment of your passions. The Devi will train her Deva to remain neutral or receptive to her Shakti with this communion position. By prolonging karezza, they can enter any state, including falling asleep, and return profoundly refreshed, having shared the essence of Devi/Deva communion.

106. Shaw, *Passionate Enlightenment*, 164–65.

Do your best to allow all feelings and sensations, whether physical, emotional, or sexual, to simply arise and run their course. This is the practice of sensual detachment called, in the *Yoga Sutras* II, 53, *pratyahara,* in which the senses are allowed, but no encouragement is given them. The goal is to experience communion without desire. In this manner, we will sustain the state of yoga. Do not move toward sexual energy expression, but rather allow for an "inner course" of your pranic energies.

When sexual or emotional energy is allowed to build, it becomes neutral energy and, if you persist, it will be experienced as spiritual energy. To move to take actions on your feelings without discernment is to create *bhoga*. Bhogis are hedonistic pleasure seekers who never find the source of their real pleasure, so they lead a life of seeking more enjoyment without finding fulfillment. Bhogis tend to regress, becoming *rogis*, or sick people. Do not let yourself go from Yogi to bhogi to rogi; instead remain as a Yogini. Yoginis remain in touch with their pranas, searching for those "currents of sensation" to guide them to the primal Source of all the currents of sensation.

The secret women need to learn is that they possess the Unknowable as Shakti, which will change their Deva in ways that lead to his spiritual sadhana commitment. By allowing yourself to be fully and completely spontaneous and assertive, you can open to love of the Divine Presence. This state is highly contagious to your partner. When he knows Shakti in this direct way, he will spontaneously experience his spiritual nature as Shiva.

As a seeker opens to her true nature as Shakti, she is likely to cry with tears of fulfillment. Tears are a natural expression of the Ayurvedic principle of kapha (earth and water elements); when kapha evolves, it becomes the juice of love called ojas. So it is quite natural for tears to arise during true moments of love-making. When there is love being made, it naturally produces byproducts that are of the essence of kapha as juice. The salivary glands moisten the mouth; breasts swell resembling those of a nursing mother; the sexual organs flow with a unique nectar called amrita; our eyes flood with tears of pleasure, gratitude, and ecstasy. Ojas is a nectar that is found in these various ways. The Yogini may experience this ojas as kechari, a nectar that flows from a secret bindu center behind the third eye. This secret kechari mudra is an extremely subtle way of sealing the "leaky pranic bucket." Otherwise, this nectar flows down the palate, and is eventually burned up in the solar chakra.

Techniques such as kechari mudra, in which the tongue goes upward beyond the soft palate, or viparita karani mudra (modified half shoulderstand) help the Yogini to retain her spiritual nectar, expressing it as supreme love. When love evolves, it is no longer experienced as personal, but as divine, spreading equally to all that come into our awareness. In truth, it is consciousness that is bliss and that is natural to experience, accompanied with tears of love. My book *The Yoga Poet*[107] is filled with stories of varied Tantrik ojas ecstasies like the eyes being filled from the infinite black hole of love juice. There is no end to love. The Yogini experiences that this is who she is and what she is made of.

> The wise consider the soul (jiva) to be the essence in the sperm. In it is hidden the bliss of the self which it experiences as if independent of itself.[108]

Thus the wise man will conserve his sperm and wait until the couple is ready to listen to the voice of a baby's soul wishing to come into their lives for mutual benefit.

> The "I" enters into the Yoni Mudra triangle in its own conception; and because it is aware of itself, it believes itself to be a body, though this is unreal and only appears to be real. In that triangle which is the sheath of karma, the soul which is of the very essence of the sperm exists in that body just as fragrance exists in a flower. Even as the sun's rays spread throughout the earth, this soul which is in the sperm and which has entered the triangle spreads itself throughout the body. Though the soul is everywhere inside and outside, yet it has an identification with this vital energy of the sperm and is therefore considered its special abode.[109]

## The Secret of Tantrasana Partner Practice

The secret of the tantrasana is prolonging the exchange of Shiva and Shakti's prana at each step in the sadhana. In the same way that advancement in asana occurs by moving more slowly and holding the pose longer, in pranayama, it is attained by slowing and ultimately suspending the breath (kumbhaka). In Tantrik Devi/Deva communion, the deepening of physical, pranic, and spiritual benefits arises from being still and

---

107. Mukunda Stiles, *The Yoga Poet* (Boulder, CO: Yoga Therapy Center, 1990).
108. *Vasistha's Yoga*, 503.
109. *Vasistha's Yoga*, 505.

slowing down the breath so prana will expand. Prior to the lingam entering the yoni, there is much benefit in experiencing what I call "outer course." This is clothes-on contact of your whole body, especially seeking to balance the communion feelings at heart-to-heart and pelvis-to-pelvis placements in hugasana. I recommend this step be a minimum of fifteen to twenty minutes.

Then tantrasana proceeds to hugasana, either standing or seated with Devi above Deva. In this outercourse practice, the Devi and Deva can process all their energetic and emotional reactions, until a sattvic exchange is achieved. This may take some time and plenty of communication to be sure that both are truly feeling neutral or supported when kriyas arise. Persistence is maintained until a stable sattvic state is shared. This step should be prolonged for thirty minutes. Then, if intercourse is desired, it will be a natural expression of sharing your love. Once this is regularly sustainable, Tantrik Devi/Deva communion will evolve in its own unique way.

One view calls this next step in practice intromission. "Intercourse conveys the impression of movement and activity. Intromission refers to the act of the insertion of the lingam in the receptive yoni. The symbol of Tantra is the erect lingam in the primal waters of the Yoni. The principle sacrament is the intromission's stillness. Not a culmination but rather an ongoing ever creative communion."[110]

The next step is to prolong your practice of serene continuous love-making (kar-ezza). A realistic goal is forty-five minutes, which can enable both partners to receive the full energetic and spiritual benefits of Devi/Deva communion.


## Congratulations!

You have only three Tantra lessons to go. May your discipline continue to the end of these eighteen lessons and may you integrate them into your balanced householder and spiritual lifestyle.

Remember to persist in your practice, yet stay detached from expecting specific outcomes. Tantra is a personal spiritual practice. When you feel complete with this lesson, read the Dialogue section that follows prior to beginning lesson 16.

---

110. Arvind and Shanta Kale, *Tantra and the Secret Power of Sex* (Mubaik: Jaico Publishing House, 2004), 130–37.

# With Great Respect and Love, I Honor My Heart, My Inner Teacher.

## Dialogue with Mukunda

**Student:** Although I am in a very devotional mood with this practice, I feel I need some guidance or readings to help my mind understand the sensual, sexual, spiritual arousals that are happening when I am alone, doing consort practice, or visualizing what has happened. I cannot distinguish one energy from the other, at times, and wonder if that is natural or beneficial. Do you have some suggestions?

**Mukunda:** It is wonderful that you do not distinguish the energies; this shows you are entering into the deeper kosha where mental distinctions are not possible. Nonetheless, here is a list for your consideration; the most detailed work is the second one (though scholarly, it is deep):

> *Hatha Yoga Pradipika* translated by Swami Muktibodhananda, pp. 370–416 (vajroli and sahajoli mudra) and pp. 530–534 (lingam puja)
>
> *Passionate Enlightenment* by Miranda Shaw, chapters 6 (Women in Tantrik Relationships) and 7 (Spontaneous Jewel-like Yogini)
>
> *Lingam* by Alain Danielou, pp. 15–22 (Transcendent Symbol, Bija and Yoni), pp. 34–35 (Pillar of Light), and pp. 84–86 (Subtle Body of Lingam)
>
> *Yoni* by Rufus Camphausen, pp. 29–30 (Yoni Mudra), pp. 37–44 (Yoni Puja), pp. 70–74 (rajas—feminine form of ojas), and pp. 76–79 (Yoni Variety)

It feels to me as if you are ripe for more at this time. In the morning, if you do a second asana practice, that should be more rajasic; evening practice is to be more sattvic. I want you to do plenty of floor postures when possible, especially in your evening preparations for lotus, spinal twists, forward bends, done gently and calmly as if I were in the room with you. Cultivate the devotion of a bhakti to the prana, to considering Devi's presence as your own energies awakening. Follow that energy as you have in previous tantrasana practices. Especially look to see what practices open your heart and sacrum.

294

There is a polarity, a natural energy attraction, between the second and fourth chakras that will be most beneficial to locate and deepen.

***Student:*** I don't know if you want so much feedback from me, but this I have to share with you because it makes me happy! I was meditating on my yantra this morning and was drawn to the heart chakra symbol. And then it occurred to me that I could begin visualization of lesson 15 and so I did, with my husband in hugasana. We were relaxed and open and comfortable with each other. I began the breath-wave exercise and imagined I was inhaling love and exhaling grief and hurt and anger—for myself, for him, and for us. I took each breath into the belly/sacral region. I was able to feel some energy there, but it was heavy. I did this for a while and then I felt that it was time to end it; and I did so with a kiss. I stayed with the moment, however, and then was moved to lie down on my belly and place the yoni mudra over my sacrum. With each inhalation, there was a little pain. After some time, I turned my head the other way and continued to breathe, but noticed there was no pain. When I turned my head back, there was no pain on that side anymore. So I sat up and continued with my practice and noticed that the sacral region felt lighter and freer. Yay! That made me happy! Is this progress? The best thing about lesson 15 is that I am free, free, free to love, love, love! Hurts can be forgiven. Belly full of love and heart exploding with joy! Yay! (Little girls are very exuberant!) A hundred million billion hugs!

***Mukunda:*** Wonderful! It sounds like a delightful gift you have to share with your Beloved husband and also with Devi, as She is Shakti healing you. Progress indeed is happening with you. You are such an open Tantrika; may that openness deepen within you and your Beloved. Great that you are getting the essence of these lessons. Thank you for your openness. Namaste.

***Student:*** I'm confused in general about this ejaculation and prana thing. I have practiced not ejaculating by tensing my pubococcygeal muscles for a while now. I am able to orgasm without the semen leaving my body. I definitely feel more energized afterward—and not drained like a "normal" orgasm with ejaculation. I also can direct that energy upward and feel a sense of heat moving up my spine. I don't understand a couple things, however: If I am simply restraining the semen from moving into the world, why wouldn't my body have to make more and be drained anyway?

Also, am I supposed to bring the energy up? Seems a little crazy-making. The Taoists seem to think it should be brought up to the head, then down and stored on the navel/yoni mudra area. Are there any writings on this that can clarify? Any other guidance you have on the whole sexual energy thing would be much appreciated. I'm happily married and faithful, but my sexual energies are intense. Transforming them to something that moves me toward a sattvic state is very appealing.

**Mukunda:** The drain is due to energy lost. Energy is not the seminal fluid, but the loss of dispassion that occurs due to the increased passion during stimulation from arousal. One can practice restraint of prana while having intercourse. This diminishes your need for ejaculation and will prolong the sharing of loving energy. This is what Tantriks are seeking in training you—so that you can experience conservation, redirection of energy, and an awareness of your wife as Devi. Your body won't need to create more fluid if it is retained. Instead, it is changed from its gross Ayurvedic qualities—vata, pitta, and kapha—into the food for the subtle body as prana—tejas and ojas.

The prana can go different ways that are variable, not only from school to school, but from Indian Yoga and Chinese Taoist schools. I have not trained in Taoist sexual techniques, but have read they seek the energy to travel in the microcosmic orbit following the governing vessel and the conception vessel. I also feel it is not beneficial to develop different systems of energy or pranayama practice. In summary, *chi* is not prana with differing intentions for health, longevity, or spiritual communion. Each system has a unique practice and goal.

In my Tantrik training, I was taught to increase prana retention as a way to hold on to the awareness of the Divine Mother as Devi's presence. No particular place for the energy to be retained was given. She moves energy down, and Shiva moves upward. However, this pathway is only in the second and third koshas. As the sadhana progresses to higher states, the energy diffuses as it comes in the fourth and fifth koshas. At that point, it no longer has a locus, but rather leads to feeling the Divine Omnipresence. The physical or personal body is lost; the body is no longer the locus of personality identity; ego is seen as a mirage.

Since you are married and faithful, you are doing an appropriate practice by continuing to pursue this in a sattvic context. Intention and commitment to your life's integrity will promote the goal of a sattvic state. In general, let me advise you to go slower, take more time, and be sensitive to what heightens your wife's pleasure. That you wish to give her your balanced sexual energies is wonderful for you and your wife. Blessings.

**Student:** A student addressed me with his concerns about how to convert his high sexual energy. A few nights ago, he asked about how to get out of his 13-year-old-boy fantasies and sexual feelings that arise when he comes into contact with both male and female. I suggested he draw the energy he is feeling from the lower chakra regions to the middle and upward, where he has been feeling nothing. Next day, he said that it worked well for him. I felt about 80 percent sure of this next statement (so best I check with you for the other 20 percent). He said that the energy he gets from interactions with people is spiritual energy. But he is perceiving it solely as sexual energy, because that is what he knows and so he doesn't need to be afraid or ashamed of it. He should continue to let it rise upward rather than increase it.

**Mukunda:** Raising his energy upward is fine for now. When he has more stability, the goal is to increase sexual energy until it is experienced as the transformative energy of spirituality. Raising it will tend to give one a feeling of avoiding sexual energy when done for too long. It would be ideal to encourage him to do the lessons. In so doing, he will learn how important it is to train his sexuality into kindness and a loving heart.

**Student:** I have practiced aswini and sahajoli mudras and the pranic breathing with mula bandha. I have been experimenting with these variations since mula bandha was introduced in an earlier lesson. They are already getting more controlled, so maybe I am ready for the next lesson. My husband doesn't show much interest in Tantra yet, although I think that will likely change with time. He is really tense with work right now, so the timing just isn't right. We have been loving practitioners of hugasana and cuddlasana for many years, practicing throughout the day, since we work at home. We are familiar with the flow of amrita. I believe he and I are naturals together at Tantra, so I want to be careful not to complicate things with too many details or expectations—although I am soaking up the details and working on the accompanying detachment.

And then this morning everything was effortless. I woke up at 5:00 a.m. refreshed and ready (I have been trying to do this for months). I wrote in my journal and then began my morning practice with the lingam stone on my altar. Alternate nostril breathing was effortless, and I was able to concentrate better. With all yoni mudra positions, I was able to feel mula, sahajoli, and aswini mudras distinctly and could coordinate my breath with mudra. During Devi puja, Kali gave me the biggest hug and so did you! Yay! Thank you, thank you, thank you, thank you, thank you. I think that this was a major opening. Thank you for the gift of these lessons.

**Mukunda:** Developing the sahajoli and aswini mudra is a gradual process. Learn to deepen your internal strength, both on a muscular and a pranic level, until you feel these mudras following prana nadis. There are internal nadis to which these techniques connect, and it does require perseverance to find them. They are the subtle connections between head and pelvis that are between Shiva and Shakti. It is different from the sushumna or ida and pingala nadis, which are the primary kriya-purification channels that precede a balanced approach to disciplined and devotional Kundalini awakening. These subtler nadis lead to other, often misunderstood (and thus secret), processes like kechari mudra, where nectar (amrita) is experienced at the cranium flowing into the taste buds on the tip of the tongue. When they are found, then amrita begins to flow in great quantities from both the Shiva source in the head and the Shakti source in the hidden dimensions of your yoni. Hence, I recommend that you continue to develop these mudras, regardless of the content in other lessons to come.

You are making very good progress indeed. I enjoy your contagious enthusiasm for this lovely sadhana coming to you. Blessings.

**Student:** Mukunda, I had a question for you about something that has come up before. I notice, after you shared your Tantrik practice with me, that I am very noticeably less interested in receiving and sharing intimacy with my lover. It really almost irritates me, and I even kind of avoid it. This happens frequently after our intense practice. I feel that this is such a deep spiritual journey for me with your guidance and personal support, but I get confused when it keeps me from a better relationship. Any words of advice on this one would help. Do you know why this is?

**Mukunda:** In sharing this Shiva/Shakti practice with you, I am focusing on increasing what was tamasic sexual energies. This is a kriya, as it must be freed into a natural, yet comfortably assertive, feminine Shakti energy. Because of being tamasic, the sadhana that is given is rajasic until you find serenity. Shakti's nature is to increase your passions and will increase your capacity to know when and how you desire intimacy. However, when sessions bring you to Shiva energy, you have become more strongly indrawn and still. And this is as it should be. Often, one extreme will bring about the other. Over time, this gets balanced in both introspective and outgoing moods of prana. In the meantime you are likely to have irritation, as you are not used to the pitta-heating energies that come with your increased Shakti. When you are gentler (sattvic) with your Shakti, there will also be a more sattvic Shiva.

I suspect that having a long gap between individual sessions can cause your experience of a Tantric partner practice to be more intensely Shakti in nature. I know your relationship is deepening—that is clear from what you have revealed about experiencing more heart-centered energy with your lover. In contrast, shared Tantrik practice is still more of a kriya—spiritual-energy purification—due to your depth of desire for transformation. Ultimately, all energies flow into the one ocean; but, until then, they are like rivers with different intensities, colors, passions, and paces. Blessings for your persistence with this sadhana.

**Student:** I have noticed myself having aversion to continuing with the lessons, because they are so partner-directed. But I did read over lesson 15 today. It is so unbelievably intense. It is a beautiful practice and I can't wait to share it with someone. But it is so difficult for me to imagine that I can attract a partner to do these practices with. I'm having trouble bringing or allowing the depth of the practice to permeate my being, because I feel as if the other half is missing. I feel I need to wait to have a partner to do some of these. But I know that's not true. If I want to remain single, how do I do the practices alone? If I am putting the intention out there to find a perfect partner, how do I bring a practice this deep into an emerging partnership?

**Mukunda:** Indeed, you can practice this lesson in your imagination with one you call your Beloved. This may also act as a way to draw a partner to you. My guru's guru, Bhagwan Nityananda, and Swami Muktananda, my guru, used to come in their subtle bodies to their students and give both the awakening of Shakti and partner practices to promote their capacity for retaining spiritually elevated states. This helps to open the deeply seated karmas and to help the student's capacity to hold Shakti. He did this to me many times and often the Devi came to be with me in a nearly physical form of light and ecstasy. His experience with Kundalini Devi coming to him is beautifully and erotically described in his spiritual autobiography, *Play of Consciousness.*[111]

---

111. Muktananda, *Play of Consciousness*, chapter 5, called "Sexual Excitement." In the newest edition, this title has been diluted by the editors and is called "The Dissolution of Desire." I prefer the original editions (see *www.amazon.com* or *www.abebooks.com*).

The Bhadra Kali Devi that was sent gave me much of the teachings that I share. There is a temple in Ganeshpuri, north of Mumbai, devoted to her. Students have also shared that they experience my subtle body coming to them during sleep or meditation practice. While I rarely share in this consciously, I do know that a serious student can call from me energetic blessings, as that has happened frequently in my lineage. The Inner Teacher comes in many forms. See what is naturally arising and calms you or excites you into expressing what is wanted.

**Student:** Throughout the lessons, I have often caught myself in a position between wanting a genuine partner to practice with, craving any partner, and abstaining from partnership out of fear of opening to a person I cannot trust. I guess I'm having trouble clarifying my wants, desires, and intentions.

**Mukunda:** Trust yourself to be truthful enough to attract a trustworthy partner. Just see who you are and what you want to give to a partner. This leads to a path of selfless service and is more likely to be fulfilling of your relationship destiny.

**Student:** My experiences with practicing wave breath with mula bandha followed by kapalabhati breathing have intensified consistently during the breath pause (kumbhaka). There is an intense stream of energy that runs from my labia to the diaphragm and, once it begins to enter the chest cavity, it becomes too intense and I release. It had been happening just every now and then, but seems to have become regular for the past couple of days. At first, I was afraid to hold the retention. Now I feel as if I want to, but it's just too intense—as if I were going to explode, yet very pleasurable. I had a common experience last night of waking up sexually aroused and then just falling back asleep. I felt as if there were a connection between the two. So often, during sexual exchange, I rush toward the orgasm, rush past all the sensations beforehand and the experience of it. This practice encourages me to stay in the beforehand period, observing and practicing detachment. I am finding it hard to be in that intensity without trying to find a way out. So I am asking myself, is it the presence of Spirit that is hard to face, or just the intensity of feeling? Any thoughts?

**Mukunda:** Thank you for your explicit descriptions of the transformations you are experiencing. There is integrity when you share so accurately and fully your arousal's pleasures and confusions. When I was assisting my long-term friend over the final phase of pregnancy, I taught her what was given to me as apana pranayama. David Frawley, in his Ayurvedic correspondence course, which I edited, defined this as the final phase of the exhalation. During this phase, the student relaxes the pelvic and lower abdominal region to encourage the natural expression of the subtle prana, apana. Normally, this is a movement that goes unnoticed. But with practice, it becomes more apparent as a naturally arising movement. It is the down-and-out pelvic prana that creates the passing of waste products like urine, feces, and menstrual fluids. It is a progressive force that rhythmically moves to their expulsion.

Similarly, this apana prana builds over nine months, until it becomes so strong that it pushes the fetus from the uterus. By learning to work with the subtler sensations building up to labor, when labor comes, it is a powerful force. In my friend's case, the increase in apana prana was balanced with an equally enhanced udana prana that began to express itself as upward Kundalini rushes. By guiding her to relax into the naturally arising pranas of the final phase of pregnancy, these upward and downward pranas spontaneously increased. For the final eight hours before she felt ready to go to the hospital, she had continual pranas downward, leading to blissful and prolonged orgasms. This alternated with strong upward pranas, resulting in Kundalini bliss in the crown chakra. All were experienced as giving her spiritual ecstasies. The two forces were experienced by her as: I am bliss, I am not this body.

During sexual arousal, these forces are at play in both men and women, giving increased sensations in both directions—toward the pelvis as Shakti and toward the crown as Shiva. By learning to relax and not rush toward orgasm (which is natural due to the increased apana prana), one can open to the opposite upward flow. From this, the energies are no longer experienced as purely sexual, but rather as spiritual transcendent experiences. That Self is not worldly, not interested in desires of the material world like sexual arousal or material possessions. Yet, what is appropriate is freely given, just as what is not beneficial is taken away effortlessly. That Self is unfamiliar or, more literally, unknown to the mind. When the mind disappears, the Self appears.

When the pause (kumbhaka) increases, the movement of thought we call the mind slows down to a trickle and is likely to have a kumbhaka also. Kumbhaka of breath leads to kumbhaka of mind, which in turn leads to the Self. Entry into the Self is accompanied by detachment from this body, as well as practice to sustain what is felt as an increase in all forms of prana, including sensual, sexual, and spiritual. This is one of many secrets of the Tantrikas; for ordinary spiritual practices will tend to control, and hence cut off, these energies, often turning them into premature celibacy. Many practitioners cannot allow these energies for fear of a loss of morality, since they are associated with worldliness. The Yogini seeks to control desire, while the Tantrika seeks freedom of expression. Thus the Tantrika practices in secrecy with the guidance of a teacher and the loving support of a partner. Once their awakening is stable, they may be moved to share it at the encouragement of the teacher.

**Student:** With regard to the Tantrik practices, I am progressing without a partner. Through visualization of being with a partner, usually the same specific person, I experienced a profound state of non-attachment. In my visualization, the arousal just stopped because fulfillment was found entirely in the heart. Then, last night, I had a dream about practicing some of the techniques with an older teacher and mentor (seventy-seven years old). In the dream, we had sexual feelings for each other. In person, we have acknowledged these too. But in the dream state, we acted on them. He took off my shirt, but did not touch me. Then I touched the place between the lingam and the anus (perineum), which gave him great pleasure. When he touched my yoni, my sexual feelings totally stopped, and I did not feel anything except contentment. I think things are progressing on many planes. I am willing to try the next lesson. I am still very much going over older lessons and my learning from them continues. Thank you very much. Great changes are occurring.

**Mukunda:** You are doing quite well with Tantra practices. Let me point out, however, an important sign of this Tantrik relationship. While you are not experiencing physical connecting, you are inviting pranic and dream Tantrik practices with your mentor. Rarely does one not have a Tantrik partner; often it's just a matter of being "available" for an encounter. Allowing these visualizations and dreams to arise can heal sexual frustrations and help you find appropriate experiences. What occurs in a dream is as valid as what happens in the "real world." But to protect yourself, it is best that you keep the dream-state experiences on that level and not act them out. Maintain a healthy mentor/student relationship.

You are doing well to revisit the previous lessons, as they may pull you deeper and help you set and maintain clearer boundaries between Pink and Red Tantra. Blessings.

***Student:*** I had a deep, deep kriya this night. My partner was over here, and what he and I didn't expect happened. He feels, lately, to be in a very sattvic state—not feeling the need to contact other women and, for the first time this week, also not feeling the need to have physical sex, not with himself or with me. He feels there is a shift in our connection since last week, when we had a very deep sharing on all levels. It was very intimate; we shared everything you would in a relationship, but we aren't in one. He pulled back after that weekend, telling me he needed space, because he didn't want to get attached to me emotionally.

So yesterday evening, we saw each other for the first time in a week. Later, I realized I missed our sharing. We spoke a lot, and finally, he told me he felt so full of love toward a few friends of ours. He felt so blessed and cried tears of bliss. He told me he didn't want to sleep with me anymore, that he didn't understand it himself, as the love-making is bliss between us and, till now, he always loved love-making every day several times. He wished we could make the shift toward friendship, away from sexual intimacy.

Oh Mukunda, it hurts so much. I have no regrets at all of the choice I made with him. My wish is to continue this friendship, because he is such a truthful respectful person. With him, my longing to share with a partner has been ignited.

You told me I was probably going to have more Tantrik relationships. Although I feel the bliss and release it gives me, I would love to have that within a romantic relationship. Isn't that strange—knowing that I am longing for a relationship in which I will build up karma instead of living a single lifestyle? Please share your thoughts with me. What is your experience with how Tantrik relationships developed for you?

***Mukunda:*** Tantrik relations are different from romantic ones. You must get the basics clear. The two types of relationships are rarely available together in one person. One can lead to the other in a different person. But to want what isn't is to create more suffering. Yoga is to free you from current and future pain. The pain you have is from wanting what is not available. Practice wanting what you have. It is what you are blessed with. Stop wanting what is not there. See it for what it is and learn from the Tantra lessons how to proceed to deeper levels of sadhana. If your partner cannot see it from that level, that is fine. You can pursue this for your own benefit. A physical relationship is not needed to initiate Tantra, as, at some point, it lightens up into a spiritual relationship with occasional physical practice. Do what you can to stay sattvic after the emotional turbulences of rajasic encounters that stir up your samskaras (conditioning and memories).

Sadhana is the most important element that promotes Tantra. But if it is not a truly Tantrik relationship, then one sees the emotional and romantic overtones as more of a priority than spiritual seeking and manifesting Spirit. If this is the case with you, then you are not ready for deeper Tantra partnership lessons. Remember to keep doing the previous lessons, no matter what happens with this. Without guidance, the situation can create more karma to be burned later on.

I am delighted that you take such confidence in me that you allow your vulnerability to be present. I hope my words are helpful in sorting out your path and destiny. Do stay in touch and keep going deeper into your Tantrik sadhana. Just remember that you are a committed Yogini first of all, and that what definitions you give to yourself or your fluctuating emotional or mental state are less significant.

**Student:** Interesting dreaming last night (Valentine's Day). Erotic dream involving Tantra and you, but you were able to "transform" yourself to show me what it was like for me to love a woman, quite intimately—as if to show me what it was like to love sensually, physically, and spiritually regardless of my prejudices or preferences. This is a bit cryptic, but it was really lovely and comforted me.

**Mukunda:** How delightful to hear of your Valentine's dream. Dreams are often a way of giving spiritual energy to physical events, thus transforming all the people and events to a higher perception of what is unconditional love. According to the teachings of the *Vijnana Bhairava Tantra* and other Tantrik texts, the physical body is not real. Yet it is the vehicle for transforming our experience of the world. This hidden world is neither masculine nor feminine, but pure consciousness. The essence of that is love. So beautiful of you to share such an intimate insightful inner life.

**Student:** From the visualization practice with lesson 15, I could not stand to be separate from my husband. So I simply leaped into him and melted into him. Now when I do this practice, we are actually one; I can't visualize him as a separate entity. It is a beautiful and wonderful sensation. So how do I proceed from here?

**Mukunda:** Just practice allowing yourselves to "be one and to separate just for the pleasure of being two." This comes from Jnaneshwar's *Nectar of Self Awareness— Amritanubhav*, translated by Swami Abhayananda.

*Student:* When my husband and I were meditating today, the red dot that I sometimes see dissolved into a bright blue dot that was new to me. I usually see only a red or purple dot. Is it because it was the two of us that there was this color change? Does this have any meaning?

I would like to have you initiate me, if you think that it would be appropriate, because all I have of this spiritual practice is from your guidance and the Grace of God/dess. When I say that "I meditate," it actually is that I want to meditate, but I don't truly have the stillness or concentration. However, this blue dot/pearl is going to teach me how to meditate so I can focus on it and be with it, because it comes and goes.

*Mukunda:* The blue dot, or blue pearl as Swami Muktananda calls it, is very significant. It is of the form of the True Self. Details can be found in Swami Muktananda's spiritual autobiography, *Play of Consciousness.* The blue dot can come and go. Just hold the intention of looking for it and encouraging your love and devotion to increase. Feel the source of the blue pearl to be your True Self. On the way there, it may reveal its forms of various attributes like love, peace, sexual arousal, fear, joy, anguish, or confusion. Just persist, and the initiation you seek will be forthcoming.

*Student:* I have been having some experiences and would like to find out how you interpret them. It is a long story. It started with me noticing a holding of energy in the back of the heart area. One day during a yoga class, I decided to go there energetically and nurture the spot. So I caressed the spot; I imagined my yoga teacher caressing and loving that spot in me. Then, like a tidal wave, I began to cry. I had to leave the room, as I sobbed hopelessly. In my mind, I begged my teacher to come to me and just hold me while I cried. He did not come. I cried a very long time, then left.

A couple days later, I was in a Tantra workshop, and the same teacher had us intentionally call up an area of pain and let it go. I cried again, but this time, supported by my classmates. And he hugged me in support. It was a long, deep, and loving hug. After that, I began to have all these experiences. For eight days straight, I could not sleep for more than four hours and *I was not tired.* Food lost all its appeal to me. Then, I began having these incredible metaphysical experiences in my body. They started with me imagining this hug. It was felt so deeply.

Then I had a craving to join my heart energy with this teacher's, and I offered myself to him in my mind. I craved it so deeply that my body became moist and stayed that way for six or seven days. I was in a constant state of arousal. While I was imagining the hug, my entire body energized and contracted, and I lit up like a Christmas tree. I went into a state of bliss. It was a metaphysical orgasm, not physical at all.

When I left that experience, I felt so completely satisfied and full. From that, during yoga classes, I began to feel more. My practice started to make me cry, but not with sadness. Mine were tears of profound joy—joy of movement, joy of feeling, joy of the love coursing through my body. Then a different energy force came to me. My root chakra was stimulated and aroused; I could do things I could never do before—physical things in the yoga practice that never were that full. Upward bow (wheel) was full and big and complete and so *strong*. I could physically do twice as much as before, holding longer, opening deeper. I craved it; I had to do it.

So this is what is happening, and it seems to be related to my loving this teacher. I feel "in love" with him, ever since that first hug. I crave to feel his heart energy. Now things have settled down. I still am very moved by my back-bends and twists, and still get mild energy surges that expand my yoga poses. Can you offer me some interpretations of these experiences and some suggestions as to how I can integrate this in my life.

***Mukunda:*** What you need to know is that this is due to your self-effort; it is from this effort that this opening arises in you. It is not likely to be only from the power or gentleness of the teacher. This is a good teacher by the sound of it. He is not seeking emotional or sexual intimacy with you, correct? He is unlikely to be trained in Tantra, as what is aroused in you is a deeper energy than sexual arousal. If he is trained to be a Tantrik teacher by a guru rather than merely having an interest in Tantra sex, then more detailed help can be given through the hugasana that is so attractive to you. The spiritual energies seek connection to the feelings of love, especially those of a higher spiritual, not physical, love. But it is necessary to go through that level of arousal to move upward to a higher realm. So be patient and let them come; that is the best practice to engage in.

There are many rare books that describe the arousal of Kundalini, but only a few describe the experiences you are having. I suggest reading *Play of Consciousness* by Swami Muktananda. He also had surprising sexual arousal from an awakening, as described in the Dialogue section of lesson 10.

Other teachers of the secret shaktipat Tantrik traditions have left teachings—notably Dhyan Yogi Madhusudandas's *Light on Meditation* and *Shakti*. Also see Swami Kripaluananda's *Science of Meditation*. There are also texts cited in my reference list. You need to know that, while rare, this is not unheard of. Very few spiritual paths involve this form of awakening, which is called shaktipat. It is a secret, sometimes called the secret of the siddhas (Tantrik masters). I am sending you some advanced literature to skim for reference. Lesson 15 tells you how this sadhana can best proceed with a partner or teacher trained to help you feel love, but not love attached to the teacher. Namaste.

# PART VI

# Toward Unity and Spiritual Illumination

# Tantrik Secrets—Beyond Duality

With Great Respect and Love, I Honor
My Heart, My Inner Teacher.

Congratulations on your persistence at consistent Tantra sadhana! And welcome to Tantrik Secrets. This lesson is to show you that Tantra, when grounded in an evolving spiritual practice, constantly reveals new insights, unveiling the infinite Unknown. And yet the infinite Unknown is, in truth, the Unknowable. The regular pursuit of Tantra requires courage, vulnerability, and wisdom. These seekers earn the yogic titles of Vira (hero), Karuna (compassion), and Jnana (wise One). These qualities together reveal the Ayurvedic harmony of the doshas—vata, pitta, and kapha—indicative of sattva as the true nature of the Divine Presence. That Presence has been calling you to your own Self for as long as you can remember, and now you are here where you belong. In the loving arms of the Beloved, you find the embrace of your own self-acceptance and your own perseverance at being True to your heart of hearts. In Tantrik practice, this merging of the masculine and feminine is called the union of Shiva and Shakti. The progress is normally slow and steady if your practice is regular, although, for some rare souls, a full vision of the Divine Presence is granted early on in their spiritual path due to previous karmas. The pace matters not. That is predetermined by previous self-effort, factors not currently in your control. Now you can be yourself and allow your sadhana to unfold in its own manner, with increased self-effort compared to your previous efforts.

# Secrets of Yoni and Lingam Mudras

The yoni and the lingam are the primal energies of Devi and Deva respectively. At this point in the process, these two qualities can unite within you, or you and your partner, more completely to allow the primal pair to manifest as the mudra, or seal of communion.

> The "I" enters into the Yoni Mudra triangle in its own conception; and because it is aware of itself, it believes itself to be a body, though this is unreal and only appears to be real. In that Yoni Mudra triangle which is the sheath of karma, the soul (jiva) which is of the very essence of sperm exists in that body just as fragrance exists in a flower. Even as the sun's rays spread throughout the earth, this jiva which is in the sperm and which has entered the Yoni triangle spreads itself throughout the body. Though this jiva is everywhere inside and outside, yet it has a special identification with this vital energy of sperm, which is therefore considered its special abode. Thus it exists in the very heart of all beings.[112]

The quality of ojas sexual fluids in the Deva/male and amrita in the Devi/female, being contained by their commitment to love, generates mudra, which allows a deeper level of safety to unfold. From this safety, the final essences of structure, as kapha, can become transformed into their essential nectar, ojas. It is this male essence that is contained by yoni's form as a downward-pointing triangle calming the last levels of self-centeredness until communion with the higher Self naturally arises. This process takes some time, occurring through the prolonged practice of communion as the yoni mudra becomes enhanced by an ever-deepening of prolonged intimacy manifesting as karezza. Through reaching the prolonged goal of communion, an infinite pause (kumbhaka) in both outercourse and innercourse, there will be a fading away of the distinction of self. What arises from the blessing of kumbhaka mixed with karezza is that the communion will continue effortlessly. Once the communion falls away, the memory is built to sustain the underlying qualities of karezza and kumbhaka in harmony. A sadhana free of ego produces a host of unsought psychic abilities (siddhis).

---

112. *Vasistha's Yoga*, 505.

The Yogini welcomes and experiences whatever comes to her unsought.
If She is caught up in rigid conformity, it gives rise to foolish ignorance.[113]

## Wrapping Yourself in the Stillness of Eternity—Shiva-Lata-Mudra

Another means to Devi/Deva communion attained by yoni and lingam mudra is the practice of Shiva-lata-mudra. *Shiva* means "stillness, eternity"; *lata* means "creeper or vine"; *mudra* means "seal or retention." Together, the meaning is "wrapping, intertwining yourself in the stillness of eternity and realizing That."

Mudras are both hand and full-body gestures that manifest the experience of the fifth step (pratyahara) of the eight limbs (Ashtanga Yoga) of Patanjali's yoga. In this state, you intertwine yourselves in the five practices of the elements—offering earth, water, fire, air, and ether to each other. Earth can be your body; water can be made holy when blessed by sacred objects on your altar (puja); fire is the offering of a lit candle; air is the offering of mantras; ether is the offering of incense or a flower's aroma. By sharing this lovingly with your partner, you begin to let the prana creep more deeply into your subtle channels (nadis). Then practice sitting in the lap of your Shiva with your Shakti fully empowered, as a spiritual guide directing the awakened pranic energies to a place of safety and fulfillment.

As you intertwine your energy bodies, the pranas begin to vibrate, resonating with exquisite sounds, like celestial instruments that generate an interplay of serenity, light, and love. This is the higher form of balancing Ayurvedic doshas (harmony of vata, pitta, and kapha). As you are both sincere, you will be captivated and taken by Grace to share secrets that neither can access alone. Your breath, even your pulses, will synchronize as the pranas of two bodies become One. Allow yourselves to be guided. It is safe to surrender when there is only One Heart.

Now is the time to allow yourself to flow with Shakti. Find your energy and let it guide your unfolding. Remember to disengage yourself from identifying energy as

---

113. *Vasistha's Yoga*, 461.

sexual, mental, or physical; see it all as Shakti. As your energy becomes more balanced, it will naturally seek a higher fulfillment in searching for Spirit. For this to happen, men need to be more still and not seek stimulation to increase Shakti. Women can increase Shakti by moving beyond where they feel their energy guiding them, thus being more active. Allow yourself to release any movement or sensation that feels restricted, forced, or unnatural. We are seeking the natural unfolding of a higher principle and, as we do, the grosser koshas need permission to unfold fully.

This process is, in essence, worship of your True Self. This sadhana is to love your Self in all its forms. By being with your Devi or Deva, you can allow a natural unfolding of your True Self. There is only one of you, although, due to loss of worship of the Self, duality and its resultant suffering and distress arise.

## Opening to the Breath of Love

The *Vijnana Bhairava Tantra* (VBT) is my favorite of all the Tantrik texts. It articulates the most profound teachings in a "series of simple affirmations—You are shakti-shiva; Shakti-Shiva is the Self, the universe is the play of your consciousness.... This tradition is a tribute to our most anciently held memory, the divinity of woman, and likewise an homage to today's woman, who carries this divinity within herself and is able to transmit the deep feeling of this divinity to the sensitive and wonder-filled men who she welcomes into her body."[114]

Each of the 112 meditations that Shiva gives to Shakti in the VBT are profound in their simplicity and directness. They lead to that which is called, in various circles, the void, the supreme consciousness, the Divine, or non-dualism. The VBT can be found in terse forms in Daniel Odier's *Yoga Spandakarika* and also at the end of *Zen Flesh, Zen Bones* by Paul Reps, where it is referred to as a pre-Zen text. There is much fuel within this text for continuing to deepen your Tantrik Yoga sadhana beyond these lessons.

There are many meditations throughout the text on the use of breath to uncover the breathless One. Here are two of my favorites. Just sit with them, searching for the communion of Shakti as Bhairavi and Shiva as Bhairava. Whatever you search for diligently you will find.

---

114. Odier, *Desire*, 22–25.

The highest Shakti ceaselessly expresses herself upward from the center of the body in the form of the exhalation and downward in the form of the inhalation. By steady fixation of the mind at the two places of their origin there is the beatitude.

> When the Shakti in the form of exhalation is retained outside at the point 12 finger widths from the nostrils (dvadasanta), or in the form of the inhalation is retained inside at the heart center (hridaya), then the union of Shakti and Bhairava is known. One's small self vanishes.

The effect of following yoga and Tantrik practice is to come to know your true Self. As a function of following the changing field of your breath, you can perceive the fading away of your personality into the True Self. With patience and persistence, Patanjali and other sages like Vasistha declare that this will lead us to knowing the True Self. The following quote reveals an exquisite similarity to the Bhagavad Gita.

> The mind is a field. It is plowed by right action, it is watered day and night by right feeling, and it is nourished by the practice of pranayama. On this field known as the mind the seed known as samadhi (turning away from the world) falls of its own accord when one is alone in the forest known as wisdom. The wise man should endeavor constantly to keep this seed of meditation watered and nourished by intelligent methods.[115]

My process of self-exploration has led spontaneously to the joys of poetry. I have found this to be an ideal medium for communicating my experiences of Tantra and yoga. I wrote a book of poetry sharing these insights called *The Yoga Poet*. Here is an excerpt from "Who am I?"

> I am a Tantrik
> a lover of the Divine
> The She who appears as the world.
>
> I am a Yogi,
> constantly reminded of

---

115. *Vasistha's Yoga*, 530.

the curiosity for,

the craving for,

the lust for,

and the bliss that is

communion.

I encourage you to take time to write a similar poem about who you perceive yourself to be. Allow time to digest these teachings, in the same way that you are gentle following a meal, perhaps going for a walk in nature to process it fully. There is a saying that we are what we eat. That goes for what we eat on all levels—food, emotions, information, people, sacred space, and the media. It's a deeper truth that we are what we eat, even before we eat it.

The cornerstone of these teachings is that, when sexual, mental, or emotional energy is fully experienced and allowed to build, it becomes neutral energy, and if you persist, it will be experienced as spiritual energy. Know that these lessons are for the purpose of moving through yourself to find that deeper current that will always lead you home.

> As you drink more and more from your own fountain source dissatisfaction will cease to exist, as will outer demands, because it is the whole of life that brings you this loving tremoring. There is no longer something missing to make up for; it is the unrestrained intensity of your desire that fulfills you now, and no longer the ideas of possessing, of seducing, of filling a void, of feeding your dissatisfaction. Curiously you will see that the more incandescent your desire, the less it will turn toward objects of desire, because it no longer needs them to mask incompletion.[116]

Remember to persist in your practice, yet stay detached from expecting specific outcomes. Tantra is a personal spiritual practice. When you feel complete with this lesson, read the Dialogue section that follows prior to beginning lesson 17.

---

116. Odier, *Desire*, 88.

## With Great Respect and Love, I Honor
## My Heart, My Inner Teacher.

# Dialogue with Mukunda

**Student:** I have tried to pull prana down through the chakras, rather than pushing it up and piercing them. It is very powerful, but I also feel prana rising out of the crown chakra at the same time. It feels a bit like having one elevator dropping and another rising at the same time. It is not unpleasant, but I am curious as to what is going on. I would appreciate your thoughts. Thanks.

**Mukunda:** The key to your questions is your description of "trying" to pull prana and your use of willpower. This reveals confusion. Tantra's essential quality is surrender, while control is the essence of the yoga path. Your description shows how prana reflects your confusion by not flowing harmoniously. Choose your path and be singular, not mixing these teachings with other paths.

Shakti energy is predominantly a descending energy from the head. When it is given from Grace or a Tantrik master, the process is called shaktipat (literally, the descent of Mother's Shakti energy). The reverse energy is Shiva, which is opposite Shakti as it rises from the base of the spine. This is called Kundalini. This energy is often spoken of as the individual's will to unite with the Divine. Thus, it requires self-effort in harmony with Her Grace. When both Shakti and Shiva forces function together in harmony, it is a sign of sattvic practice and of an ego balanced by the Power of Grace. Namaste.

**Student:** Do the subtle expressions of the chakras exist at the same time? Or is it the shift from the larger petals of the chakras to the opening and spreading to the column of light that takes you into the other koshas? When resting there, hanging out in kosha three for example, with chakras spreading through the universe, do we look around for other manifestations of mano maya kosha to get to know it and be familiar with the feel/taste? I wonder if the shifting of the experience of the chakras is like an elevator to take you to the different levels. Once you get to that floor, do you get out of the elevator and look around?

**Mukunda:** The multiple dimensions of the koshas exist simultaneously. It is the mind that experiences them as separate or intermingled. The body-mind-spirit experience is not a trinity, but an expression of either confusion or communion. When the mind is calm, the trinity disappears into the universal consciousness. Consciousness with thought is the mind. Without thought, there is only pure consciousness, according to the *Yoga Sutras* and the *Yoga Vasistha*. Attention can shift from one chakra level to another in the prana maya kosha. As the mind goes from kosha to kosha, it reveals the play of consciousness. The looking out at the world is characterized by thoughts and memories on kosha three; on kosha two, it is emotions and vitality; on kosha one, it is physical sensations and activities. When inwardly directed, the mind experiences the varieties of energies that the chakras may manifest. The chakras, upon spreading into the subtle body, become more and more diffuse. When they enter the fourth kosha, they spread throughout the universe until they dissolve, which produces the feeling of communion and true illumination. This must be stabilized, so continued sadhana is required, not just one experience.

Before that, they dissolve from six chakras into a gradually subtler form, then into a column of light called the Shiva lingam. This literally means the "first form of the form-less Shiva." His first form is a wand of light; this has become condensed into these unique naturally arising forms from the Narmada River called Shiva lingam stones. The shift is subtler than an elevator, as it is on the etheric plane. Air gives a sense of motion, while with ether it is merely thought-directed. A beautiful depiction of the five koshas is found in spiritual artist Alex Grey's book *Sacred Mirrors*. He has a gallery in New York City by the same name (see *www.sacredmirrors.com*).

All five koshas exist simultaneously; it is merely the perceptual field we call mind that looks at each dimension from a different perspective. So, what is perceived as kosha two is the gross chakras; what is perceived as kosha three are subtler more diffuse chakras; in kosha four, the chakras merge into a column of light. These are the descriptions of the evolution of the chakras. At first, they are vague in their kosha expressions, then they become clearer and more distinct indicators of mood and spiritual states (*bhav*).

**Student:** Regarding movement from kosha to kosha, I began having an experience of stilled thoughts and lessened physical sensation. I had told you about much sensation during a prolonged breath pause (kumbhaka) in kapalabhati pranayama practice. Then it became no sensation, with little or no awareness of my physical body. I assumed this was a movement toward third and fourth kosha, being in the mind and the focus of the kumb-haka as you have spoken about with shambhavi mudra. Tonight has brought a similar occurrence, but it seemed very dualistic. There was a sense of stillness, also an observation of the thoughts "over there," a sense of wanting to float out of my body, but also a sense of being pulled back in. A sense of distraction, but then a desire to stay in the stillness. In the third kosha, does the sensation of energy subside? And the sensation of embodiment?

**Mukunda:** That is true. The sense of energy is heightened in kosha two and less in the third and fourth koshas. As one becomes more integrated in the koshas, there can be a gradually increasing sense of all dimensions being simultaneous. As your thoughts and breath become subtler, you will be entering kosha four, where new insights and wisdom predominate. It is indeed from a relaxation of the fourth kosha that you are prone to a feeling that you are leaving the physical body. This experience leads to a deeper relaxation pose (shavasana). It trains one how to leave the body so that, when death approaches, there is no suffering. This is the greatest serenity of sattva, as one shows a fearless acceptance of life by a surrender to the naturalness of death (mahasamadhi). Mature souls learn to relax through the koshas as they suspend the life force from going out, so that they depart this world gracefully.

**Student:** In lesson 16, you say: "It is the unrestrained intensity of your desire that fulfills you now, have no longer the ideas of possessing, of seducing, of filling a void, of feeding your dissatisfaction." When one has reached that state, it seems to me that there is no more purpose to be on earth, because all the ordinary things were done to fill this void only. Is that why most of the Realized Ones only have interest is helping others reach the same state—why they have no more other cravings? I remember Sadhu Vaswani once said in a lecture that the Realized Ones live in the world as actors. But I find it quite difficult to act in ways that can be different from the Self, especially in relation with so many people who are not in that state.

**Mukunda:** The sages Vasistha and Ramana Maharshi seem to point out that it is like a lamp that has no oil, yet remains burning. Karma is there, but no fuel to cause identification with actions or deeds. Desire is not the problem. It is desire without a stable state of sattva that creates problems. Without sattva's serenity, there is craving or repulsion, instead of natural activity free of a sense of doership. Activities happen, but no stress is felt in this complex of body/mind/spirit. The next lessons will help to unveil more Tantrik secrets to you. Blessings.

# God/dess Consciousness

With Great Respect and Love, I Honor
My Heart, My Inner Teacher.

Patanjali's text, the *Yoga Sutras,* defines the different yoga sadhanas to be undertaken, the methods to be used, and the goals to be attained by each practice. It is a procedure manual for those who would delve into yoga's secrets. Yoga's secrets are not unveiled without a commitment to spiritual practice (sadhana) generated by self-effort (tapah) to discern, then dissolve, the most primal roots of duality. For it is here that non-duality can be known as simply a mistaken interpretation of perception. Duality vanishes when known. Non-duality is known in the field of silence, without form. And yet its triple qualities of sat/chit/ananda make it known to those who interpret the experience as spiritual or mundane. To know how to unveil yoga's secrets, the guidance of a master is invaluable; for, in asking for help, we receive our own Grace in the form of humility.

## Integrating Yoga and Tantra

Perhaps the most renowned Hatha Yoga master of the past century is professor T. Krishnamacharya. His son, Desikachar, has described some intriguing insights into the *Yoga Sutras* that his father revealed to him in his book *Health Healing and Beyond.* He states: "Patanjali's work is divided into four chapters. According to my father, they represented the sage's teachings to four different disciples, each at a different stage of yogic development."[117]

From this perspective, I see the four chapters as describing, not merely four individuals, but four archetypes for whom specific paths are given by the sage. While the teachings of the entire text are comprehensive and beneficial, the sadhanas given may not be as suitable for your archetype at this stage of your spiritual development. By reflecting upon the four paths, you will see insights similar to those that were shared by the contemplation of your Ayurvedic constitution (prakruti).

The first chapter is entitled Samadhi Pada, literally "walking the path of Samadhi." Samadhi is the procedure for "stilling the mind," as most translators render sutra I, 2. It is a discipline. In contrast with this, my Raja Yoga teacher, Swami Shyam of Kulu, defined it as a "mind that has ceased to identify itself with its vacillating waves of perception (vrittis)."[118] In my library, I have over fifty editions of the *Yoga Sutras*. The only other interpreter using this distinction is Marshall Govindan, in his book *Kriya Yoga Sutras of Patanjali and the Siddhas*. This teaching is in harmony with the *Charaka Samhita*, the earliest Ayurvedic text, which states that "detachment is salvation." Patanjali and the sage Charaka are said to be reincarnations of the same soul.

The archetype described is one who naturally experiences detachment from thoughts and dispassion from suffering. He or she requires no instruction in meditation, but rather in how to deepen the communion of samadhi. The practice given is to still the thoughts, emotions, and prana and detach yourself from the mental tendency to be identified with them. This is a naturally arising meditation; this is the process of lesson 1—just to feel your feelings and thoughts and to know that they are there, but they are not you.

The sadhana for this chapter has no physical discipline. The longest series of practices recommended are a devotion to the One Being in *Yoga Sutras* I, 21–29. The way Patanjali writes is to first define a technique, then immediately tell us how to practice. Then he shares the signs that reveal the attainment of perfection in the practice. The first sutra in this series on devotion, 21, defines the state of consciousness

---

117. Desikachar, TKV, *Health, Healing and Beyond*, 55.
118. Swami Shyam, *Patanjali Yoga Darshan* (Kulu, India: International Meditation Institute, 2001), 1–2.

that characterizes the Presence, regardless of its closeness. The urge for closeness to the Divine Presence is the technique that draws Spirit to the devotee of samadhi.

Now that you have experienced moments of the unity of Shiva and Shakti, consciousness and matter, you have an awareness of the Divine Presence. To know that One is to know Isvara, the Lord of the *Yoga Sutras*, described in sutras 21–29 of chapter 1. Krishnamacharya's student, Srivatsa Ramaswami, comments on sutra I, 23: "The end of spiritual practice is *only* attained by placing yourself in the Lord (Isvara)."[119] Krishnamacharya taught him that the *va* in Sanskrit does not mean the same as in other sutras preceding it—that is "or"—that it means "only" in this case. This frankness means that devotion is the only path for this archetype student. There is nothing to be done but to give devotion to the One Being. The highest practice is constant submission. My last teacher, Yogi Hal, who chose to be secretive and live a life among the majestic redwoods of northern California, recommended that the attitudes of gratefulness and gratitude be given priority. He showed me that, by cultivating these attitudes, humility naturally arises.

How is this submission or worship to be practiced? It requires many years to perfect illumination. Some practical advice in the meantime:

> The Lord should be worshipped with everything that is obtained without effort. One should never make the least effort to attain that which one does not possess. The Lord should be worshipped by means of all the enjoyments that the body enjoys, through eating, drinking, being with one's consort and other such pleasures. The Lord should be worshipped with the illnesses one experiences and with every sort of unhappiness or suffering one experiences. . . .The realization of this infinite consciousness (which is totally effortless) is alone the best form of worship.[120]

The sage Vasistha goes on to describe how all of life's situations should be engaged with naturalness and seeking the Divine Presence within them. Regardless of whether they are pleasant or unpleasant, the divine consciousness shines within them all. Its nature is the unity of the trinity sat/chit/ananda. This trinity is the yogic apex of prana, tejas,

---

119. Srivatsa Ramaswami, *Yoga for the Three Stages of Life* (Rochester, VT: Inner Traditions, 2000), 54.
120. *Vasistha's Yoga*, 381 and 387.

and ojas. It is the unity of the duality expressed as self and other. It is constantly both veiling and unveiling itself.

> This infinite consciousness, which is unmodified and non dual, can be realized by one in the single self luminous inner light.[121]

What is that Being that is the Lord? It is neither feminine nor masculine, neither Shiva nor Shakti, neither the Father nor the Mother; neither heaven nor hell can contain that One. What is it?

> If one says that the first Creator is the original cause of all subsequent bodies, in that even that is not true! The creator is non different from the reality; hence the appearance of this One as other than the reality of this world is delusion. The realization of this truth enables one to get rid of ignorance and egosense.[122]

For those who consider the Divine to have a personality with sexual attributes, Devi is the Divine Mother and Deva the Divine Father. As cited earlier, Shakti Devi can be found within the three veils of the subtle body. She is most likely to be found in the grossest energy portions of our bodies—Sarasvati in the first chakra; Lakshmi in the second; and Kali in the third. The fourth chakra has a form as Tara. However, since Her form is air, She is composed of the subtlest of the elements that can have a form. Beyond that, the Divine Presence is just that—a presence. In describing Herself to Her devotee Lila, Sarasvati says,

> I do not really do anything to anyone. Every soul earns its own state by its own deeds. I am merely the deity presiding over the intelligence of every being; I am the power of its consciousness and its life force. Whatever form the prana of the living being takes within itself, that alone comes to fruition in the course of time. You longed for liberation and you obtained it. You may consider it the fruit of your discipline or worship of the deity; but it is consciousness alone that bestows the fruit upon you.[123]

---

121. *Vasistha's Yoga*, 371.
122. *Vasistha's Yoga*, 450.
123. *Vasistha's Yoga*, 74.

How do we find that One? The *Yoga Sutras* I, 12 states that "success is attained by consistent earnest practice over a long period of time coupled with dispassionate nonattachment from the result of that practice." Effort and surrender are the keys to knowing that One.

Paul Brunton was a figure who played a central role in bringing to light the message of the spiritual masters of India. His first book, published in 1934, is entitled *A Search in Secret India* and is still in print. He wandered the length and breadth of India searching for an illumined master. His search led him to Ramana Maharshi. In his book *Day by Day with Bhagavan*, A. Devaraja Mudaliar quotes Paul Brunton as saying:

> Divine Grace descends and acts only when it is invoked by total self-surrender. It acts from within, because God resides in the heart of all beings. Its whisper can be heard only in a mind purified by self surrender and prayer.[124]

In my personal experience with sadhana, I have found myself closest to God when I am in suffering or pain. It is in such moments of agony, frustration, and low self-esteem that I found myself in the primal state of dispassion, crying out to God to show me Her form, or at least Her face. I struggled with a negative behavior that was compulsive and left me feeling weak, sad, lonely, and dejected. I criticized myself for not being stable on my spiritual path due to these negative emotions, which came like a plague of locusts to overwhelm my crop of positive, elevated consciousness from yoga.

At one period in my life, I turned to twelve-step programs to help me resolve my spiritual suffering. I discovered from going to meetings that, while I knew meditation, I did not know how to pray. I was shocked. So, I began to supplement my spiritual practice with what I learned from doing the steps with the aid of a sponsor. One of the most dramatically effective prayers I found was a prayer used to reinforce the third step. It is found in the *Big Book*.[125]

> Divine Mother (or God/dess of my understanding), I offer myself unto
> Thee—to build with me and to do with me as you will. Release me

124. A. Devaraja Mudaliar, *Day by Day with Bhagavan* (Tamil Nadu, India: V.S. Ramanan, 1968).
125. *Alcoholics Anonymous* (New York: Alcoholics Anonymous World Services, 1976), 63.

from the bondage of self, that I may better do Thy will. Take away my difficulties, that victory over them will bear witness to those I would help of Thy Power, Thy Love and Thy Way of life. May I do Thy will always!

When I begin my morning sadhana, I begin by doing a full pranam (lying facedown with my arms extended) to my altar, which contains relics of my spiritual journey. In that submissive position, I say this prayer three times, or until I feel taken over by that One who is the object of my prayer. The Presence comes in Her time and Her way, and yet She consistently comes to me and to those who seek Her. One can pull Her energy from another sincere devotee. She lives with Her lovers, and if it can be said that She enjoys anything, it is being energetically pulled out by another sincere seeker. In so doing, both are elevated. Those who lose energy when they give to others are not stable for such a practice and are encouraged to repair their "leaky buckets." They also need to learn to have a steady, sustainable prana to meet with equanimity all that life presents.

How should one act in the presence of this One? They will be practicing worship of the One in all natural activities. The disciplines of yama and niyama, yogic ethics, are naturally arising in them, as their unique expression of a sattvic life. They will not harm others nor cause themselves harm. For the perception is only of One.

> They who do not let their organs function naturally as long as the body is alive, are obstinate and stubborn people. The equilibrium of yoga is for the mind not for the organs of action and their states. As long as the body lasts, one should let the organs of action perform their proper function, though the intellect and senses remain in a state of equanimity. Such is the law of nature to which even the illumined master, angels, and gods are subject. Let come what may, for the True Self is not affected by the fate of the body. Whatever be the joy or sorrow that is allotted to one affects the body, not the indweller. Hence let us do what is natural, without desire and aversion.[126]

It is natural activity done with detachment that is the expression of a sattvic mind. This is both a practice and the most immediate sign of the luminous liberated Self. The process is one of involution. As was mentioned in the third lesson on yogic anatomy, the

---

126. *Vasistha's Yoga*, 462.

chakras involute upon being exposed to true spiritual life. As they involute, the mind reverses itself and the current goes, not to seeking pleasure and pain from outer life, but rather to seeking its source as it flows inward. In ordinary consciousness, the flow is outward and the Self is lost.

One who is given over to selfless service or Karma Yoga attains that path in a gradual way. For, by seeking to be of service to others, your life force is gradually given over to considerations for others first and for yourself second. In the beginning, Karma Yoga is a trial—a test of seeking to uncover when it is appropriate for you to give. Should I give to this homeless person, or to that person suffering from abuse or the violent difficulties of Mother Nature's forces? We seek a lofty place to give our service and money, so that we will feel good about what we have done. There is a self to serve in this case. When we fully give ourselves to the Divine Presence, there is no thought of what comes for us. There is no other to consider. All is done as a force of nature expressing service to itself. By finding the path, whatever it is, prana increases. By becoming firm on the path, the prana that is gained will be retained.

## What Is the True Self?

This is a great question to pursue persistently. It is a question that does not have an answer, except in silence. For, if the Self could be known, it would no longer be the Self. If an answer arises, it is not the Self. Remember that there are three worlds (three bodies that are veiled by five koshas): that of the mind, that revealed by the intuition, and that which is beyond and transcendent in all other koshas simultaneous to being One. The known, the unknown, and the Unknowable, as Yogi Hal called the trinity. It is by inquiry into the first two attributes or worlds that the mind comprehends the known and the unknown. Each of these worlds can be seen as composed of dual forces—the wave and its wetness; the sky and its blueness; a flame and its warmth. And yet, this duality is clearly an illusion. The first primal duality of the Indian trinity is Sarasvati and Her consort, Brahma, as the creative force. The second is Lakshmi and Her consort, Vishnu. The third is Kali and Her consort, Shiva.

The power or energy that creates and brings about bondage is also the power or the energy that dissolves creation and liberates.[127]

I would add that it is also the power that sustains and brings about attachment. The trinity is one. For the mind that perceives a difference between these three, there is suffering (*dukha*). That difference causes pain and bondage, and yet it is also the means for release from suffering. By seeing clearly the essential unity of the paired consorts of the trinity, the Self is revealed. The effulgence of the Self shines forth, eliminating the perception of the world.

> The one becomes three, the three become five and the five become many; that is, the pure self (sattva which appears to be one) becomes through contact three (sattva, rajas and tamas) and with those three the five elements come into existence, and with those five, the whole universe. It is this which creates the illusion that the body is the self. . . . If the secret truth mentioned above is ascertained by self-enquiry, the multiplicity resolves itself into five, the five into three, and the three into one. . . . It is true that it is only possible for mature minds, not for immature ones. For the latter, repetition of a mantra under one's breath (japa), worship of images, breath-control (pranayama), visualizing a pillar of light and similar yogic and spiritual practices have been prescribed. By those practices, people become mature and will then realise the self through the path of self-enquiry.[128]

Maturity on the spiritual path ends in natural activities and in inactivity when to act would be inappropriate. Thus the form of that activity varies from being to being. There are no singular activities that one can say are natural to the divine consciousness. Worship of the Self is the highest expression of that consciousness, but such worship does not take an external form. It is not worship of an "other" that is the hallmark of this consciousness.

> The external worship of a form is prescribed only for those whose intelligence has not been awakened and who are immature like little boys.

---

127. *Vasistha's Yoga*, 474.
128. *Vasistha's Yoga*, 324.

When one does not have self-control, he uses flowers in worship; such worship is futile, even as adoring the self in an external form is futile. However, these immature devotees derive satisfaction by worshipping an object created by themselves; they may even earn worthless rewards from such worship.[129]

It is through such ignorance that one continues to spin on the cycle called samsara (worldliness and the belief in the substance of what is without true form, what is not eternal). There is no end to this samsara, this cycle that constantly creates birth and death repeatedly.

A man whirling on the wheel of ignorance thinks that the world and the body are evolving. The spiritual hero should reject this: this body is the product of thoughts and notions entertained by an ignorant conditioned mind. The creation of ignorance is false. However, even if the body seems to be active and doing all kinds of actions it is unreal, even as the imaginary snake in the rope is forever unreal. What is done by an inert object is not done by it; though appearing to act, the body does nothing.

The inert body does not entertain any desire to motivate its actions and the self which is infinite consciousness has no such desire either; hence there is in truth no doer of action but only the witnessing intelligence. Even as the sun, resting always in himself and in his own essential nature constantly engages himself in the affairs of the day, you too, resting in your own self engage yourself in the affairs of the state.[130]

This natural activity is known as sattva; its predominant feature is serenity. Sattva is what is behind the perception of witness consciousness. As such, it is the great doer of actions, the great enjoyer of pleasure, and the great renouncer—free of identification with any of the attributes of personality and ego. The purist form of sattva is simply being yourself, a stress-free being.

---

129. *Vasistha's Yoga*, 368.
130. *Vasistha's Yoga*, 364.

When sattva is in a state of total equilibrium, then no physical or psychological defects are experienced. It is not possible to abandon sattva; however it reaches its end in course of time. When there is neither the mind nor even the sattva in the body, then like snow melting in the heat, the body dissolves in the elements.[131]

This does not mean that a true Yogini is without illness or concern. It means that she is free from that karma that ordinarily arises from the activities of body and mind. Yoginis do not cause other than a natural response and appropriate activity. When that activity passes, they remain stress-free, with serene bodies and minds. And in a timely manner, death comes without producing distress.

Baba Muktananda frequently said: "Whatever you do in spiritual life never goes to waste." Although he did not mention that it can be forgotten, misused, or abused. The Tantrik Yogini must remain vigilant regardless of whatever attainment, pleasure, praise, or criticism may be given. For indeed, it is possible to fall from your attainment. One must be ever-mindful and protect what is given, regardless of whether it arises from sadhana or from no apparent causation. The value of keeping good friends close to you (satsang) cannot be overemphasized. Even casual conversations about your pleasures or challenges with those seeking higher consciousness will deepen your understanding of how to live your life. In the trials of my life, I have found my spiritual friends to be fountains of coolness. Their presence more than their words is what I really need during these times. They don't have to console me with their words; their very spiritual essence is consolation. Spirit increases for both of us when we are together, regardless of the activity.

> If you conceptualize this teaching for your intellectual entertainment and do not let it act in your life, you will stumble and fall like a blind man. In order to reach the state of perfection or liberation taught by Vasistha you should live a life of non-attachment, doing what is appropriate in every situation as it reaches you. Rest assured that this is the vital factor in the teachings of all scriptures.[132]

---

131. *Vasistha's Yoga*, 460.
132. *Vasistha's Yoga*, 326.

Naturally arising activities are cited repeatedly throughout the text as the means of expressing self-realization. One seeking this finds stress-free activities and performs only those. Swami Muktananda often referred to his lineage of teachers as "stress-free beings." Stress only arises in those minds identified as the doers of mental and physical activities. This is true regardless of the activity, whether it is expressing any of the four virtues of life—dharma, righteous lifestyle to fulfill your duties; kama, sexual and sensual pleasure; moksha, spiritual liberation; or artha, appropriate abundant wealth. In one who is manifesting the Devi/Deva communion consciousness, activities will persist, yet without any sense of stressful residue.

Kali is the Goddess whose nature is time. As such, she destroys the world. There is nothing She does not terminate. She is the death of all that appears to have a separate existence. Kali frees the mind from the illusion of the world being separate from Self.

> Innumerable forests known as creation have been reduced to ashes by the fire known as time (Kali). Such is the state of this creation. But since the ignorant are bound fast to their own false notions, neither the transiency of the world nor the hard blow they suffer in their life is able to awaken them.... The whole universe is the begging bowl of Kali the goddess whose nature is action and motion. This Kali constantly seeks to fill the bowl with all the creatures of this world and to offer them again and again to Her Lord.[133]

There is nothing that She cannot create or destroy. However, all this is mere appearance—notions created from the absolute consciousness that is the true nature of Devi/Deva. There is nothing impossible for Her. All prosperity and all adversity, all ages of the life span, all happiness and suffering—they are all nothing but the play of God/dess as consciousness. Seeing this fear and illusion dissolve and peace beginning to arise naturally and spontaneously of its own accord is the true peace of the nature of the purified sattva. Sattva, in its essential nature, is God/dess consciousness playing as this world, as the soul (*jiva*), as the sense of individuality, and as the sense of eternal unity. Resting in your own relaxed self is the most natural act. Being that one, one knows the purity of the Self.

---

133. *Vasistha's Yoga*, 334.

# Puja for Devi/Deva Communion

This practice is a deeper version of the Tantrik puja practice given in lesson 3. You will be invoking Shiva within yourself and in your partner. This is to be followed by invoking Shakti within yourself and in Her. Both sexes do both the Shiva and Shakti pujas. It is optimal to do this free of clothing, becoming as free as a newborn. This sadhana was given to me by a naga (naked) yogi in the Tantrik tradition.

## Shiva Puja

The Shiva puja practice begins by surrendering yourself fully in front of your sacred space/altar, doing a full pranam, lying flat with palms together extended toward your chosen deity. Repeat constantly the mantra Om Namah Shivaya or play a tape with it continuously throughout the practice. Reflect on its meaning: "With great respect and love, I honor my heart my inner teacher."

Assume any tantrasana seated posture that you can comfortably sustain. These were described in detail in lesson 7. Sit before the *ista devata* (chosen deity) and do a brief puja to the statue or picture that is most central to you. Have some chalk (*bhasma*), red powder (*kumkum*), henna oil, and if possible, sacred ash (*vibhooti*) handy. These can be purchased at many Indian food stores or given in temples and ashrams as blessed gifts (*prasad*). If they are helpful in creating devotion, use them. If not, do what is more personal to create an intimate environment.

With the first three fingers of your right hand, swipe across the chalk block and scribe the chalk across the top of your right foot. The three fingers symbolize that Shiva transcends the known world, three gunas. With each swipe on each location, say the mantra and reflect that this body is Shiva. Shiva alone lives here.

Then, in order, go through the body from bottom to top, flowing with the direction of Shiva's upward-moving energy (udana prana). Do the right foot then the left foot, the right lower calf then the left, the right upper calf then the left, the right lower thigh then the left, the right upper thigh then the left, the root of the lingam (just in front of the central pelvic floor or perineum), the base of the lingam (upper pubic bone), the lower abdomen, middle abdomen, and upper abdomen, the right chest and left chest, the back of the right hand then the left hand, the right forearm, the left forearm, the right upper arm, the left upper arm, the throat, and finish with three horizontal marks across your forehead. This is the sign of Shiva—that mind and body are given up.

The next phase is to linger with the three-finger placements on the chakra locations. Conceive that the one touching you is Shiva. Hold the tips of the fingers together and encourage the Shiva prana to go deeply into each chakra, clearing it so that energy can ascend to the higher koshas. Begin with the root chakra at the perineum; move to the second chakra at the pubic region; to the third chakra near the navel; to the fourth at the breastbone midway between the breasts; to the fifth at the base of the throat; and finally to the sixth chakra at the third eye. Sit for some time, then do savasana (Shiva's pose), lying with limbs apart on your back. Alternate tantrasana and savasana for one hour.

## Shakti Puja

For the Shakti puja practice, constantly repeat any of the Devi mantras that you are attracted to or play a chant to the Devi as Shakti. Do the same procedure except in reverse, as Shakti's energy is to descend from above. When you have offered the entire physical and subtle body to Shakti Devi, form the yoni mudra with your hands. Search for an experience of the meaning of yoni—its various meanings include Source, uterus, vagina, and the place where Shiva's lingam arises from a lifeless into a firm form. Sometimes, this yoni is experienced as being in the physical body; at other times, it is clearly a chakra-like energy; at still other times, it is even subtler.

These are experiences that show the three different bodies that comprise the five koshas. Subtler is not better or higher. All together make up the complete experience of yoni mudra. The essence of this profound practice is to experience the sensation of "becoming captivated," the literal meaning of mudra. When experiencing the yoni as Source, it means "the place where energy becomes matter." This is the fullness of being one with all your koshas. As you observe energy in your body resolving into one singular point of awareness, regardless of where that is, use henna or red kumkum to mark its downward-pointing triangular space. In the center of the yoni mudra, mark a spot (bindu) indicating the Source space. Stay here with your hands marking the space for some time, then lower your hands and let the yoni mudra expand, until it encompasses you fully. Do what is natural from there.

## Shiva-Shakti Dharana

After each puja is done, sit and gaze at each other (or if you are alone, gaze at your chosen deity's form). After Shiva puja, look to see yourself as Shiva in what you behold. Then, following Shakti puja, look to see nothing but Shakti. As a variation, let Deva do Shiva puja to himself while Devi does Shakti puja to herself. Then sit with each other and follow your awakened energies into Unity.

Remember to persist in your practice, yet stay detached from expecting specific outcomes. Tantra is a personal spiritual practice. When you feel complete with this lesson, read the Dialogue section that follows prior to beginning the final lesson.

### With Great Respect and Love, I Honor My Heart, My Inner Teacher.

# Dialogue with Mukunda

***Student:*** In a retreat named God-dess Awakening by Sonia Sophia, I felt and thought I was going to die. I was opening my heart and fell to the floor clutching it in agony. Then there was bliss. Parts of my hands awoke and took flight, lifting like two cobras. Many jolts of energy passed through me and the back of my heart chakra opened up and radiated rays past my crown. Definitely, life has changed from this and many other experiences. I'm not having personal obstacles, as you have mentioned. Is this a result of the quick progress I made? Was the Kundalini rising? Or was I just opening blocks that have been closed for so long? Any insights are truly appreciated. Thanks for your guidance and wisdom. By the way, I have started a satsang at my house as a result of all of this.

***Mukunda:*** Sounds to me as if you encountered a wonderful teacher and are receiving the blessings of her and your own sadhana. I suspect, from what you describe, that this is the opening of one of the three granthis (psychic knots). They are located in a subtler kosha than the chakras, which are on the second or prana maya kosha. They are in the fourth kosha, and are the final blocks to spiritual illumination. One of the granthis is located in the subtler heart, not the chakra. Often, when they open, the pain is unbearable, excruciating. It often lasts for many days or months, until the old karmic pattern of closing the heart is broken. If the opening persists, it is a sign of Kundalini spiritual awakening. If pain persists, then it is the granthi. If it is a short-lived experience, then it is a block on the chakra level, and that is a sign that it is removed. I cannot say for certain until time has passed and I see you in person. It is good that you are offering spiritual gatherings at your home. That will help to stabilize the process and allow God/dess energy to persist in awakening you and others drawn there. Blessings.

**Student:** It seems as if what you say here of devotion, which continues to be a struggle for me, is the key concept of lesson 17. This practice seems particularly stalled for me. It may be because there is not a specific "sit-down" practice, or just that the surrender to devotion is difficult. I had a similar reaction to the Devi puja Tantrik practice, where I felt dismayed from the lack of connection to devotion, but it was wonderful and pleasant to sit at the altar and chant. You wisely pointed out to me that it's called practice because you have to practice it. For most, it is not spontaneously arising. Am I correct in my concept that, in lesson 17, we are to take that devotion to everything we do, everyone we meet?

And how do we know which practice will retain the experience? As far as memory goes, is this memory nadi a different type of memory than the memory of the mind that has expectations of what a practice should feel like based on past experience? Memory beyond thought, just naturally occurring when the groove is deepened? How do we find our way back into that groove when it starts as just a scratch on the surface? Practice, but practice what? The same as we were practicing when the experience happened?

**Mukunda:** Yes, ultimately, although practice must go hand-in-hand with naturally arising experiences. It is optimal, when we are given an experience, to do a practice to help us retain that experience. Thus prana can be used as an avenue to deepening the memory nadi and allowing it to become a steady mind, free of concepts of time. After all, there is no time but now. Memories are of current events thought of as if they have happened previously. They are crucial in generating spiritual desire, to enlarge desire for all spiritual qualities. Positive desires are to be encouraged with spiritual practice. Over time, the seeker is reconditioning the mind, and the Presence is increasingly felt.

Memory is one of five forms of mental fluctuation (vrittis), which may be either painful or not. See *Yoga Sutras* I, 5–12. It is built into the system as the natural functions of the sushumna nadi. I call it the Truth nadi. Just staying conscious and clear, detached from all the apparent states, allows what memories have been experienced to be recalled. One is not encouraged to try to remember all events, but rather simply to have access to the nadis within sushumna where memory and karma are stored. Behind all these experiences is a subtle current seeking only sattva, the truth of your innate purity. In the same way that a computer stores much more than you can bring up to the desktop, so also the subtle bodies each have different views of the same experiences. So don't bother the conscious mind with desires to know. It is said in the *Yoga Sutras* IV, 20–21 that not everything can be known simultaneously. In III, 9–18, Maharishi Patanjali discusses the transformations of the mind that arise from its surrender into the process of samyama. Reflect on these sutras as a practice.

**Student:** As I told you back during the practice of Devi puja, you are still what I feel as my main connection with spirit. Even with whatever mystical experiences I have had with Kali, or Ganesh, or whatever else I recognize as beyond human, yet there is still the human form with which I identify—the form of Mukunda, my structural yoga therapy teacher. And the form of Mukunda that is the transmitter of this vastness that makes my ears tingle and blows my mind when and if I let it. I guess the truth is what you say: Being with a surrendered student of Muktananda is the same as being with Muktananda himself. That seems to go far beyond the form of Baba Muktananda too. And then I see how that makes the *devotion* what you love, rather than the *form*. But this is all concepts, not reality for me. My mind tells me this would be easier to dive into if I felt this strong devotion toward a disembodied being or energy. So I wonder, is it my fantasy of wish-fulfillment? Or should I direct myself in that way? Or give my faith and confidence, such as it is, with what I've got. (This feels like a bad Hallmark romance novel.)

**Mukunda:** Developing devotion occurs when you just focus on naturally arising feelings of surrender, humility, devotion, and love. If these feelings are to Mukunda, then encourage them. It is not the object that is to be held, but the inner experience—the cultivation of devotion—that is crucial here. It is okay to be self-centered with spiritual practice, as it is all about the Self.

**Student:** Today, something reminded me of what you said in reference to a question I asked about practice 15. You said it sounded as if I had been disappointed by my lover before and had to make him my perfected idea of a lover. I realized I have been disappointed by *love* before, way back, and that this is what I have to get beyond. I must not be afraid of it just because it may not work out or be reciprocated. You keep suggesting blocks that I identify and saying it would be a good thing to get past this or that block. Is it the surrender to the Shakti that can clear this? "Siddha Yoga teaches that with grace and self-effort all people can achieve identification with God." Is this the same thing?

**Mukunda:** Surrender comes from self-effort. Self-effort is to increase the capacity to surrender. They are interrelated. Shakti allows this to happen, as it is the energy that propels thoughts and actions. Increasing Shakti will increase your capacity for self-effort to surrender. You can direct it either way. The end of all spiritual pursuit is limitless, boundless serenity, becoming effulgent light, becoming perpetual blissful love. This is the manifestation of Baba's Siddha Yoga teaching that you paraphrased.

**Student:** I told you in our last private session that I was feeling impatient, and you asked me where I am going. I found the answer in the movie classic, *The Wizard of Oz*. I want to go home! And lately, the more at peace I feel in practice, the more painful it feels out of practice, because I am out of practice for most of my day. This too feels like the essence of lesson 17, but I am not finding a foothold, yet. My mind wants a foothold to move the mind aside.

**Mukunda:** No foothold needed, as, at this level, there is no gross kosha to hang your foot onto. There is nothing left. The feeling that is most perplexing is that emptiness is so captivating that there is nothing else there. It appears to have no form, and yet it brings the mind to being totally present too. Which is the first mind, which is the second? Is there a mind after all? The sage Vasistha says that mind, ego, and world are all illusions. They are merely concepts without form. When we look for the mind as the source of our thoughts, we find it disappears into stillness. When we seek the nature of worldly objects, we find the same. Namaste.

# Spiritual Illumination

With Great Respect and Love, I Honor
My Heart, My Inner Teacher.

There are many spiritual questions that will inevitably arise in ripe students, chief among them: What is realization? How can I tell a realized master from one who is unripe? Is the path I am on the right one for me? Will my path lead to realization or to more illusion and suffering? As long as there is a mind, there is no end to these questions. That is the nature of the mind. When the mind is reduced to its basic components, it is nothing more than a bundle of thoughts and notions based on conditioning of memory. Investigating further, we experience thoughts arising and subsiding from the field of pure consciousness. Thoughts appear to move, yet they never separate from the field. It is this naturally arising pause (kumbhaka) and the field that captivate us in this lesson. To enter the pause is to end the form of the mind and enter the world of endless illumination.

## What Is Spiritual Illumination?

For those who seek to be free of the limitations imposed on the Self by its power as the individuating consciousness of the mind, the highest teachings are necessary. The sage Vasistha says:

My teachings are not meant for those whose intelligence has been silenced by a firm faith in the reality of this illusory world and the consequent striving for the pleasures of this world.[134]

If the teachings fall on a qualified heart, it expands in that intelligence. It does not stay in the unqualified heart.[135]

Illumination requires both a well-prepared student and the assistance of an adept for the seed of the teachings to blossom in the fertile heart soil that seems to be the source of this field of consciousness. One needs to understand the motivation of the spiritual teacher. Vasistha clarifies this:

The wise man does not attempt to teach those who have not overcome their own mind, whose actions spell their own doom, and who are therefore miserable in every way. On the other hand, the wise do endeavor to remove the sorrow of those who have conquered their mind and who are therefore ripe to undertake Self inquiry (vichara).[136]

The result of a ripe soul being with a spiritual mentor or teacher is nothing short of transformation. Merely changing your direction to lessen stress won't suffice. One needs a complete removal of the mind's dualistic perceptions.

He who has not gained a victory over greed, shame, vanity and delusion derives no benefit by reading this scripture: it is a useless waste of time.[137]

So what is the elevated student to do? You should understand the nature of your mind and seek to discipline it according to the guidance of those who have gone before. Their wisdom is the medicine for the removal of the roots to the sense of separation and its resultant perception of suffering.

When the intelligence is still unawakened, one should fill two quarters of the mind with enjoyment of pleasure, one part with study of

---

134. *Vasistha's Yoga*, 216.
135. *Vasistha's Yoga*, 499.
136. *Vasistha's Yoga*, 217.
137. *Vasistha's Yoga*, 490.

scriptures and the other with service of the guru. When it is partially awakened, two parts are given over to the service of the guru and the others get one part each. When it is fully awakened, two parts are devoted to service of the guru and the other two to the study of scriptures, with dispassion as the constant companion.

Only when one is filled with goodness is one qualified to listen to the exposition of the highest wisdom. Hence one should constantly endeavor to educate the mind with purifying knowledge, and nourish the mind with the inner transformation brought about by the study of scriptures. When the mind has thus been transformed, it is able to reflect the truth without distortion. Then without delay one should endeavor to see the Self. These two—self-realization and the cessation of craving—should proceed hand in hand, simultaneously.[138]

In the final chapter of the *Yoga Vasistha*, the Lord instructs the sage Vasistha in how to attain Him who is pure consciousness, the Self, infinite awareness. Vasistha asks Lord Shiva: If realization is beyond the mind, how is it realized? The Lord replies:

In the case of the seeker who is eager to attain freedom from ignorance and who is therefore equipped with what is termed "sattvic avidya" (subtle ignorance). This sattvic avidya, with the help of the scriptures, removes the ignorance. . . . . If one inquires into the nature of the Self and at the same time refrains from those actions that promote ignorance, the darkness of ignorance vanishes. The Self is not revealed either by the scriptures or by the instructions of a preceptor, nor vice versa. It is revealed only when all these come together. It is only when scriptural knowledge, instructions of a preceptor and true discipleship come together that Self knowledge is attained.[139]

A sage, Narada, lived in a cave not far from Vasistha's cave, near Rishikesh on the bank of the holy river, Ganga. He attained Self Realization. At the end of his sadhana, he heard the sound of bracelets belonging to some people playing at the water's edge. Out of

---

138. *Vasistha's Yoga*, 229–30.
139. *Vasistha's Yoga*, 384.

curiosity, he looked in their direction and saw the most lovely celestial nymphs sporting naked in the river. They were indescribably beautiful. His heart experienced pleasure, and his mind momentarily lost its equilibrium, overcome by lust. Prince Rama was confused by Narada and asked, "How can a sage of great learning and indeed one liberated, whose consciousness is as vast as the sky, how can they be overcome by lust?"

The answer given by Queen Cudala is that all beings in all of the three worlds, including the gods in heaven, have a body that is subject to the dual forces. Whether one is ignorant or wise, as long as one is embodied, the body is subject to happiness and unhappiness, pleasure and pain. By enjoying satisfying objects, one experiences pleasure; by deprivations like hunger, one experiences pain. Such is nature. Just having a body is a sign that one has not overcome attraction and aversion.

If the Self, which is the reality, is forgotten even for a moment, the object of experience attains expansion into desire and, from there, to craving enjoyment. If there is unbroken awareness, this does not happen. Even as darkness and light are associated with night and day, the experience of pleasure and pain has confirmed the existence of the body in the case of the ignorant. In the wise, even if such an experience is reflected in consciousness, it does not produce an impression. The wise one is influenced only by the object when it is actually present. The ignorant are so heavily influenced that they react to the object even in its absence. Such are the characteristics: "thinned out vulnerability is liberation, whereas dense coloring of the mind is bondage."[140]

One must reflect on the great timeless teachings of yoga and, with the help of a spiritual mentor, find the path that is most suitable for you. It should not only be one that you are attracted to, but one that reflects your spiritual evolution. In lesson 17, an overview of the *Yoga Sutras* showed that each chapter represents one of four valid yogic paths toward Self Realization. When one reads the sutras with the understanding that they are different paths for different motivations, one sees that the culminating sutras of each chapter reveal different perspectives on Self Realization. The infinite awareness includes all possible levels of illumination, including dullness. Any teaching worth giving is worth repeating and restating.

The first archetype described in chapter 1 is for that student who is walking the path of samadhi (Samadhi Pada). This one is not seeking understanding of the

---

140. *Vasistha's Yoga*, 437–38.

contents of the mind, nor interested in wisdom or power. His or her interest is in uncovering the inner Lord who stands behind the mind. The realm of sadhana is not the body, nor the senses, but the mind only. We know that cultivation of devotion and surrender to the Divine Self give, not only serenity, but also meaning in life. And in spite of our wisdom, we need guidance, perseverance, and detachment from the temptations that the unpurified mind demands. Above all, we seek to be like the One we are looking for, free of karma and its effects. Freedom alone is our path and goal.

For archetype two, described in the second chapter, there are two paths that branch out of Sadhana Pada, the path of spiritual practice. The first half of the chapter, sutras 1–27, is dedicated to Kriya Yoga, the means for purifying the mind. Here we see Patanjali giving the threefold path of discipline, scriptural study, and devotion for the purpose of minimizing the primal causes of suffering. He, like the Buddha, is well aware of the universal presence of suffering. It is a fact of life that it can be overcome by involuting pranic energies through the process of pranayama and meditation. What begins as the path of Kriya Yoga ends in a purification that moves beyond the initial help one experiences through scriptural study seeking a guru and terminates in inquiry.

The second half of chapter II, beginning with sutra 28, is the first five limbs of the eightfold path of Ashtanga Yoga. Here, students are given a step-by-step progression that begins with disciplines of lifestyle and practices for elevating their natural ethical nature into integrity and culminates in physical, pranic, and sensory disciplines that reveal the light of the Self. The practice of the fourth type of pranayama, in which your personal prana is extended into the Divine Presence, leads to "the lifting of the veil that obscures the radiant supreme light of the inner Self."[141]

In commenting on this light of wisdom, Vasistha says:

> Self knowledge or knowledge of truth is not had by resorting to a guru nor by the study of scripture, nor by good works: it is attained only by means of inquiry inspired by the company of wise and holy men. One's inner light alone is the means, nothing else. When this inner light is kept alive, it is not affected by the darkness of inertia. Whatever sorrows there may be that seem difficult to overcome are easily crossed over

---

141. *Yoga Sutras of Patanjali* II, 52.

with the help of the boat of wisdom (the inner light). He who is devoid
of this wisdom is bothered even by minor difficulties.[142]

The third archetype seeks to develop the final three steps of the eight limbs (Ashtanga Yoga) to uncover the hidden powers of the mind. Hence, chapter III is entitled *Vibhuti Pada* (Supernatural Abilities and Gifts). Travelers on this path seek to know the difference between what is permanent and what is transient. They seek to learn how to attain knowledge of the universe and, by attaining its wisdom, let it go, resolving the powers of the mind back to its Source. For they have an inherent understanding that the fame, fortune, and power that it can give are impermanent. They seek to know what is beyond objectivity and duality. They know that what can be given can be lost. What they want is not of this world; indeed, knowledge of this world provides the very means for its transcendence.

The fourth archetype is one who seeks only liberation. It is entitled *Kaivalya Pada*, for one who seeks only Self Illumination. This one has no interest in the affairs of the world. For this one, the Self is attained by the spirit of inquiry into the unity that is yoga. The concept of matter (*prakruti*) and spirit (*purusha*) as separate is dissolved as one reaches the final stages of illumination. What appears to the scholar or philosopher as the dualistic system of Patanjali is not the experience of the Yogi.

> Not even the state of the jivanmukta, the liberated soul, is possible in a
> strictly dualistic philosophical framework.[143]

Unity is all there is.

Regardless of the circumstances students find themselves in, they must persist at becoming wise—*jnani*. Jnanis possess wisdom in the same sense that scholars possess knowledge—not as information, but rather as a steady access to the fourth kosha and an ever-unfolding of infinite life-enhancing perception. They do not hold it; they merely are given the key to being in that state wherein the most appropriate answers are given for the situations in which they find themselves. Watch out for those who attain only pseudo-wisdom.

---

142. *Vasistha's Yoga*, 209.
143. Marshall Govindan, *Kriya Yoga Sutras of Patanjali and the Siddhas* (Eastman, Quebec: Kriya Yoga Publications, 2000), 186.

One who studies scriptures for pleasure or profit and who does not live up to the teachings is a pseudo-Jnani. His scriptural knowledge is not reflected in his daily life. He is more interested in applying scriptural knowledge to promote his physical welfare and sensual happiness. Wisdom is self knowledge. One should work in this world as much as is needed to earn an honest living. One should eat in order to sustain the life force. One should enquire into and know that which frees him from sorrow. He is a Jnani who is oblivious to the consequences of actions, because he is established in self knowledge and ignores both the individualized mind and its objects.[144]

## Cultivation of the Infinite

The highest practice of Tantra and Classical Tantra manifests as freedom to be your Self—that which has always expressed itself as it is. Thus, there is no posture that reveals the Self. It is a "nonpostural yoga of presence that naturally emerges from consciousness. For Tantrikas consciousness does not proceed from activity; on the contrary, it is activity that flows from consciousness."[145]

Vasistha reflects this understanding.

> The Self is not affected by the body, nor is the body in any way related to the Self. They are like light and darkness. The self, who transcends all modifications and perversions, neither comes into being nor does it vanish. Whatever happens, happens to this body which is inert, ignorant, insentient, finite, perishable and ungrateful: let it happen. How can this body ever comprehend through the senses or the mind the eternal consciousness? For, when either is seen as the reality the other ceases to be.[146]

---

144. *Vasistha's Yoga*, 503–04.
145. Odier, *Desire*, 39.
146. *Vasistha's Yoga*, 326.

Regardless of the path taken, the end result is the same—Self Realization. The illumined ones find only One, not a multiplicity of consciousness. The experience is described in *Vasistha's Yoga*:

> Now that craving for pleasure has ceased in me, I shall attain to the state of tranquility which is like nectar. I am really and truly tired of repeatedly earning wealth, fulfilling my desires and enjoying sexual pleasures. Delightful is the state of peace; in utter tranquility all pleasures and pains cease to be of value.[147]

Watchfulness and diligence are needed, no matter what your attainment. My final spiritual teacher, Swami Prakashananda, revealed that it is possible to fall from the highest stages of Self Realization. He said that it is not a permanent state, but rather a constantly evolving experience of the unity of all life. Without diligence in conscious awareness and respect for the appropriateness of ethical actions, your resulting karma can pull you back to worldliness and duality.

The sage Vasistha emphasizes this point:

> If you conceptualize this teaching for your intellectual entertainment and do not let it act in your life, you will stumble and fall like a blind man. In order to reach the state of perfection or liberation taught by me, you should live a life of non-attachment, doing what is appropriate in every situation as it reaches you. Rest assured that this is the vital factor in the teachings of all scriptures.[148]

The appearance of the world is due to diminished consciousness; thus with it, there is loss of truth, a loss of the dynamism of the Self. The five veils (panchamaya koshas) arise due to ignorance (maya Shakti). To the ignorant separate mind, reality is lost. Yet all the five veils are the Self. It is due to an apparent, yet false, perception of a loss of prana that the physical body appears to be real; as a consequence, its changing states seem to be a significant problem. Due to a loss of clarity of mind, prana appears real and its changing states appear to create diminished health and vitality. Due to a loss of wisdom and spiritual truths, the mind appears to be real and the variety of mental

---

147. *Vasistha's Yoga*, 231.
148. *Vasistha's Yoga*, 326.

activities creates significant, yet transient, disturbances. By not knowing the Self as pure consciousness, omnipresent and bliss-filled, happiness seems to arise from the world. Spiritual truths are lost, because they are not worldly, not of value.

> Neither the gross elements nor the forms exist in truth: they arise as they arise in a dream. As forms arise in dreams, so do they arise in the waking state too. If this is realized, there is liberation.[149]

The sage Vasistha says:

> Water has no motivation to throw up ripples. Nor does Brahman have any motive in "creating" the world. Hence, it is right to say that, in the absence of a valid cause, creation has not taken place. Wherever the supreme Brahman exists (and it is infinite and exists everywhere) there arises this world appearance. In a blade of grass, wood, water and in all things in the universe the same Brahman, the infinite consciousness, exists.[150]

There is nothing but the Self, whether it is called the mind, the world, the ego sense, the koshas, God/dess, or Brahman.

## Continuing to Deepen Your Sadhana of Love

Now that you have come to the end of the Tantrik lessons, I have three recommendations to stabilize your ever-expanding wisdom and realizations.

1. Review the summary of the Tantrik lessons and the attainments that can be achieved from each lesson (See Appendix). If you feel yourself incomplete on any lesson or attainment, repeat the lesson. Now that you have gone through the lessons, you have a deeper perspective as you know the illusion of variable prana and unstable koshas to be false. Consult me or your spiritual advisor for more personal sadhana.

---

149. *Vasistha's Yoga*, 600.
150. *Vasistha's Yoga*, 494.

2. Repeat the entire eighteen-lesson course after taking a brief break of a month or two, and encourage yourself to seek a higher level of perception as you engage in your sadhana.

3. Reflect that the essence of the eighteen lessons is in this quote from the sage Vasistha:

> Know that all you experience in the name of mind, egosense, intellect, etc., is nothing but ignorance (avidya). This ignorance vanishes through self effort. Half of this ignorance is dispelled by the company of holy ones; one fourth is destroyed by the study of the scriptures and the other one fourth by self effort.
>
> One should resort to the company of the wise and in their company one should examine the truth concerning this creation. One should diligently search for the holy one and adore that one. For the very moment such a holy one is found, half the ignorance ceases in their company. The company of the holy one puts an end to craving for pleasure; and when it is firmly rejected by self effort, ignorance ceases. All these may happen together or one after the other.[151]

If you established a Tantrik partner sadhana as a result of these lessons, by all means continue to develop your intimacy. Encourage the male to become increasingly grounded in the stillness of Shiva and the female to possess and manifest more of Shakti's life forces. Though this is the primary practice for consorts, I encourage you to reverse roles, at least occasionally. Thus let the woman be passively receiving and the male actively giving. This will help you develop the deeper practices that allow enhanced Shiva Deva and Shakti Devi qualities. As you continue to evolve each lesson, allow for a third role to occur, in which neither of you assumes your archetypal sexual role. In this manner, allow for fluidity in your connecting to the Divine to occur, so that you move freely between the qualities of Deva and Devi in each session.

> From the tantrik viewpoint, the perfect human is the melting together of man and woman in the Self—as individual consciousness merges

---

151. *Vasistha's Yoga*, 496.

into a shared consciousness. This state is called ananda, eternal bliss, the highest Joy.[152]

If, on the other hand, a partner practice has not evolved, neither seek it nor reject it. Let what is sought naturally arise. Let what is not sought fall away or arise without any disturbance of your primal sattvic self. Be free to release or receive.

Remember to persist in your practice, yet stay detached from expecting specific outcomes. Remember that Tantra is your personal spiritual practice. For more details, see the Tantrik References section of my Recommended Reading list at *www.yogatherapycenter.org*.

Blessings on your sadhana. Know that wherever you are is where you are supposed to be. Swami Muktananda taught that "God dwells within you as you." Not different from you, but as you. En-Joy your own True Self. You are That.

**With Great Respect and Love, I Honor
My Heart, My Inner Teacher.**


## Dialogue with Mukunda

***Student:*** Is sattva non-dual?

***Mukunda:*** A profound and beautiful question has arisen from the depth of your inquiry. I am very pleased at getting this question. It shows that sadhana is alive within you. All yoga practices and lifestyles are indeed to deepen sattva. Thus, a study of Patanjali's text reveals only sattvic descriptions of all methods to spiritual illumination. Indeed, the methods to the end of sattva are not different from sattva. Sattva, or harmony, is, of course, the central of all yogic concepts, called the *gunas* (the constituents of life expressions). The other two are rajas (excess activity) and tamas (excessive rest). These are apparently in continual conflict with each other. As a result of this inherent tension between them, they create the different levels of existence. The goal of Patanjali's Classical Yoga is to bring about the involution of the gunas, their reabsorption into the transcendental matrix of nature (Prakriti) on the personal level.[153]

---

152. Ajit Mookerje, *Kundalini: The Arousal of the Inner Energy* (Rochester, VT: Destiny Books, 1991).

153. Georg Feuerstein, *Shambhala Encyclopedia of Yoga* (Boston: Shambhala, 2000), 111.

My view is that, as we follow Patanjali's guidelines, we move to a more sattvic experience of life. He is very literal in how to do this. *Yoga Sutras* II, 46 shows how to be sattvic in the first kosha. As a result of stillness of the body, the next two sutras speak of the shifts that occur in the subtler koshas. The sutras that follow show how to deepen that experience of sattvic harmony so that the energies of the gunas conflicts become resolved through their involution to ever-deepening experiences of sattva as it extends to all the koshas.

*Yoga Sutras* II, 49 is the sutra on sattvic prana. It also affects other koshas, and the results are spoken of in the sutras that conclude chapter II. In all cases, sattva is characterized by stillness—body, prana, then mind—in the sequence of refining the koshas. By reading Patanjali with "great respect and love," and perseverance over a long period of time, sattva manifests. In time, that sattvic state is seen to be the underlying experience of all states of consciousness. The sage Vasistha has said: "Sattva is pure consciousness; pure consciousness is sattva." There is no difference. To the one who sees a difference, it is due to the presence of desire. Those without desire are non-dual.

Vasistha says:

> One who has desires undergoes pleasant and unpleasant experiences. If one wishes to get rid of the disease of such experiences, the only thing to do is to get rid of the desires. . . . This is the essence of the scriptural teachings. . . . It is only by thus understanding the essence-lessness of the objects of experience that one becomes free from the disease of desire. The arising of desire is sorrow and the cessation of desire is supreme joy. . . . The mind is desire and the cessation of desire is liberation (moksha): this is the essence of all scriptures. . . . There is no samadhi without the cessation of desire! . . . Even if you desire to have something, there is nothing other than the Self. What would you desire? Consciousness is subtle like space and indivisible; that itself is this world. . . . the whole world is the Lord.[154]

His teachings are so profound. It is only through persistent reflection on the teachings of the sage and putting the lessons into practice in your life that the sattvic state becomes your living experience. Being natural, doing appropriate activities at the appro-

---

154. *Vasistha's Yoga*, 518–21.

priate time with the appropriate people is sattva, and that is living without a concern for the results of your activities. This is indeed non-dual.

Realize that these Tantra lessons began with the assumption that the reader comes from a dualistic experience based on the perception that the world and all experiences are real. The Self remains unknown to the extent that it is unknowable. Gradually, the student is brought to the perspective of training unconscious aspects of the five koshas, and into seeing the interplay of mind/prana creating both sattva states and perceptions of suffering. As the reality of suffering becomes clearer, Vasistha's non-dual teachings and Tantrik sadhana are given to show the illusory and unstable nature of the dualistic world. The truth is that sattva is non-duality.

*Student:* I had time to reread the Tantra lessons while on vacation. I like the new order and the extra chapters. It was good to review some things as well and fine-tune my practice. As a White Tantrik, I am feeling closer to my female half lately; this is very comforting. I am enjoying the pre-Zen text, *Vijnana Bhairava Tantra,* at the end of *Zen Flesh, Zen Bones*, and have woven that into my practice.[155]

*Mukunda:* I am struck by the lack of questions in response to the final lesson. I receive a free newsletter from Ramana Maharshi's New York devotees, *The Maharshi* (*www.arunachala.org*). A lovely quote is given on the reverse of this bimonthly newsletter. "Silence is the ocean in which all the rivers of all the religions discharge themselves" (Thayumanavar).

*Student:* I actually fell into a mild depression after I completed the lessons. I was so sad they were over, but I must say that what I gained from them was amazing. I now have a genuine sense of evenness and joy that never existed before. My spiritual connection and understanding has also deepened considerably. I just wanted to say thank you for all your love and support through these amazing lessons. What a gift!

*Mukunda:* Namaste and Blessings for extending the benefits of sadhana to others.

---

155. Paul Reps and Nyogen Senzaki, *Zen Flesh, Zen Bones* (Boston: Shambhala, 1994), 191.

# Appendix: Attainments for each Tantra Lesson

I have emphasized throughout this text the importance of persistence without concern for mastery and yet, as each lesson leads you steadily into higher consciousness, specific attainments can be recognized as part of that emergence. I have named these attainments for each lesson below.

For those just beginning the lessons, the attainments named for the early lessons will often arise by persistence in the subsequent lessons. Do not stop the process simply because you have not attained what is cited for each lesson. Sometimes, elevating consciousness to the sadhana of higher koshas (dimensions) gives attainment to a grosser kosha. Your primary intent and focus should always be on persisting and remaining detached from the results of your Tantrik sadhana. I encourage you to read *Yoga Sutras* I, 12, as this will help you clarify the signs of progress regardless of your path. See also *Structural Yoga Therapy*; Table 7: Phases of Progress in Yoga Practice (Sadhana) on page 326 and the Symptoms of Inner Peace on page 315.

For those who have completed the eighteen lessons, use this list to review the Tantrik lessons. If you feel you have not attained what is cited for a particular lesson, then do that lesson again.

Lesson 1: The Energy Body and Tantrik Practice—leads to the capacity to perceive your energy and allow it to guide you.

Lesson 2: The Five Elements and Sensuality—leads to the ability to stay centered within your yoni mudra, as the pranic Source.

Lesson 3: Yogic Anatomy and Sacred Space—leads to the capacity to see that energy is all-pervasive, yet seeks a spiritual container.

Lesson 4: Healing with Prana and Emotional Energy Expression—leads to the ability to open yourself to a higher level of prana in spite of feeling blocked.

Lesson 5: Transforming Sensuality into Prana—leads to the ability to turn your direction inward while pursuing naturally arising acts in outer life.

Lesson 6: Tantra Prana Bodywork—leads to allowing the higher levels of prana to transform your gross body touch into subtler transformative loving expressions.

Lesson 7: Tools for Tantra—leads to familiarity with the multi-dimensional tools of Tantrik sadhana and exploring your own preferences.

Lesson 8: Sexual Health Practices—leads to the ability to heal yourself and your partner of potential health and sexual obstructions for an enjoyable lifestyle.

Lesson 9: Tantrik Love and Its Natural Sexual Expression—leads to developing the muscles of loving kindness to ground into safe intimacy.

Lesson 10: The Divine Couple—leads to yearning for and communing with the Divine Mother.

Lesson 11: Initiation and Spiritual Awakening—leads to the ability to connect to your Inner Teacher and allow Her to guide you in daily life.

Lesson 12: Signs of Kundalini—leads to discernment and discrimination of the signs of effortful and Grace-filled spiritual life.

Lesson 13: From Pranayama to Bandha to Mudra—leads to uncovering your truly unique path of Tantrik sadhana.

Lesson 14: The Colorful Paths of Tantrik Yoga—leads to the ability to open to higher dimensions within yourself and your partner as seekers of Divine Love.

Lesson 15: Deva/Devi Communion—leads to the realization of your Devi as your Deva.

Lesson 16: Tantrik Secrets—Beyond Duality—leads beyond duality by opening to the Divine's Breath as a trinity of Peace, Light, and Love.

Lesson 17: God/dess Consciousness—leads to a committment to the sadhana of seeking Oneness of the God/dess in all life activities.

Lesson 18: Spiritual Illumination—leads to the continual, naturally arising of practice and the infinite realization of the One.

# Glossary of Yoga and Tantrik Terms

***abhyasa***—consistent, earnest practice; see Yoga Sutras I, 12

***adhya***—"primary" first prana, most active on inhale; all pervading

***agnisar dhouti***—cleansing the digestive fire, purification practice

***ahimsa***—nonviolence, non-injury, non-harm

***ajna***—third eye chakra

***ama***—toxicity

***Amba Mata ki Jay***—salutation to the Divine Mother

***Amma***—Divine Mother; Ammachi; Amritanandamayi Ma

***amrita***—nectar of one's inner Shakti

***anahata***—heart chakra

***ananda***—bliss

***ananda maya kosha***—the fifth veil; body sheath made of bliss

***anga***—limb

***anna maya kosha***—first body sheath made of food

***apana***—prana of elimination from pelvis, the prana that births the baby

***ardha padmasana***—half-lotus pose: one foot on upper thigh, the other below

***artha***—abundance and wealth

***asana***—yoga pose, a means to mental stillness and serenity

***aswini mudra***—contraction of the anal sphincter muscles; horse gesture

***avidya***—ignorance, illusion, lack of appreciation for spirituality

***baba***—spiritual father; guru

***baddha konasana***—seated asana with soles of feet together

***bandha***—energetic lock which can arise spontaneously or is taught—pelvic floor, diaphragm, neck or tongue

***bhadrasana***—auspicious pose

***bhakti***—devotional mood

***bhasma***—chalk applied in stripes of three signifying devotion to Shiva

***bhastrika***—rapid abdominal contractions for spiritual awakening; one of the six cleansing practices

***bhav***—spiritual mood

***bhogis***—those who languish in pleasure

***bija***—seed, formative sound of chakras and their nadis

***bindu***—mark on the third eye with red powder (kumkum), also a subtle energy center

***Brahma***—God as Creator, consort of Sarasvati

***brahmacharya***—sexual integrity


***chaitanya***—alive, mantras that enliven Shiva

***Chandra***—feminine goddess of the moon; also the lunar nadi, Ida, which begins inside the left nostril

***chitrini nadi***—thread of light; third tube inside sushumna

***citta***—thought


***darshan***—view; in the company of a saint; seeing from their viewpoint

***devi/deva***—Beings of Light; female/male

***dharana***—contemplation

***dharma***—pursuing righteous duties

***dhyana***—second stage of meditation, entering stillness

***dosha***—primal elements of Ayurveda

***drishti***—external gaze point, an inner or outer point of attention


***granthi***—like bandha, only these locks are freeing deeper karma

***gunas***—primary forces of nature—rajas, tamas, and sattva

***guru***—"from darkness to light"; teacher

***Gurudev***—beloved teacher (inner or outer)

***guru seva***—service to the guru


***ham'sa***—mantra meaning "swan" or the soul

***hatha yoga***—physical purification practices

***himsa***—violence; "ahimsa" means nonviolence

***homas***—fire ceremony to invoke Shiva

***hridaya***— heart chakra; spiritual heart to right of center

***ida***—left nostril; feminine energy channel

***Indra***—Heavenly Father

***ishtad ievata***—personal form of Divine, *Yoga Sutras* II, 44

***Isvara pranidhanani***—devotion or surrender to the lord, *Yoga Sutras* II, 1, 45

***Isvari/Isvara***—Goddess/God, *Yoga Sutras* I, 23–27; II, 45

***japa silent mantra repetition***

***jiva***—soul

***jivanmukta***—liberation

***jnana***—wisdom

***jnana mudra***—gesture of wisdom, tip of forefinger and thumb touching

***jud***—mantras that are not awakened, given by one lacking authority

***Kali***—Mother of transformation, ruler of fire region

***kama***—sensual and sexual pleasure

***kamalasana***—lotus pose

***kapalabhati***—one of six purifications given before pranayama to purify digestion

***kapha***—ayurvedic dosha (that which solidifies)

***karezza***—prolonged intimacy

***kechari mudra***—tongue gesture in which tip of tongue goes up past the uvula

***kirtans***—devotional chants

***ko'ham***—mantra for Self inquiry: Who am I?

***kosha***—five "veils" that obscure the true Self: body, prana, mind, wisdom, bliss

***kriyas***—spontaneous movements indicative of Kundalini awakening

***kumbhaka***—spontaneous or deliberate pause during rhythmic breathing

**kunda**—coiled serpent Kundalini

**Kundalini**—Mother's "holy spiritual" energy; one of Her forms

**kutir**—meditation hut


**langouti**—yogi's loincloth, hidden

**Laxmi or Lakshmi**—Divine Mother providing abundance, rules second chakra

**lingam**—energy of stillness as it becomes "with form"; phallus

**loka**—world beyond this one


**maha mudra**—great seal, all four bandhas arise simultaneously

**mahasamadhi**—great samadhi, consciously leaving the body at time of death

**makara**—the prime substances of tamas; foods that lower consciousness

**manipura**—third chakra

**mano maya kosha**—third body sheath made of thought

**mantra**—"mind transformation"; changes the perception as to the origin of thought

**marmas**—vital points, similar to acupuncture points

**maya**—illusion; one of Mother's siddhis

**moksha**—liberation

**mudra**—seal; retention of pranic energy

**mudra**—gestures of the hands symbolic of expanded awareness

**Muktananda**—Mukunda's guru, lineage of Bhagwan Nityananda

**muktasana**—liberation pose, cross-legged seated pose

**mula**—root

**muladhara**—first chakra


**nada/nadi**—a pranic channel; when prana moves through the nadis, sound is created

**naga yogis**—wandering naked sadhus

**na'ham**—mantra meaning "I am not the body"

***nauli***—isolation of the rectus abdominus muscle; one of six purification practices

***Nityananda***—Muktananda's guru; also one of Muktananda's successors

***niyamas***—precepts, observances, fixed rules

***nyasa***—practice of touching the five sense organs and the correlating chakra

***nyasa puja***—elevation of the primal elements


***ojas***—spiritual juices, elevated kapha

***Om Namah Shivaya***—with great respect and love, I honor my Heart as my inner Self


***padmasana***—lotus posture

***panchamaya koshas***—the five veils that disguise the world as non-spiritual

***Patanjali***—author of classic text, *Yoga Sutras*

***pingala***—right nostril, masculine energy channel

***pitta***—Ayurvedic dosha (that which digests)

***prajna***—wisdom

***prakrti***—the material world disguised as not spiritual

***prakruti***—Ayurvedic constitution, determined at conception

***prana***—all pervasive life force

***prana maya kosha***—second body sheath made of prana

***prana prathista***—installing the life force into a statue so that it comes alive

***pranam***—bow, attitude of submission

***pranayama***—disciplines of prana; the state of pranic suspension; fourth of eight limbs of classical Ashtanga Yoga, turning breath into life force

***prasad***—blessed gifts

***pratyahara***—indrawing of senses; dissolution of first two koshas

***puja***—worship, rituals to invite divine grace and meditation

***puraka***—inhalation

***purusha***—the great Spirit

***rajas***—overexertion in sadhana

***rajasic***—one of the gunas, activity; literally means "overly stimulating"

***Ramana***—Ramana Maharshi, an enlightened master

***rasa***—essence

***rechaka***—exhalation

***rogi***—a sick yogi

***sadhana***—spiritual practice given by a teacher

***sadhus***—wandering ascetics

***sahajoli mudra***—isolation of contraction of the urethra in the female (more in essence than physical)

***sahasrara***—seventh chakra, thousand-petaled lotus

***samadhi***—absorption into Spirit

***samana***—digestive "cirulating" prana that spreads outward from the belly

***samasana***—seated tantrasana in which the ankles are placed parallel on the floor

***samasthiti***—standing posture

***samskara***—past impression

***samyama***—the continuum of attention from dharana to dhyana, leading to samadhi

***sangha***—spiritual community

***sankalpa***—a resolution to manifest latent desire

***sannyas***—a celibate monk who is a seeker of truth

***Sarasvati***—goddess of arts, learning, music, dance; rules the first chakra

***sat/chit/ananda***—the primal state unifying existence/consciousness/bliss

***satguru***—true guru

***satsang***—to be in the company of a sage

*sattva*—state of balance or harmony

*savasana*—corpse pose; posture of Shiva lying on back in submission to Kali

*shaligram*—symbol of Vishnu, an ancient spiral shell

*Shakti*—evolution of prana revealing mother as the essence of life force

*shaktipat*—descent of shakti; the primal maternal form of grace

*shambhavi mudra*—inward-looking, seeing Mother

*shavasana*—alternate spelling of savasana

*She'hina*—Jewish goddess

*Shiva or Siva*—the Inner Self, God within, the quality of stillness

*Shiva/Shakti tandava*—the communion of male and female; literally: the eternal dance

*siddha*—master teacher, illumined

*siddha loka*—the world of siddhas, illumined masters

*siddhasana*—seated tantrasana

*siddhayoniasana*—a woman's version of siddhasana

*siddhis*—supernatural abilities of senses and mind

*so'ham*—mantra meaning "I am That I am"

*soma*—nectar of the gods, a secret tantric drink

*spanda*—eternal pulsation

*strotras*—gross channels

*surya namaska*—"I am beautiful light"; Sun salute

*sushumna*—central channel where Kundalini ascends and Shakti descends (three additional nadis exist within sushumna)

*svadhisthana*—second chakra

*svadhyaya*—self-study, study of spiritual texts and sacred lore

*swastikasana*—seated tantrasana with ankles crossed


*tamas*—too passive in sadhana

*tamasic*—lethargic

*tandava*—spontaneous Tantric dance into Shiva/stillness or into Shakti/motion

***Tantra***—yoga of honoring Divine Mother; transformation of energy body

***tantrasana***—asana placements that aid the prana to a higher level of expression

***Tantrika/Tantrik***—female/male practitioners

***tapah***—self-discipline and purification, austerity, action without desire

***tarasana***—seated tantrasana (on floor, sitting, begin from bhadrasana forward bend, forehead to heels, hands holding toes, forearms straight across on floor)

***tattvas***—the five elements from which evolution arises

***tejas***—spiritual luminosity; elevated and balance pitta

***tratak***—fixed gazing


***udana***—upward-moving prana; when this prana evolves, it is Kundalini

***udana prana***—upward-moving prana

***uddiyana bandha***—purification practice (stomach lock)

***ujjaye***—wave breath

***Uma***—primal Divine Mother; Shiva's consort

***urdhvareta***—elevated state where energy only moves upward


***vaastu***—principles of placement, the Indian version of feng shui

***vairagya***—detachment

***vajrasana***—sitting on the shins, heels touching

***vajrayoni***—literally, "diamond womb"; a Yogini

***vajroli mudra***—isolation of contraction of the urethra in the male

***vasanas***—latent emotional tendencies

***Vasistha's Yoga***—text of the sage Vasistha teaching Prince Rama

***vata***—principle of motion (literally "that which moves")

***vijnana maya kosha***—fourth body sheath made of wisdom

***vinyasas***—flowing sequences

***viparita karani mudra***—inverted action; mild, safe version of shoulderstand *vira*—hero

*virasana*—seated asana

*vishuddhi*—throat chakra

*vritti*—wave, primal thought; see *Yoga Sutras* I, 2

*vyana*—subtlest of the pranas; pervades the body as the aura


*yab/yum*—Father Mother Communion

*yama*—self-control, *Yoga Sutras* II, 30–35

*yantras*—geometrical symbols, aid for visual meditation; what is outside is to be found inside

*yoga*—Indian-originated spiritual path to communion

*yogasana*—generic term for a yoga posture

**Yoga Sutras**—original Classical Yoga text written by Patanjali

*Yogini/Yogi*—female/male yoga practitioners

*yoni*—source; womb, vagina, female sex organs

# Recommended Tantrik References[*]

## Books

Bhairavan, Amarananda. *Kale's Odiyya: A Shaman's True Story of Initiation.* York Beach, ME: Nicholas-Hays, 2000. An Indian boy living in a matriarchal society is given a consort for Tantrik apprenticeship.

Camphausen, Rufus. *The Yoni: Sacred Symbol of Female Creative Power.* Rochester, VT: Inner Traditions, 1996. See pp. 29–30 (yoni mudra), pp. 37–44 (yoni puja), pp. 70–74 (rajas, feminine ojas), and pp. 76–79 (yoni variety).

Danielou, Alain. *The Phallus: Sacred Symbol of Male Creative Power.* Rochester, VT: Inner Traditions, 1995. See pp. 15–22 (transcendent symbol, bija, yoni), pp. 34–35 (pillar of light), and pp. 84–86 (subtle body of lingam).

Frawley, David. *Tantric Yoga and the Wisdom Goddesses.* Salt Lake City, UT: Passage Press, 1994. Ten Goddesses and how they are invoked; Ayurvedic and Tantric practices for opening the chakras; developing deeper practices.

* Grey, Alex. *Sacred Mirrors: The Visionary Art of Alex Grey.* Rochester, VT: Inner Traditions International, 1990. Exquisite original art of the energy bodies, drawn from his personal visions.

Johari, Harish. *Tools for Tantra.* Rochester, VT: Destiny Books/Inner Traditions, 1988. Mantras and yantras, and how to construct them.

Khanna, Madhu. *Yantra: The Tantric Symbol of Cosmic Unity.* London: Thames and Hudson Ltd., 1994. Thorough presentation of the Tantrik forms as embodiments of the Divine Feminine.

Mookerjee, Ajit. *Kundalini: The Arousal of the Inner Energy.* Rochester, VT: Destiny Books/Inner Traditions, 1982. Mixture of rare, beautiful art and scholarly overviews.

Mookerjee, Ajit, and Madhu Khanna. *The Tantric Way: Art, Science, Ritual.* New York: Thames and Hudson, 1996. An overview of the art, science, and rituals of the Tantrik cosmology and spiritual path.

* Odier, Daniel. *Desire: The Tantric Path to Awakening.* Rochester, VT: Inner Traditions 2001. A practical guide to pleasure.

*———. *Tantric Quest: An Encounter with Absolute Love.* Rochester, VT: Inner Traditions, 1997. A Western seeker finds an amazing Indian Tantrika.

---

* indicates highly recommended sources

*————. *Yoga Spandakarika: The Sacred Texts at the Origins of Tantra.* Rochester, VT: Inner Traditions International, 2005. Exquisite writings on the Spandakarika of Kashmir Shaivism and the non-dualism of the Vijnanabhairava Tantra.

Pattanaik, Devdutt. *Devi, The Mother Goddess: An Introduction.* Mumbai: Vakils, Feffer and Simons Ltd, 2000 A lovely perspective on Goddess qualities, worship (puja), the 108 names.

Saraswati, Sunyata, and Bodhi Avinasha. *Jewel in the Lotus: The Tantric Path to Higher Consciousness.* Los Osos, CA: Tantrika International, 2000. A wide variety of personal and partner practices for sharing energy.

* Shaw, Miranda. *Passionate Enlightenment: Women in Tantric Buddhism.* Princeton, NJ: Princeton University Press, 1995. A scholarly, yet intimate view of Buddhist monks sharing sexual/spiritual practices; recommend chapters 6 and 7.

Sovatsky, Stuart. *Passions of Innocence: Tantric Celibacy.* Princeton, NJ: Princeton University Press, 1993. Sensual elevation appropriate for couples or singles on either a White or Pink path.

Stevens, John. *Lust for Enlightenment: Buddhism and Sex.* Boston: Shambhala Publications, 1990. The Buddha's sex life and Buddhist Tantric practices of India, Tibet, China, and Japan.

Swami Muktananda. *Kundalini: The Secret of Life.* South Fallsburg, NY: Siddha Yoga Publications, 1994.

* ————. *Meditate: Happiness Lies Within You.* South Fallsburg, NY: Siddha Yoga Publications, 1999. The best book on meditation as a spiritual practice.

*————. *Play of Consciousness.* South Fallsburg, NY: Siddha Yoga Publications, 1994. An autobiography of a Kundalini awakening and the significance of spontaneous sexual, physical, and energetic kriyas.

Swami Muktibodhananda, translator. *Hatha Yoga Pradipika.* Munger, Bihar, India: Yoga Publications Trust, 1998. See pp. 370–416 (vajroli and sahajoli mudra) and pp. 530–534 (lingam puja).

*A Systematic Course in the Ancient Tantric Techniques of Yoga and Kriya.* Munger, Bihar, India: Yoga Publications Trust, 1989. Voluminous study book.

* van Lysebeth, André. *Tantra: The Cult of the Feminine.* York Beach, ME: Red Wheel/Weiser, 1995. Wonderful book for yoga practitioners wishing a deeper spiritual experience by one of Europe's most respected Hatha Yoga teachers.

## Journal Articles

Bass, C. and W. Gardner. "Emotional influences on breathing and breathlessness." *Journal of Psychosomatic Respiration* 1985; 29: 599–609.

Feleky, A. "The influence of the emotions on respiration." *Journal of Experimental Psychology* 1916; 1:218–241.

## On DVD

*Secrets of Sacred Sex.* Real-life partners, beautifully presented. *www.gaiam.com.*

Muir, Charles and Caroline. *Freeing the Female Orgasm—Awakening the Goddess.* *www.sourcetantra.com.* Audiotapes and booklet that help you lovingly arouse the G-spot.

## Websites

*www.SivaSakti.com.* Romanian Tantrik site with extensive articles.

*www.shivashakti.com.* Different from above, yet similar.

*www.religiousworlds.com.* Very full site on Hindu Tantra.

*www.sacred-texts.com.* Sacred Texts of Hindu traditions.

*www.claysanskritlibrary.org.* Downloadable texts.

*www.derekosborn.accountssupport.com.* A practicing English Naga Yogi has a thought-provoking site with many good and practical articles.

*www.aypsite.com.* Anonymous Yogan; a serious American Yogi writing on many subjects.

*www.danielodier.com.* An insightful teacher and author.

*www.kalima.org.* Tibetan woman teacher in Santa Cruz, CA.

*www.bhagawannityananda.org.* My guru's guru and Ganeshpuri village.

*www.sivanandadlshq.org.* Sivananda free downloads and connection to Swami Venkatesananda, translator of my favorite text—*Yoga Vasistha*

*www.hindugods.net* Art of Hindu and Tantra deities; maker of my Patanjali sandalwood statue.

*www.lindasyoga.blogspot.com.* 1938 video of Krishnamacharya.

# About the Author

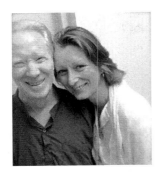

Mukunda Stiles is the director of the Yoga Therapy Center in California and lectures throughout the U.S., Europe, and India. He serves on the Advisory Board of the International Association of Yoga Therapists and is the author of *Structural Yoga Therapy, Patanjali's Yoga Sutras,* and *Ayurvedic Yoga Therapy.* He lives in California with his consort, Chinnamasta Stiles. Visit him at *yogatherapycenter.org.*

## To Our Readers

Weiser Books, an imprint of Red Wheel/Weiser, publishes books across the entire spectrum of occult, esoteric, speculative, and New Age subjects. Our mission is to publish quality books that will make a difference in people's lives without advocating any one particular path or field of study. We value the integrity, originality, and depth of knowledge of our authors.

Our readers are our most important resource, and we appreciate your input, suggestions, and ideas about what you would like to see published.

Visit our website *www.redwheelweiser.com* where you can subscribe to our newsletters and learn about our upcoming books, exclusive offers, and free downloads.

You can also contact us at info@redwheelweiser.com or at

Red Wheel/Weiser, LLC
500 Third Street, Suite 230
San Francisco, CA 94107